MEASUREMENT and the MEASUREMENT of CHANGE

A PRIMER FOR THE HEALTH PROFESSIONS

Denise F. Polit, PhD

President, Humanalysis, Inc., Saratoga Springs, New York
Professor, Griffith University, Centre for Health
Practice Innovation, Brisbane, Australia

Frances M. Yang, PhD

Assistant Professor of Epidemiology,
Medical College of Georgia
Department of Biostatistics and Epidemiology
Georgia Regents University, Augusta, Georgia

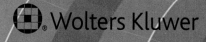 Wolters Kluwer

Philadelphia · Baltimore · New York · London
Buenos Aires · Hong Kong · Sydney · Tokyo

Acquisitions Editor: Christina Burns
Product Development Editor: Katherine Burland
Editorial Assistant: Zack Shapiro, Dan Reilly
Marketing Manager: Dean Karampelas
Production Project Manager: Cynthia Rudy
Design Coordinator: Holly McLaughlin
Artist/Illustrator: Jonathan Dimes
Manufacturing Coordinator: Karin Duffield
Prepress Vendor: Absolute Service, Inc.

9 8 7 6 5 4 3 2 1

Printed in China

Library of Congress Cataloging-in-Publication Data

Polit, Denise F., author.
  Measurement and the measurement of change : a primer for the health professions / Denise F. Polit, Frances Yang.
    p. ; cm.
  Includes bibliographical references and index.
  ISBN 978-1-4511-9449-4
  I. Yang, Frances, author. II. Title.
  [DNLM: 1. Epidemiologic Methods. 2. Health Care Evaluation Mechanisms. WA 950]
  RT48
  610.73—dc23
                                                                                              2014042604

Dedication

To our husbands and sons, who are wonderful beyond measure.
Alan and Alex
Solon and Oliver

Acknowledgments

This book depended on the inspiration from and support of many individuals who nurtured our interest in measurement as a field of scholarly inquiry, and helped us during its preparation. Many colleagues and students contributed ideas for this book, and to all of you we are very grateful. A few people deserve special mention.

Faculty at Griffith University in Australia planted the seed for writing this book, and Drs. Cindy Jones and Leanne Aitken played particularly valuable roles. Dr. Peter Airasian was motivational and inspiring. Other important advisors and mentors, especially for content relating to item response theory, include Drs. Richard N. Jones, Jeanne Teresi, Paul Crane, Laura Gibbons, Dan Mungas, and Gerald van Belle.

We also extend our thanks to those who helped to turn the manuscript into a finished product. The staff at Wolters Kluwer has been of great assistance to us. We are indebted to Christina Burns, Kate Burland, Cynthia Rudy, and all the others behind the scenes for their fine contributions.

Finally, we thank our family and friends. We know that our family's support of this project required considerable patience.

Reviewers

Tanya Altmann, MSN (Ed), PhD
Associate Professor of Nursing
Sacramento State University
Sacramento, California

Joel Anderson, PhD
Assistant Professor
University of Virginia
Charlottesville, Virginia

Christina Baggot, RN, PhD
Assistant Professor
University of California–San Francisco
San Francisco, California

Lanell Bellury, PhD, RN, MN, BSN
Associate Professor
Mercer University
Atlanta, Georgia

Michelle Block, PhD
Associate Professor
Purdue University Calumet
Hammond, Indiana

Stephanie Blundell, MSN-Ed, DNP/FNP in progress
Assistant Professor, Nursing
Fresno Pacific University
Fresno, California

Diane Breckenridge, BSN, MSN, PhD, ANEF
Associate Professor and Director, Nursing
    Workforce, Strategies for Success Program
La Salle University
Philadelphia, Pennsylvania

Barbara Brewer, PhD, MALS, MBA
Associate Professor
The University of Arizona
Tucson, Arizona

Mary Jo Bugel, PhD
Assistant Professor
Rutgers School of Nursing
Newark, New Jersey

Shari Burns, MSN, CRNA, EdD
Director and Associate Professor
Midwestern University–Glendale
Glendale, Arizona

Jeanie Burt, BSN, MA, MSN
Assistant Professor
Harding University
Searcy, Arizona

Eloise Carr, BSc (Hons), MSc (Nursing), PhD
Professor
University of Calgary
Calgary, Alberta, Canada

Stephanie Chalupka, MSN, EdD
Associate Dean for Nursing
Worcester State University
Worcester, Massachusetts

Adeline Chu, PhD
Assistant Professor
University of Houston–Victoria
Victoria, Texas

Lynne Connelly, PhD, RN
Director of Nursing
Benedictine College
Atchison, Kansas

Constance Dallas, PhD, RN, FAAN
Associate Professor
University of Illinois
Chicago, Illinois

JoAnn Daugherty, PhD
Faculty
California State University San Marcos
San Marcos, California

Jane Dixon, PhD
Professor
Yale University
New Haven, Connecticut

Heather Fenton, EdD, MSN, RN, CNE
Assistant Professor of Nursing
Northeastern State University
Tahlequah, Oklahoma

Kathleen Fitzgerald, PhD, RN
Associate Professor
Lewis University
Romeoville, Illinois

Boyd Foster, PhD
Associate Professor
Gonzaga University
Spokane, Washington

Betsy Gulledge, PhD
Associate Dean
Jacksonville State University
Jacksonville, Alabama

Susan Hayden, PhD
Assistant Professor
University of South Alabama
Mobile, Alabama

Marilyn Hodgins, BScN, MN, PhD
Associate Professor
University of New Brunswick–Fredericton
Fredericton, New Brunswick, Canada

Brenda Hosley, PhD
Clinical Associate Professor
Arizona State University
Phoenix, Arizona

Catherine Kane, PhD
Associate Professor of Nursing and
    Psychiatry
University of Virginia
Charlottesville, Virginia

Rebecca Keele, PhD
Associate Professor
New Mexico State University
Las Cruces, New Mexico

Erin Killingsworth, PhD
Assistant Professor
Samford University
Birmingham, Alabama

Laura Kimble, PhD
Professor
Mercer University
Atlanta, Georgia

Mary Lopez, PhD
Assistant Dean, Administration and Research
Western University of Health Sciences
Pomona, California

Hayley Mark, PhD, MPH, RN
Assistant Professor
Johns Hopkins School of Nursing
Baltimore, Maryland

Frederick May, PhD
Associate Professor, Nurse Educator Track
    Coordinator
University of Indianapolis
Indianapolis, Indiana

Maureen McLaughlin, PhD
Assistant Professor
Georgetown University
Washington, DC

Sarah Newton, PhD, RN
Undergraduate Program Director and
    Associate Professor
Oakland University
Rochester, Michigan

Catherine Pearsall, PhD, FNP, RN
Associate Professor
St. Joseph's College
Patchogue, New York

Lusine Poghosyan, PhD, MPH, RN
Assistant Professor
Columbia University
New York, New York

Preface

This book focuses on the measurement of health constructs, particularly those constructs that are not amenable to quantification by means of laboratory analysis or technical instrumentation. These health constructs include a wide range of human attributes, such as quality of life, functional ability, self-efficacy, depression, and pain. Measures of such constructs are proliferating at a rapid rate and often without adequate attention paid to ensuring that standards of scientific rigor are met.

The book is designed for use by a wide range of health professionals who want to make thoughtful decisions about the measurement of health constructs. This audience encompasses many researchers and clinicians because measurement is vital to high-quality science and to excellence in clinical practice. In this book, we offer guidance to those who develop new instruments, adapt existing ones, select instruments for use in a clinical trial or in clinical practice, interpret information from measurements and changes in scores, or undertake a systematic review on instruments.

This book is not aimed at a particular health discipline. To illustrate measurement concepts, we have included examples of measures and classification systems used in many health fields, including medicine, public health, nursing, psychotherapy, epidemiology, physical therapy, and nutrition science. This book will be useful in graduate-level courses on measurement or research methods and will also serve as an important reference and resource for researchers and clinicians. To this end, we have taken pains to create a thorough index and have also included a glossary of key terms.

Practical Approach

As the title indicates, this book is designed to be practical. No book on measurement could avoid some statistical presentations, but because it is a "primer," it is not aimed at readers with extensive statistical backgrounds. Thus, the book is a "gentle" introduction to and overview of complex measurement content. We do expect readers to have a basic understanding of statistics and statistical inference. However, statistical content in this book serves primarily to enhance conceptual understanding rather than to guide computations, which in any event are almost never done without computer software. We offer guidance relating to software for some measurement parameters, primarily for users of SPSS.

This book draws on measurement theory and approaches from a variety of fields. We have combined recent advances from psychometrics, clinimetrics, and other fields in a manner that we believe has not been achieved in other health measurement books. We acknowledge the important contributions of several international work groups that have tackled the issue of health measurement, but in some areas, this book breaks new ground.

Key Measurement Domains

This book offers guidance on how to develop new instruments using both "classical" and "modern" approaches from psychometrics, as well as methods used in clinimetrics. Much of this book, however, concerns the evaluation of instruments in relation to three key measurement domains: reliability, validity, and responsiveness. In terms of reliability, we offer strategies and advice with respect to the reliability of a score, and the reliability of a *change* score. Two chapters are devoted to the topic of interpretability—how to make sense of information from measurements. Although the discussion of measurement properties and interpretability applies to virtually all types of health measurement, we focus primarily on patient-reported outcomes (PRO) in the chapters on instrument development.

This book does not give advice about *specific* instruments, although we mention numerous instruments as *examples* of measurement concepts. It would be impossible to catalogue all instruments, not only because they are too numerous but also because new ones are created daily. We offer information useful to those who want to select instruments according to their measurement properties; we explain what those properties are and how to draw conclusions about their soundness.

In a book of this length, and in light of it being introductory in nature, there are many measurement topics we have not been able to cover. For example, we have included only a cursory overview of generalizability theory because most instrument developers do not conduct G studies. We do not address issues relating to health econometrics. We also do not cover diagnostic classification models (DCM), which are powerful and complex statistical models that have been developed for educational measurement in the past 20 years, because these models are aimed primarily at educational assessment and curriculum development.

Teaching–Learning Package

Measurement and the Measurement of Change comes with a selection of ancillary materials designed to aid effective teaching and enhance students' progress and comprehension. Resources that can be found online at thePoint—http://thepoint.lww.com/PolitYang—include the following:

- PowerPoint Presentations
- Journal Articles

We hope that this book will serve as a useful guide to many health care professionals, and we hope that this book will contribute at least in part to improvements in health research.

Denise F. Polit, PhD
Frances M. Yang, PhD

Contents

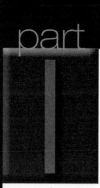

part

I

INTRODUCTION

chapters

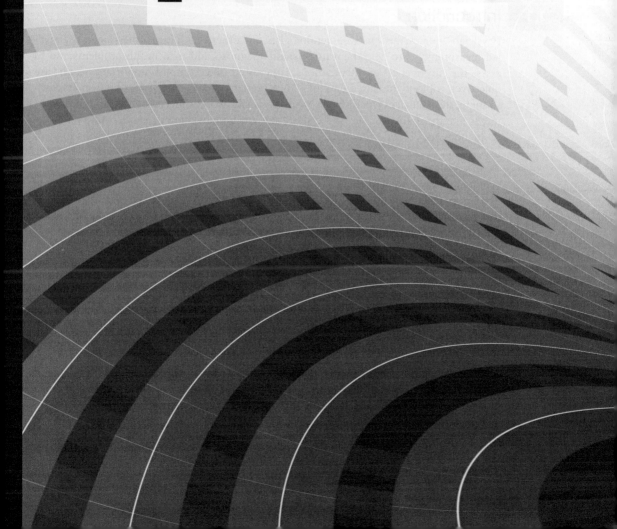

1

Basics of Measurement

Chapter Outline

1.1 Introduction

Physicians, nurses, therapists, epidemiologists, and other health care professionals use myriad measurements to help them understand, diagnose, and treat health problems and to assess the effectiveness of interventions. How could we accomplish important health care objectives without measurements of blood pressure, cholesterol levels, body mass, grip strength, sleep efficiency, and so on? We don't usually worry much about whether measurements like these are accurate and capture the attribute of interest. We depend on sphygmomanometers, blood tests, weight scales, dynamometers, and polysomnographs to yield numerical values that are trustworthy and meaningful.

So why, then, does an entire book need to be written about measurement? If every relevant health measurement could be obtained by using sophisticated technical instruments and equipment, there would be little need for this book. However, many important indicators of health status cannot be measured through technology and biophysiologic instrumentation. Here is just a small sample of constructs that require alternative approaches:

- Pain in patients with arthritis
- Confusion in older adults
- Fatigue in patients with cancer
- Alcohol dependence in a general population
- Postpartum depression in new mothers
- Patient satisfaction in hospitalized patients

Measurement instruments for each of these nonphysical constructs (and thousands of others) have been developed, and there are often numerous instruments for each construct. How does one select a good instrument to measure characteristics not amenable to high-tech instrumentation or lab analysis? Also, on what basis does a researcher decide that a new instrument needs to be created?

In thinking about measurement issues, six important questions need to be addressed, which we illustrate with an example. Suppose you selected the World Health Organization Disability Assessment Schedule 2.0 (WHODAS 2.0; Üstün et al., 2010) to measure the functional ability of patients with spinal cord injury. You administer the 36-question scale to a group of patients. Patient number one receives a score of 80 on an initial visit and a score of 75 on a 3-month follow-up (higher scores reflect greater disability).[1] Key measurement-related questions regarding these scores include the following:

1. Is the score of 80 at baseline the right score value for this patient? Is it possible that the score *really* should be 78? Or 83?

2. Is the scale truly measuring the construct *functional ability*? Or is it measuring something else?

3. What does a score of 80 *mean*? How can it be interpreted? Is it high or low for patients with spinal cord injury?

4. Does the change from 80 to 75 reflect a true change, or does it merely reflect a random fluctuation in measurement?

5. Does the change from 80 to 75 correspond to a commensurate improvement in the patient's degree of functional ability?

6. What does a 5-point change *mean*? Is the improvement large enough to be considered clinically significant?

Unfortunately, researchers have developed hundreds (even thousands) of health instruments without providing potential users with good answers to these questions. This book discusses mechanisms for addressing such questions and for evaluating whether the answers engender confidence in the scientific merit of an instrument. As these questions suggest, this book is about both measurement and the measurement of change.

1.2   The Importance of Measurement Quality in Health Care

If a digital thermometer gave a reading of 96.7° F one minute and 99.3° F the next minute for the same patient, that thermometer could not be trusted to guide clinical decision making. Clinicians make decisions on the basis of measures of nonphysical attributes as well, and so confidence in the quality of those measurements is crucially important.

Researchers undertaking clinical trials often include measures of attributes such as *functional ability* and *quality of life* as primary or secondary end points. Topnotch measuring tools are essential for coming to the right conclusions about the effectiveness of health care interventions. Effect sizes can be underestimated solely because of low-quality measures. The most rigorously designed randomized controlled trial (and meta-analyses of such trials) can yield misleading information if the measurements are substandard. Evidence-based practice requires sound measurement.

The importance of using instruments with excellent measurement properties has been expressed in guidelines written by the U.S. Food and Drug Administration (USFDA, 2009). This agency has established standards for medical product development to support labeling claims. High-quality measures are needed to support claims of treatment benefit of both pharmacologic and nonpharmacologic interventions.

There is also an ethical aspect to having high-quality measurements. If we administer flawed measurement scales to patients, we are burdening them needlessly and risk giving them ineffective health care advice.

---

[1]Referenced here are the WHODAS raw scores, as described in Üstün and colleagues (2010). Guidelines for score transformations can be obtained at http://www.who.int/icidh/whodas/index.html.

1.3   Basic Measurement Definitions

In this book, certain terms will be used repeatedly, so some definitions will hopefully help to enhance communication. Definitions of key terms used in this book, those that are bolded, are included in the Glossary.

A **construct** (in the context of health care phenomena) is an abstraction that is inferred from human behavior or human attributes. This broad definition of *construct* means that attributes such as blood pressure, heart rate, and body temperature could be considered constructs. The central focus of this book, however, is measuring health-related constructs that are not directly measurable or observable using medical equipment and instrumentation—they are abstractions that are *constructed* on the basis of observable phenomena. When we use the term *construct* in this book, this is the type of abstraction to which we are referring. Such constructs are sometimes referred to as **latent traits** (i.e., human traits that are not manifest or directly observable but that can be inferred from people's behavior or their responses to a set of questions).

To be useful to clinicians, patients, administrators, or policy makers, constructs have to be *operationalized* (i.e., made amenable to measurement). **Measurement** involves assigning numbers to represent the amount of the construct that is present using a specified set of rules. *Rules* are necessary to promote consistency and interpretability. Rules for measuring constructs such as weight and body temperature are well-known, but even with these constructs, the rules are not universal (i.e., there are metric and nonmetric systems). Rules for measuring constructs such as nausea or quality of life must be invented. Instrument developers must specify the criteria for assigning numerical values for the construct of interest, and then the rules must be evaluated to see if they are *good* rules. It is not enough to have rules—the rules must yield quantitative information that corresponds to different amounts of the targeted trait. The measurement process ideally enhances understanding about the nature of the construct as well as about the person being measured.

When researchers or clinicians invent a set of rules to gauge a construct, they create a **measure** of the construct, often in the form of a formal instrument. An **instrument** is a device used to make a measurement (e.g., a patient-reported scale with multiple questions). Measures are designed to be quantitative analogs of constructs. Measures can be derived through various mechanisms, such as by asking questions or making observations (see Chapter 2). For health constructs, a particularly useful type of instrument is a **composite scale** that involves combining information from multiple questions (**items**) into a single numerical value that places people on a continuum with respect to the target attribute.

Measures yield **scores**—numerical values that communicate *how much* of an attribute is present or whether it is present at all. Scores can differ in many respects, one of which concerns their **level of measurement**.

1.4   Levels of Measurement

As we may recall from Statistics 101, there are four levels of measurement:

■ **Nominal measurement** involves assigning "scores" based on categorical classifications. For example, for classifying binge drinking, the score could be 1 for those who are binge drinkers (typically defined as having five or more drinks on the same occasion in the past 30 days) and 0 for those who are not. Nominal measurements are often dichotomous, but not always. For example, the World Health Organization has created and regularly updates a measurement classification for the construct "cause of death." The International Classification of Diseases (ICD) system involves nominal measurement with over 100 categories.

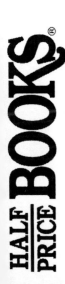

HALF PRICE BOOKS ®

Half Price Books
1835 Forms Drive
Carrollton, TX 75006
OFS OrderID 20958559

Thank you for your order, Tess Allen!

Thank you for shopping with Half Price Books! Please contact service105@hpb.com. if you have any questions, comments or concerns about your order (111-4074404-8736252)

Visit our stores to sell your books, music, movies games for cash.

SKU	ISBN/UPC	Title & Author/Artist	Shelf ID	Qty	OrderSKU
S338358603	9781451194494	Measurement and the Measurement of Chang Polit PhD FAAN, Denise F.	HLTH 7.3	1	

SHIPPED STANDARD TO:
Tess Allen
2158 CUMBERLAND PKWY SE APT 9206
ATLANTA GA 30339-4571
c8x90r7ywzzvv6j@marketplace.amazon.com

ORDER# 111-4074404-8736252
AmazonMarketplaceUS

■ **Ordinal measurement** involves rank ordering categories to represent incremental amounts of an attribute. The ranked categories cannot, however, be presumed to be equidistant from one another. For example, staging of severity in breast cancer (ordered stages from Stage 0 to Stage IV) is ordinal measurement.

■ **Interval measurements** have equal distances between points on a scale, but there is no rational (true) zero point signifying the absence of the attribute. For example, on the Fahrenheit scale, temperature is an interval measurement. The difference between 50° F and 60° F is the same as the difference between 60° F and 70° F, but 0° F does not represent the total absence of heat.

■ **Ratio measurements** have equal distances between points along a scale *and* a true zero. For example, in measuring urine output in milliliters per hour, zero is a possible score, signifying the total absence of urine output.

For measuring the type of constructs of concern in this book, this four-level distinction is usually not necessary. It is rarely important to distinguish interval and ratio measurements in the context of evaluating measurement properties, and so we will refer to scores for both levels as **continuous**.[2] Many of the scores discussed in this book are continuous; that is, they take on a range of values that designate incremental amounts of the attribute. There have been debates and controversies about whether composite scales and indexes constructed with traditional scaling methods are truly interval measures or are better described as ordinal measures (see Cano & Hobart, 2011; Streiner & Norman, 2008). For the most part, we will treat scores from multicomponent summated scales as continuous, but we will return to the issue about the measurement level of composite scales in Chapter 6.

In many cases, continuous measures are converted to nominal or ordinal classifications that have powerful clinical relevance. For example, birth weights (measured in ounces on a ratio scale) are often converted to ordinal classification: very low, low, and normal birthweight. Such classifications will be discussed in Chapter 16.

1.5 Purposes of Measurement

In health fields, measurements can serve a number of purposes. In an often cited paper, Kirshner and Guyatt (1985) developed a classification for health status measures based on measurement purposes.

■ *Discriminative.* A discriminative measure is used to examine differences between individuals and groups with respect to health-related characteristics. Discriminative measures are frequently used in cross-sectional studies to describe a health construct at a particular point in time for a population. For example, the U.S. National Health Survey, which is administered to thousands of randomly selected people annually, includes a six-question scale to measure "serious psychological distress." Scores on this scale can be used to examine differences between groups of people who were or were not in psychological distress at the time of the survey.

■ *Predictive.* A predictive measure is used to predict a health outcome, and usually the goal is to correctly classify people. Screening and diagnostic instruments typically have primarily a predictive purpose—they are used to identify people who either have or will develop a condition, problem, or outcome of interest. For example, the Malnutrition Screening Tool is used to predict risk for malnutrition in hospital and nursing home settings (Ferguson, Capra, Bauer, & Banks, 1999).

---

[2]Note that we depart from a strict mathematical definition of continuous, which would require the possibility of a measurement intermediary between two numerical values (e.g., between 8 and 9).

■ *Evaluative.* An evaluative measure is used to assess the benefits and outcomes of a health treatment or clinical regimen. Such measures are useful in clinical trials and also in everyday clinical situations to monitor stability, improvements, and deterioration. For example, the Clinical COPD Questionnaire (CCQ) is a disease-specific symptom severity scale that has been used to monitor change over time in response to treatment among patients with COPD (van der Molen et al., 2003).

Kirschner and Guyatt (1985) argued that it is imperative to know the intended purpose of a measure prior to developing or using it because the underlying purpose has implications for its development and evaluation. They offered some important thoughts about how an instrument's purpose affects various decisions during its development, and their classification has been especially influential in the development of quality of life measures (e.g., Hankins, 2008). Others, however, have argued that most instruments serve multiple purposes (e.g., Streiner & Norman, 2008), and therefore, such classifications are not especially meaningful. For example, a scale to measure depression might be used to describe a general population (What percentage of people is depressed?), to predict (Which patients with depression are at highest risk of self-harm?), and to evaluate (Was a mental health intervention effective in reducing depression?). De Vet, Terwee, Mokkink, and Knol (2011) noted that it may be better to think of discriminative, predictive, and evaluative *applications* of instruments rather than of separate classes of instruments.

1.6 Disciplinary Perspectives

Interest in the measurement of constructs that cannot be measured through biophysiologic instrumentation developed more than a century ago among psychologists and educational researchers. The field of **psychometrics** was created to formulate statistical and conceptual frameworks for those who wanted to measure such constructs as *intelligence, introversion, motivation,* and so on. Much of the important theoretical and statistical work on measurement that is included in this book was developed by psychometricians.

More recently, researchers in the fields of medicine, clinical epidemiology, and other health fields recognized the need to create measures of important health outcomes that cannot be captured through biophysiologic instrumentation. Such outcomes as *quality of life, pain, fatigue, skin integrity, balance,* and so on, required creative formulations. Although psychometric contributions remain prominent in health fields, new concepts and approaches have been introduced to address the perspectives of clinicians. Some of these advances were made within a discipline called **clinimetrics**. Clinimetricians have pursued a somewhat different path than psychometricians, especially with regard to the development of new instruments. Other advances in medicine concern a new focus on the measurement of change.

In the 1980s, psychotherapists became concerned with how to evaluate the effectiveness of their treatment through measurement of such outcomes as *depression* and *anxiety*. Researchers in the field of psychotherapy have made contributions with regard to assessing the *clinical significance* of change scores.

This book describes methodologic advances in measurement that have been developed in all these disciplines.

1.7 Overview of This Book

In the next two chapters in Part I, we present additional general information about measurement. Chapter 2 discusses various types of measures and measurement sources. This chapter also describes differences between psychometric and clinimetric scales and gives an overview of the two primary measurement models that have been developed by psychometricians. Chapter 3 summarizes major *properties* of measurement (e.g., reliability, validity) and presents a taxonomy that has been adapted from an important initiative called **COSMIN** (**Co**nsensus-based **S**tandards for the selection of health status **M**easurement **In**struments) (DeVet et al., 2011; Mokkink et al., 2010a, 2010b).

Part II offers some guidance on how to develop instruments to measure key health constructs. We begin in Chapter 4 with a discussion of the many challenges that instrument developers face, regardless of what type of measure they are creating. Chapter 5 offers advice on the development of psychometric scales using the "traditional" psychometric model, classical test theory, and Chapter 6 provides an introduction to scale construction using item response theory. Chapter 7 describes the development of measures using clinimetric methods.

Part III is devoted to the *reliability* domain within the measurement property taxonomy. Chapter 8 addresses reliability parameters that relate to test–retest, parallel test, interrater, and intrarater reliability situations. Chapter 9 discusses internal consistency in multi-item scales and also indicates when parameters of internal consistency are not appropriate as a method of assessment. The final chapter in Part III (Chapter 10) describes parameters of measurement error.

Part IV is devoted to the *validity* domain. There are separate chapters for the various ways of assessing the validity of measures, including a chapter on content and face validity (Chapter 11), criterion validity (Chapter 12), hypothesis-testing construct validity (Chapter 13), structural validity (Chapter 14), and cross-cultural validity (Chapter 15). This section of the book concludes with a chapter on the interpretability of point-in-time (cross-sectional) scores (Chapter 16).

Part V covers material relating to changes in score values over time. Chapter 17 describes the challenges of measuring change in an attribute and discusses the reliability of change scores. Chapter 18 addresses the measurement property called *responsiveness*, which, consistent with COSMIN, we equate with longitudinal validity. Chapter 19 describes approaches that have been used to interpret change scores and to draw conclusions about whether score changes are *clinically significant*.

References

Cano, S. J., & Hobart, J. C. (2011). The problem with health measurement. *Patient Preference and Adherence, 5,* 279–290.

DeVet, H. C. W., Terwee, C., Mokkink, L. B., & Knol, D. L. (2011). *Measurement in medicine: A practical guide.* Cambridge, MA: Cambridge University Press.

Ferguson, M., Capra, S., Bauer, J., & Banks, M. (1999). Development of a valid and reliable malnutrition screening tool for adult acute hospital patients. *Nutrition, 15,* 458–464.

Hankins, M. (2008). How discriminating are discriminative instruments? *Health and Quality of Life Outcomes, 6,* 36.

Kirschner, B., & Guyatt, G. (1985). A methodological framework for assessing health indices. *Journal of Chronic Diseases, 38,* 27–36.

Mokkink, L. B., Terwee, C., Patrick, D., Alonso, J., Stratford, P., Knol, D. L., . . . de Vet, H. C. W. (2010a). The COSMIN checklist for assessing the methodological quality of studies on measurement properties of health status instruments: An international Delphi study. *Quality of Life Research, 19,* 539–549.

Mokkink, L. B., Terwee, C., Patrick, D., Alonso, J., Stratford, P., Knol, D. L., . . . de Vet, H. C. W. (2010b). The COSMIN study reached international consensus on taxonomy, terminology, and definitions of measurement properties for health-related patient-reported outcomes. *Journal of Clinical Epidemiology, 63,* 737–745.

Streiner, D. L., & Norman, G. R. (2008). *Health measurement scales: A practical guide to their development and use* (4th ed.). Oxford: Oxford University Press.

U.S. Food and Drug Administration. (2009). *Guidance for industry patient-reported outcome measures: Use in medical product development to support labeling claims.* Washington, DC: U.S. Department of Health and Human Services.

Üstün, T., Chatterji, S., Kostanjsek, S., Rehm, J., Kennedy, C., Epping-Jordan, J., . . . Pull, C. (2010). Developing the World Health Organization Disability Assessment Schedule 2.0. *Bulletin of the World Health Organization, 88,* 815–823.

Van der Molen, T., Willemse, B., Schokker, S., ten Hacken, N., Postma, D., & Juniper, E. (2003). Development, validity, and responsiveness of the Clinical COPD Questionnaire. *Health and Quality of Life Outcomes, 1,* 13.

2

Types of Measurement

Chapter Outline

This chapter describes some of the diversity that characterizes the health measurement landscape. The chapter begins with a discussion of sources for measuring health constructs. Next, we briefly describe options relating to measurement complexity, which concerns the methods by which scores are derived. Several typologies for multi-item measures are then discussed. One typology reflects disciplinary underpinnings (psychometrics vs. clinimetrics), whereas another concerns different theories of measurement (classical test theory and item response theory). The concluding section explains the important distinction between reflective and formative multi-item measures.

2.1 Measurement Sources

Measurements of health-related phenomena can be derived from many different sources. The least problematic measurements, with regard to measurement properties such as reliability and validity, are those that are made through biophysiologic equipment and instrumentation and laboratory analysis. As noted in Chapter 1, however, many important health constructs require different approaches.

2.1.a Verbal Reports and Patient-Reported Outcomes

Verbal reports are a very important source of information for health care professionals. Answers to carefully worded questions can yield measurements of intangible constructs that would otherwise be impossible to measure. If we want to know patients' level of fatigue, for example, the best way to obtain that information is to ask them questions; the answers can be used to create fatigue scores. **Self-report** data can be obtained in several ways. The primary mechanisms are through oral interviews between an interviewer and a respondent (either face-to-face or on the telephone) or by means of self-administration (with a paper-and-pencil questionnaire or using a digital format).

A major class of verbal reports is widely referred to in the medical literature as **patient-reported outcomes (PROs)**. PROs are often associated with the measurement of subjective states (e.g., how patients *feel*), but direct questioning can also be used to measure outcomes that would be more difficult or expensive to measure in other ways, such as nutritional intake, sleep habits, smoking behavior, and physical functioning.

Not all verbal reports are *patient*-reported outcomes. For example, verbal-report instruments have been developed to measure attributes of health care staff rather than patients (e.g., their clinical empathy). Moreover, not all self-reports from patients are measurements of *outcomes* (i.e., the result of treatment). For instance, a measure of patients' attitudes toward assisted suicide would not be considered an outcome. Moreover, not all verbal reports of patient outcomes are provided by the patients themselves. For example, for patients with cognitive or other impairments, **proxy reports** from caretakers or clinicians are sometimes used to measure patient outcomes.[1] Nevertheless, PROs are the largest class of verbal reports, and we will use the acronym in this book in many instances when the discussion applies to all types of verbal reports. Much of the content of this book focuses on the development and assessment of verbal report measures.

2.1.b Observations

In some situations, people cannot be asked for a verbal report of their attributes or behaviors. **Observations** can be used to record people's behaviors, actions, and circumstances and sometimes to capture such constructs as people's moods or emotions. Observations are especially useful with people who cannot provide verbal reports (e.g., young children, patients with dementia, patients in a coma) or for constructs that might be difficult to measure in an unbiased fashion through self-reports (e.g., informal caretakers' abuse of a patient).

Structured observational measures that yield a score involve the use of a system for categorizing, rating, and recording observations. Observers typically use a formal instrument— such as an **observational checklist**—to indicate the presence or absence (or frequency of occurrence) of certain traits or behaviors. For example, the Child-Adult Medical Procedure Interaction Scale-Infant Version (CAMPIS-IV) requires observers to code for the occurrence or nonoccurrence of 2 infant behaviors (e.g., sucking) and 10 adult behaviors (e.g., stroking the infant) in 5-second intervals (Blount, Devine, Cheng, Simons, & Hayutin, 2008). In some cases, observers indicate the *intensity* of phenomena under scrutiny using **observational rating scales**. For example, an observer using the Richmond Agitation-Sedation Scale (Sessler et al., 2002) rates the state of an intensive care unit patient along a 10-point scale from +4 (*combative*) through 0 (*alert and calm*) to −5 (*unarousable*). Observational methods are often applied during in-person sessions in which the observer watches what is transpiring in environments such as hospitals, rehabilitation facilities, nursing homes, and so on. However, permanent observational records can in some cases be maintained for later coding by means of such technical aids as videotaping.

Clinical observations are also used to measure (categorize) a wide range of nonbehavioral phenomena. For example, radiologists reading mammograms can use the Breast Imaging Reporting and Data System (BI-RADS) to rate the probability of a malignancy on a scale from *negative* to *highly suggestive of malignancy* based on their observation of mammographic breast density.

---

[1]Some scales have been developed for either self-administration or proxy-administration—for example, the World Health Organization Disability Assessment Schedule 2.0 (WHODAS 2.0, Üstün et al., 2010)

2.1.c Performance Tests

Patients' abilities and skills are sometimes measured with **performance tests** or knowledge tests. For example, the 6-minute walk test (Guyatt et al., 1985) is a widely used measure of physical functioning for patients with various cardiovascular, respiratory, or neurologic diseases. The measure is the distance walked in a 6-minute period, typically involving the use of a treadmill. Many other physical performance tests have been devised to measure such attributes as balance, mobility, endurance, and flexibility.

Tests for cognitive performance abound. In the health care field, such tests are used primarily to screen for and monitor problems in people with cognitive or memory deficits. Examples include the Mini-Mental State Examination or MMSE (Folstein, Folstein, & McHugh, 1975) and the clock drawing test (Sunderland et al., 1989).

Finally, some health researchers, especially those who focus on health promotion, develop tests of knowledge, such as patients' knowledge about nutrition or smoking. As an example, Wyatt, Sikorski, and Wills (2013) developed a 13-item scale to test complementary and alternative medicine (CAM) knowledge: the Complementary and Alternative Medicine Knowledge instrument.

Like measurements from other sources, performance and knowledge tests require assessments of key measurement properties.

2.1.d Other Measures

Although most health-related measurements of nonphysiologic attributes are either verbal reports, observational measures, or performance tests, a few others are also used to describe, screen, or evaluate people. In psychotherapy, for instance, **projective tests** present patients with vague stimuli that are open to multiple interpretations. A well-known example is the Rorschach inkblot test (Rorschach, 1927). Projective tests have been used to measure a wide array of constructs, such as psychological distress, perceptual accuracy, neurologic impairment, and personality disorders.

Some health measures are composite indexes that rely on information from multiple sources, including physiologic measurements, health records, verbal reports, and observations. For example, the Apgar score to assess newborn health status involves summing scores for five separate attributes, one of which requires a physical measurement (e.g., whether the infant's pulse is above or below 100 beats per minute [bpm]) and four of which are based on observation (e.g., whether respiration is absent, slow/irregular, or good/crying) (Apgar, 1953). Many screening instruments also fall into this category, such as patient fall risk assessment instruments. For example, the STRATIFY fall risk assessment tool (Oliver, Britton, Seed, Martin, & Hopper, 1997) incorporates information from records (e.g., whether the patient presented to hospital with a fall) and from observational ratings (e.g., whether the patient is in need of especially frequent toileting). Although this book does not offer explicit guidance on the development of such measures, the discussions about measurement properties and parameters apply to these as well.

2.2 Health Measurement Variants

Health measurements vary in several other ways in addition to the source of information. In this section, we consider variation in terms of complexity, generality, and adaptability.

2.2.a Measurement Complexity

The complexity of measurements can vary considerably in terms of the operations needed to derive a score. A *simple measure* is one that involves no manipulation of numerical values. Simple measures yield score values that can be used directly to measure the construct of interest. Many biophysiologic measures used in regular clinical settings are simple ones—the numerical value for, say, body temperature from a thermometer is typically used directly as the patient's score. An example of a PRO that is a simple measure is a single visual analog scale (VAS) to measure a patient's rating of pain on a scale from 0 to 100.

As will be discussed in later chapters, almost all measurements contain at least a small amount of error. For that reason, when it is important to minimize error, it can be useful to use *averaged values* as the scores. For example, clinical guidelines recommend that patients' blood pressure be measured two or more times on each visit and then averaged because single measurements have been found to misclassify a sizeable minority of patients into hypertensive categories (Handler, Zhao, & Egan, 2012).

Most of the measures discussed in this book are not simple or averaged measures but rather *composite measures* that require several individual measurements to be combined. As an example, dozens of composite scales have been developed to measure the construct of *self-efficacy*, which refers to a person's belief in his or her capacity to successfully achieve certain outcomes or goals. Self-efficacy is critical in many areas of health, such as in the management of chronic diseases. Van der Ven and colleagues (2003) developed a composite scale with 20 items to measure self-efficacy relating to diabetes self-care, the Confidence in Diabetes Self-Care Scale (CIDS). An example of an item is, "I believe I can adjust my insulin for exercise, travelling, or celebrations." Patients answer each item on a 5-point scale from 1 ("No, I am sure I cannot") to 5 ("Yes, I am sure I can"). The 20 item scores are summed, and higher total scores reflect greater self-efficacy.

Health constructs are often complex and complexity is often captured through scales that are multidimensional. A **unidimensional scale** is one that measures a unitary aspect of one construct. All of the items on a unidimensional scale can be added together because they are presumed to be measuring the same underlying trait. When a construct has multiple facets, it is often necessary to develop a **multidimensional scale**. Such instruments include several **subscales**, each of which taps a separate aspect of a broad construct. For instance, the Dyspnea Management Questionnaire (Migliore-Norweg, Whiteson, Demetis, & Rey, 2006) has five subscales, including one to measure self-efficacy for activity. In other cases, self-efficacy is itself conceptualized as having several distinct facets, which form the basis for separate subscales. As an example, the Children's Arthritis Self-Efficacy Scale or CASE (Barlow, Shaw, & Wright, 2001) includes items for three dimensions of self-efficacy: activity, symptom, and emotion. In instruments with several subscales, the subscales are scored separately, and thus such instruments typically yield multiple scores, which may be expressed as a score *profile*. In some cases, however, subscale scores are added together to form an overall total score. For example, the Short Form-36 Health Survey (SF-36) has eight subscales, but four subscales are combined to form an overall physical health score, and the other four are combined to yield an overall mental health score (Ware & Sherbourne, 1992). Multi-item scales and multidimensional scales are the norm in the measurement of many health constructs and have been created as verbal reports, observational measures, and performance tests.

Multi-item scales often are preferred to single-item measures for several reasons. First, many constructs are so complicated that a single question cannot capture the full range of relevant information. Single items also tend to be less reliable than multi-item scales because multiple items allow random errors of measurement to be cancelled out. Another issue is that multi-item scales can make finer discriminations among people. A single global health rating question on a 7-point scale can only discriminate seven different classifications. By contrast, a health status scale with 10 items, each rated on a 7-point scale, could take on values from 10 to 70.

One final wrinkle relating to score complexity concerns the issue of **weighting**. Composite measures often involve summing the item values to yield a total score, although sometimes, instrument developers recommend that the total score be the *average* across items so that the total score is on the same scale as the items.[2] In either case, the items are

---

[2]We are referring here to "traditional" scoring according to the classical test theory framework, described briefly later in this chapter. "Modern" methods of scale development, using a different framework called *item response theory*, involve different scoring procedures, as described in Chapter 6.

all weighted equally. Such scoring involves an implicit assumption that each item is equally important as a measure of the target construct. Sometimes, however, it is attractive to have differential weighting of items to reflect the items' contribution. Although weighting usually has been found to have little effect on a scale's measurement properties (Streiner & Norman, 2008), there may be situations in which weighting does improve predictive validity, but at the cost of increased scoring complexity and thus possibly increased error. Moreover, weights are usually developed for a specific population and may be unsuitable when the instrument is used with a different population. Thus, unitary weighting of items is typical for most composite scales.

2.2.b Generic and Specific Measurement

During the early years of developing health PROs, most scales were generic. A **generic scale** is a measure of a construct that is broadly applicable across different clinical (and sometimes nonclinical) populations. The SF-36 is a good example of a generic scale. This scale asks questions about activities of daily living (e.g., ability to lift and carry groceries), general health, vitality, pain, social functioning, and psychological state—questions that are relevant to almost everyone. The SF-36 has been used in many studies and clinical trials across health specialties and has also been incorporated into health surveys of the general population.

Beginning in the 1990s, targeted scales proliferated, especially with regard to measuring the broad construct called "quality of life." As noted by Cano and Hobart (2011), there are several different types of **specific scales**. The most common are *disease-specific scales* that are designed for use with people who have a particular disease or condition. For example, there are disease-specific quality of life scales for patients with stroke and aphasia, cancer, HIV/AIDS, and kidney disease, to name only a few. Specificity sometimes relates to health-related behaviors rather than to diseases. For instance, there are generic self-efficacy scales, disease-specific self-efficacy scales (e.g., for asthma and diabetes), and also *behavior-specific scales* that focus on self-efficacy in such health behavior areas as physical fitness, dietary habits, or compliance with a regimen. For example, Dennis and Faux (1999) developed the Breastfeeding Self-Efficacy Scale for assessing maternal confidence in breastfeeding. There are also *site-specific scales* that focus on particular parts of the body. An example is the Foot Function Index (Budiman-Mak, Conrad, & Roach, 1991), which is a PRO measure of pain and disability of the feet. Finally, there are *age-specific scales* that are sometimes adaptations of generic scales for older (or younger) populations. For example, Fertman and Primack (2009) used items from a generic self-efficacy scale as the basis for creating a scale that was both behavior specific (resisting drug use) and age specific (elementary school children).

There are advantages and disadvantages to both generic and specific scales. A key advantage of generic scales is that they permit comparisons across populations; for example, the SF-36 permits a comparison of the relative burden of disease for a wide range of diseases. Generic scales have often been subjected to more empirical testing and refinement than specific scales and so may have better measurement properties. The use of generic scales also has implications for the interpretability of scores because if they have been administered to broad or general populations, *norms* can be developed that enable people to understand what a "normal" range of values is (see Chapter 16).

There are important limitations of generic scales, however, including the fact that patients with specific conditions may not see such scales as having *face validity*; that is, the scales do not look as though they are measuring something relevant to them (Chapter 11). More importantly, however, generic scales may make poor outcome measures for evaluating treatments for specific diseases. The items on a generic scale usually do not correspond to targeted areas of improvement and thus may be inadequate for measuring change resulting from treatment or change in a condition resulting from the passage of time (e.g., deterioration). Generic scales usually fail to include items that are important to a disease while including others that are irrelevant. For example, questions on a generic symptom scale relating to "shortness of breath" or "incontinence" may have little relevance for patients with migraine headaches.

Because there are advantages to both generic and disease-specific scales, some scales have a core generic component and disease-specific *modules* that have more targeted and relevant questions for a specific population. For example, the Pediatric Quality of Life Inventory (PedsQL) has 23 items in a generic core scale and separate modules for many specific diseases such as cancer, diabetes, rheumatology, cerebral palsy, and asthma (Varni et al., 2002, 2003).

Interest in creating specific measures has been taken to another level through the creation of individualized **patient-specific measures** that allow patients to make decisions about which questions to answer. An example is the Schedule for the Evaluation of Individual Quality of Life or SEIQoL (Hickey et al., 1996; O'Boyle, McGee, Hickey, O'Malley, & Joyce, 1992). This scale asks people to nominate the areas of life that are most important, rate their level of functioning or satisfaction with each, and indicate the relative importance of each to their overall quality of life. Although these measures have high levels of face validity, they are less practical and make it difficult to make comparisons across patients. It has been suggested that such individualized measures may have greater applicability in clinical settings and in descriptive research rather than as outcomes in clinical trials (Patel, Veenstra, & Patrick, 2003).

2.2.c Static and Adaptive Measures

A **static measure** is a fixed-length measure that is administered in a comparable manner for everyone who is measured. For static composite scales, people are asked to complete an entire set of items and then a summary score is developed on the basis of responses. With such static scales, comparisons across people, and comparisons of the same people across time, depend on respondents answering all the questions on the scale (or on the use of strategies to address missing values). Most of the health-related measures that have been developed in the past few decades are static. As an example, the SF-36 has 36 fixed questions, and total scores for physical health and mental health rely on responses to the same questions for everyone. Much of this book uses static scales to illustrate key measurement concepts.

By contrast, an **adaptive measure** uses information from responses to early questions to guide the selection of subsequent questions. Dynamic adaptive measures are gaining in popularity as a way to obtain more precise information about an attribute while reducing respondent burden. Adaptive testing has its origin in measurement advances from item response theory (briefly described later in this chapter). **Item banks** (banks of hundreds of items) are now being created to store items relevant to broad topic areas. The most important example of such item banking is the Patient Reported Outcomes Measurement Information System (PROMIS®), which was developed with support from the U.S. National Institutes of Health (Cella, Gershon, Lai, & Choi, 2007). An approach called **computerized adaptive testing** (**CAT**) uses these item banks to create measurements that are tailored to individuals. With CAT, the computer uses algorithms to choose relevant questions from the item bank for each person. With such tailoring, the set of items used can be different for each patient. Nevertheless, despite item differences, cross-patient comparisons can be made because the testing places people along a dimension of interest. CAT will be further described in Chapter 6, and interested readers can find more information in the writings of Cella and colleagues (2007); Hays, Morales, and Reise (2000); and van der Linden and Glas (2010).

Most adaptive measures are administered on a computer because the software can make branching to different items seamless from the respondent's perspective. Adaptive tests based on item response theory (IRT) are also being developed for paper-and-pencil administration, however. For example, Kopec and colleagues (2013) created what they called "semiadaptive" questionnaires in five domains of health-related quality of life. Such measures require the use of *skip patterns* that respondents must follow, and this in turn runs the risk of confusion and error with some populations.

Although IRT is strongly linked to adaptive testing, IRT has also been used to develop, refine, and investigate static measures as well. For example, the PROMIS® project has developed item banks for computerized adaptive testing but has also used IRT to create static forms of many latent constructs (Varni et al., 2014).

2.3   Psychometric and Clinimetric Measures

Psychometrics refers to the branch of psychology concerned with the theory and techniques of psychological measurements, which include the measurement of abilities, knowledge, personality traits, attitudes, beliefs, intentions, moods, and emotions. Psychometrics have played a prominent role in the development, refinement, and assessment of composite scales for decades, and psychometric methods remain the dominant paradigm in the construction of health-related PROs.

In the early years of scale construction, some psychometricians used a completely empirical (statistical) approach to the construction of scales. A particularly notable example of such an approach is the Minnesota Multiphasic Personality Inventory (MMPI), a multidimensional instrument developed to measure personality structure and psychopathology. This atheoretical instrument was developed by selecting items that were endorsed by patients known to have been diagnosed with certain pathologies (Hathaway & McKinley, 1940).

Few psychometric scales being developed today have such an atheoretical origin, yet clinicians have expressed concerns about the utility of psychometrically developed scales for use in clinical practice. In particular, a prominent physician and clinical epidemiologist, Alvan Feinstein, promoted a new field called *clinimetrics* (Feinstein, 1987). **Clinimetrics** is devoted to the development and assessment of measures of clinical phenomena. Clinimetric methods, discussed in Chapter 7, differ most notably from psychometric methods with regard to the construction of multi-item scales.

Within psychometrics, different measurement theories have emerged. A **measurement theory** is a framework concerning how the scores generated by items on an instrument represent the unobservable constructs being measured. Measurement theories provide guidance about the statistical relationships between items on the one hand and a construct on the other. The "traditional approach" to scale development and evaluation—and the approach that still dominates today—is based on a theory called **classical test theory (CTT)**. A second psychometric theory that is gaining in popularity in health measurement is *latent trait theory*, which is often referred to as **item response theory**. Figure 2.1 presents a taxonomy of models for constructing scales within the two dominant frameworks of CTT and IRT; elements in the taxonomy relating to latent trait models are elaborated in Chapter 6.

2.3.a   Psychometric Scales Using Classical Test Theory

CTT (also called *classical measurement theory*) has a history going back to such statistical luminaries as Karl Pearson, Charles Spearman, and Lee Cronbach. An early application of CTT was the development of rating scales called **Likert scales**, named after the psychologist Rensis Likert. Likert's methods, which were applied to the measurement of attitudes, involved presenting people with declarative statements relating to a particular attitude (e.g., attitude toward abortion) and asking people to rate their degree of agreement or disagreement. The cornerpiece of Likert's methods was the simple addition of ordinal-level item

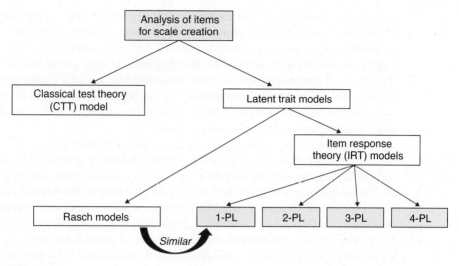

Figure 2.1

Measurement models for item analysis and scale construction. "PL" is the acronym for "parameter, logistic," as explained in Chapter 6. The numbers indicate how many parameters are estimated in the model (e.g., 1 parameter in 1-PL).

scores to compute a total attitude score. Although most health scales are not about attitudes, Likert's basic approach to scale development is widely used, and so **summated rating scales** in general are often called *Likert scales*.[3]

A basic premise of CTT is that any score from a quantitative measurement can be conceptualized as having two components, a "true" component and an error component, as shown in the following equation:

$$\text{Obtained score} = \text{True score} \pm \text{Error}$$

$$\text{Or}$$

$$X_O = X_T \pm X_E$$

The first term (X_O) is an observed score—for example, a score on a 10-item fatigue scale. The obtained score is an estimate of the **true score** (X_T), which is a hypothetical value from an infallible measure. A true score can never be known but is estimated with observed scores. The final term (X_E) is the **error of measurement**. The difference between true and obtained scores is the result of factors that distort the measurement. Factors that contribute to measurement errors are described in Chapters 4 and 10.

The basic CTT model can be applied to any type of measurement, including biophysiologic measurements, but it has been used mostly in connection with composite scales. In CTT, multi-item scales gain accuracy in approximating the true score through the aggregation of items. Traditional CTT scales rely on items that are deliberately redundant (DeVellis, 2012) in the hope that multiple indicators of the construct will converge on the true score, through triangulation, and balance out errors of measurement associated with each item.

Scale development with CTT typically begins with a conceptualization of the targeted construct and the creation of a pool of items that correspond to the theoretical understanding of the construct. Items on a CTT scale are usually ones of similar and moderate

---

[3]Other scaling approaches have been developed but have not been as widely used as that developed by Likert. These include Guttman or Thurstone scaling, multidimensional scaling, and ipsative (forced choice) scaling, to name a few. Guttman scaling is briefly described in this chapter in connection with IRT. For other scaling approaches, consult other references (e.g., Gable & Wolfe, 1993; Nunnally & Bernstein, 1994).

intensity, the goal being to have each item elicit a range of responses that can discriminate among people with different amounts of the attribute. Extreme items that are rejected by the majority of people are not useful on a CTT scale. For example, on a CTT scale to measure depression, an item such as "I am feeling blue" is more useful than an item such as "I think about committing suicide daily." Discrimination on a CTT scale is usually a result of gradations on the **response options**, which can be worded to capture frequency (e.g., always, most of the time, sometimes), intensity (e.g., strongly agree, agree), amount (e.g., none, some, a lot), or some other rank-ordered dimension.

Although careful and deliberate thought is required in developing a CTT item pool, statistical methods play an important role in the final selection of items and refinement of the scale. Following the administration of the items to a development sample from the target population, various methods of *item analysis* are used to examine how individual items perform. For example, developers typically look at the distribution of item responses, *inter-item correlations*, and *item-scale correlations*. *Exploratory factor analysis* (EFA) typically plays a role as well. The computation of an index of internal consistency called *Cronbach's alpha* is a standard feature of CTT scale development. Methods of CTT scale construction are described in Chapter 5.

CTT embodies a number of assumptions. First, it is assumed that each item is an indicator of the construct it is measuring, and that the construct *causes* responses to the item. For example, a person who is high on the fatigue construct will respond "strongly agree" to the item "I feel exhausted." Here, the latent trait fatigue *drives* that response. A related assumption is that the construct being measured is unidimensional; that is, that the subparts (e.g., items) being added together are measuring the same thing. In CTT, it is also assumed that the amount of error associated with an item varies randomly and that the error terms have a mean of zero when averaged across a large number of people. Finally, it is assumed that the error terms are normally distributed, not correlated with each other, and also not correlated with the true score.

Many resources are available for learning more about CTT. These include both recent writings (e.g., DeVellis, 2012; Streiner & Norman, 2008) as well as classic psychometric textbooks (Lord & Novick, 1968; Nunnally & Bernstein, 1994).

2.3.b Psychometric Scales Using Item Response Theory

IRT is an alternative to CTT for the measurement of unobservable constructs or *latent traits*. IRT, developed in the 1950s, has been widely used in creating cognitive and educational tests, and its use in developing measures of other constructs in health and psychology is growing.

In CTT, traits are modeled at the level of the observed test score, whereas in IRT, the models are at the level of the observed item response. The goal of IRT is to allow researchers to gain understanding of the characteristics of items independent of the people who complete them. IRT scales can use items like the ones used in CTT, such as items in a Likert format—in fact, a person completing a Likert-type scale would probably not know whether it had been developed within the CTT or IRT framework. But a person *developing* a multi-item scale must decide in advance which measurement theory is being used because the scale items and the process of item selection differs. Items on a CTT Likert scale are designed to tap the underlying construct in a similar manner, but items on a latent-trait IRT scale are carefully chosen and refined to measure different degrees of the attribute being measured.

As an example, suppose we were developing a scale to measure risk-taking behavior in adolescents. In a CTT scale, the items would likely include statements about risk taking of similar intensity, with which respondents would respond with graded responses corresponding to frequency or intensity of endorsement. The aggregate of responses would array people along a continuum indicating varying propensity to take risks.

In an IRT scale, the items themselves would be chosen to reflect different levels of risk taking (e.g., not eating vegetables, smoking cigarettes, having unprotected sex, driving a car while text messaging). Each item has a different level of **difficulty**. It is "easier" to agree with or admit to lower risk items than higher risk items. Measurements based on an IRT model result in information about the *location* of both items and people on a scale. If a pool of unidimensional items can readily be ordered into a hierarchy of difficulty, then a good IRT model fit is plausible.

IRT is best thought of as a *family* of statistical methods and theoretical models. For example, some IRT models are used with items that have dichotomous responses, whereas others can be applied to multiple choice (polytomous) items. One especially important distinction concerns the number of parameters that are analyzed during model evaluation. Item difficulty (location), for example, is one parameter. Two other parameters are an item's ability to *discriminate* and its *susceptibility to false positives* (guessing). When item difficulty is the only parameter being considered in an IRT analysis, researchers may say that they are using a **Rasch model**, crediting Danish mathematician Georg Rasch.[4] Outside of education, one-parameter and two-parameter models are most common.

The conceptual forerunner of IRT measurement is a type of scale known as a *Guttman scale*. Louis Guttman (1950) developed a scaling method that involves a small set of hierarchical items, the responses to which are dichotomous (e.g., yes/no). For example, here is a four-item version of a Guttman scale to measure self-reported distance vision (Gothwal, Wright, Lamoureux, & Pesudovs, 2009), which we adapted for simplicity:

1. I can see well enough to recognize a friend who gets close to my face.
2. I can see well enough to recognize a friend who is an arm's length away.
3. I can see well enough to recognize a friend across the room.
4. I can see well enough to recognize a friend across the street.

In a perfect Guttman scale, a person who answered *yes* to Item 4 would also answer *yes* to Items 1 through 3, and the person's score would be 4. A person who had problems recognizing a friend across the street but not across the room would presumably endorse the first three items and would have a score of 3. People who could not recognize a friend even when he or she gets close to their faces would have a score of 0. Such a scale is called *deterministic* because the person's score is determined by the highest item endorsed. Guttman scaling yields *response profiles* rather than a summed score.

IRT scales also involve a hierarchical set of items, but IRT is probabilistic rather than deterministic in that it allows for deviations from a perfect hierarchical set of responses. IRT methods describe the relationship between a person's underlying latent trait and the probability of a particular response to an item. Item difficulty and the amount of a person's trait are linked in IRT models. The higher a person's amount of a trait, the more probable it is that he or she will answer positively to a "difficult" item. And, the more difficult the item, the less probable it is that the item is answered positively by a person with a smaller amount of the trait.

In an IRT analysis, an item's parameters—such as difficulty—are summarized on an **item characteristic curve** (ICC). These curves, which are roughly S-shaped, yield information about parameters of interest. Figure 2.2 present an example of an ICC for a dichotomous item. In the figure, the total amount of the trait (analogous to total scores) is plotted on the X axis, and the probability of "passing" the item (e.g., agreeing with it) is plotted on the Y axis. For the difficulty parameter, the curve shows how much of the underlying attribute must be present in order for, say, 50% of the people to "pass" the item.

IRT is a more sophisticated approach than CTT for assessing the strengths and weaknesses of individual items, but it is more complex and cannot be undertaken with traditional

---

[4]Although there is some controversy about whether Rasch models should be considered part of IRT (e.g., Cano & Hobart, 2011), we will include Rasch models in our discussion of IRT.

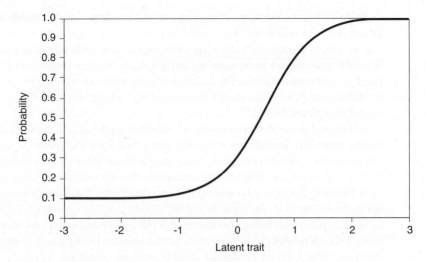

Figure 2.2
Item characteristic curve for a dichotomous item.

multipurpose software such as the Statistical Package for the Social Sciences (SPSS). For this reason, in this "primer," CTT methods that have dominated the measurement of health-related constructs are emphasized. Nevertheless, the growth of IRT scaling is indisputable, and so we offer an overview of basic IRT methods in Chapter 6 and point out features of IRT-based measures throughout the book. Those who seek greater elaboration of IRT methods should consult such sources as de Ayala (2009), Embretson and Reise (2000), and Hambleton, Swaminathan, and Rogers (1991).

2.3.c Clinimetric Measures

Scales developed through clinimetric approaches do not have an underlying measurement theory and do not depend primarily on statistical criteria for finalizing a set of items for inclusion in a scale. In clinimetric scales, judgments are used to make decisions about the clinical relevance and appropriateness of items. Clinimetric approaches have been criticized by some psychometricians who specialize in health measurement, notably David Streiner (Streiner, 2003b). Nevertheless, Alvan Feinstein, by advocating a clinimetric approach, made a substantial contribution by giving increased attention to measurement issues for clinical applications.

Clinimetric measurements, like psychometric ones, are usually multi-item composite scales. Item selection for a clinimetric measure relies heavily on judgments of what patients and (or) clinicians consider to be important. Clinimetricians typically reject the empirically driven selection of final scale items through psychometric item analysis because the resulting items are not necessarily ones that are clinically meaningful.

According to Fava, Tomba, and Sonino (2012), clinimetric scales are especially useful for measurement in certain domains, such as patients' symptoms and clinical manifestations, functional ability and disability, quality of life, allostatic load, and lifestyle preferences (e.g., alcohol use, sleep habits, dietary patterns). Although clinimetric measures follow a different development path than psychometric scales, the evaluation of their measurement properties typically follows those from CTT.

2.4 Reflective Scales and Formative Indexes

One other distinction relating to multi-item measures is important, and that is the difference between reflective and formative scales. This distinction, which concerns the nature of the relationship between a construct and the measure of the construct, is crucial for the construction of multi-item measures and also for their evaluation.

Causal language has permeated discussions on scale construction for decades (e.g., Long, 1983; Lord & Novick, 1968; Nunnally & Bernstein, 1994). In both CTT and IRT, the underlying construct is often conceptualized as the *cause* of responses on a measure. Constructs are not directly observable, and so they have to be inferred by the hypothesized effects they have on observables, such as responses to items on a PRO or behaviors witnessed and recorded on an observational scale. Psychometric scales have been coined **reflective scales** because the items are viewed as *reflections* of the construct (Edwards & Bagozzi, 2000). The items on a reflective scale share a common cause. Using terminology from structural equation modeling, items on a reflective measure are sometimes called *effect indicators* because they represent the *effect* caused by the construct (Blalock, 1964; Fayers & Hand, 2002; Fayers, Hand, Bjordal, & Groenvold, 1997).

A reflective scale can be illustrated using graphic conventions from structural equation modeling, with arrows designating a causal mechanism. Figure 2.3 uses a few items from the widely used Center for Epidemiologic Studies Depression Scale or CES-D (Radloff, 1977) to show how the underlying construct of depression can be conceptualized as affecting responses to individual scale items. In the model in Figure 2.3, depression is viewed as *causing* sleep disturbances, sadness, and crying spells, which are effects of being depressed. These items would be expected to be fairly highly intercorrelated because they all reflect the construct.

Not all multi-item instruments, however, are reflective. A multi-item measure can be conceptualized as having items that "cause" or define the attribute (rather than being the effect of the attribute). Using the terminology from Edwards and Bagozzi (2000), such measures are called **formative measures**. To distinguish reflective and formative measures, several writers advocate using the term *scale* for multi-item reflective measures and the term **index** for multi-item formative measures (DeVellis, 2012; Streiner, 2003a), and we will use that convention as well.

A formative index involves constructs that are *formed* by its components rather than causing them. Such indexes have items or components that are *causal indicators* (rather than effect indicators). The Apgar score is a widely used formative index. The five "items" on the Apgar score are distinct components that, when combined, offer a measure of newborn health

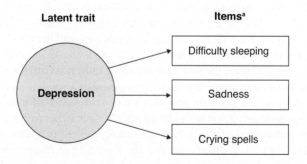

[a]Items correspond to 3 of the 20 items on the Center for Epidemiological Studies-Depression scale or CES-D (Radloff, 1977): "My sleep was restless"; "I felt sad"; and "I had crying spells." People respond by indicating how often each statement applied to them in the previous 7 days, on a 4-point scale from "rarely" to "most of the time".

Figure 2.3

Graphic representation of a reflective scale to measure depressive symptoms.

Items[a]   **Attribute**

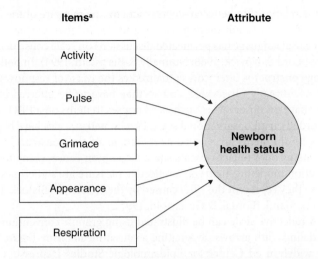

[a]Items correspond to the 5 items on the Apgar index (Apgar, 1953): Activity (Muscle Tone); Pulse; Grimace (Reflex/Irritability), Appearance; and Respiration. Each of the 5 "signs" is scored 0, 1, or 2, to yield a score on the index that can range from 0 to 10.

Figure 2.4
Graphic representation of a formative index to measure newborn health status.

status, but the items are not necessarily correlated with one another. Figure 2.4 presents a graphic illustration of the formative Apgar score. As the arrows in this diagram suggest, the five components (activity, pulse, grimace, appearance, and respiration) define a newborn's health status. Newborn well-being, as measured by the Apgar score, does not "cause" variation in pulse rate, respiration, and so on, and so the Apgar measure is not a reflective scale.

Another good illustration of a formative index is the Holmes-Rahe Social Readjustment Scale, which is a measure of stress. Psychiatrists Thomas Holmes and Richard Rahe (1967) studied whether stressful life events might cause illness and devised an index that asked patients to indicate which of 43 life events they had experienced in the past year. Examples of life event items include death of a spouse, dismissal from work, pregnancy, and change in residence. The life events are assigned different weights or "life change units" (e.g., 100 for death of a spouse, 20 for a change in residence), and the units are then added together. In the aggregate, the sum of the life change units for the 43 items define the construct of stressful life events. Clearly, the items are not effect indicators on this scale. For example, having high stress does not "cause" the death of a spouse or a residential move.

Because the items on an index are not *caused* by an underlying construct, they are not necessarily correlated with one another. In fact, items with modest correlations that capture different aspects of an attribute are usually desired in a formative index. For example, many screening tools are formative and are composed of components that independently predict an outcome of interest.

The development of reflective scales and formative indexes is necessarily different. For example, because the items on a formative index define the attribute, the specific items matter very much. If the item "I had crying spells" was removed from the CES-D scale, for example, the other 19 items could carry most of the burden of measuring depression. But if the item "Death of a spouse" was removed from the Holmes-Rahe index, the score would misrepresent the stress levels of people who had lost a spouse.

Another consequence of having noncorrelated items on a formative index is that some of the standard psychometric assessment methods associated with CTT are not appropriate.

For example, it is usually not meaningful to compute Cronbach's alpha for a formative index because this statistic measures the degree to which the items are internally consistent (i.e., intercorrelated).

The development of formative index is not discussed at length in this book, although many clinimetric measures are formative (see Chapter 7). Nevertheless, many of the methods of assessing key measurement properties are equally appropriate for scales and indexes.

References

Apgar, V. (1953). A proposal for new method of evaluation of the newborn infant. *Current Research in Anesthesia and Analgesia, 32*, 260–267.

Barlow, J. H., Shaw, K. L., & Wright, C. C. (2001). Development and preliminary validation of a children's arthritis self-efficacy scale. *Arthritis & Rheumatology, 45*, 159–166.

Blalock, H. M. (1964). *Causal inferences in nonexperimental research.* Chapel Hill, NC: University of North Carolina Press.

Blount, R. L., Devine, K. A., Cheng, P. S., Simons, L. E., & Hayutin L. (1997). The impact of adult behaviors and vocalizations on infant distress during immunizations. *Journal of Pediatric Psychology, 33*, 1163–1174.

Budiman-Mak, E., Conrad, K., & Roach, K. (1991). The Foot Function Index: A measure of foot pain and disability. *Journal of Clinical Epidemiology, 44*, 561–570.

Cano, S. J., & Hobart, J. C. (2011). The problem with health measurement. *Patient Preference and Adherence, 5*, 279–290.

Cella, D., Gershon, R., Lai, J., & Choi, S. (2007). The future of outcome measurement: Item banking, tailored short forms, and computerized adaptive testing. *Quality of Life Research, 16*(Suppl. 1), 133–141.

De Ayala, R. J. (2009). *The theory and practice of item response theory.* New York, NY: The Guilford Press.

Dennis, C. L., & Faux, S. (1999). Development and psychometric testing of the Breastfeeding Self-Efficacy Scale. *Research in Nursing & Health, 22*, 399–409.

DeVellis, R. F. (2012). *Scale development: Theory and application* (3rd ed.). Thousand Oaks, CA: Sage.

Edwards, J. R., & Bagozzi, R. P. (2000). On the nature and direction of relationships between constructs and measures. *Psychological Methods, 5*, 155–174.

Embretson, S. E., & Reise, S. P. (2000). *Item response theory for psychologists.* Mahwah, NJ: Lawrence Erlbaum.

Fava, G. A., Tomba, E., & Sonino, N. (2012). Clinimetrics: The science of clinical measurement. *The International Journal of Clinical Practice, 66*, 11–15.

Fayers, P. M., & Hand, D. J. (2002). Causal variables, indicator variables and measurement scales: An example from quality of life. *Journal of the Royal Statistical Society, 165*, 233–261.

Fayers, P. M., Hand, D. J., Bjordal, K., & Groenvold, M. (1997). Causal indicators in quality of life research. *Quality of Life Research, 6*, 393–406.

Feinstein, A. R. (1987). *Clinimetrics.* New Haven, CT: Yale University Press.

Fertman, C. I., & Primack, B. A. (2009). Elementary student self-efficacy scale development and validation focused on student learning, peer relations, and resisting drug use. *Journal of Drug Education, 39*, 23–38.

Folstein, M. F., Folstein, S., & McHugh, P. (1975). "Mini-Mental State": A practical method for grading the cognitive state of patients for the clinician. *Journal of Psychiatric Research, 12*, 189–198.

Gable, R. K., & Wolf, M. B. (1993). *Instrument development in the affective domain* (2nd ed.) Boston, MA: Kluwer Academic.

Gothwal, V., Wright, T., Lamoureux, E., & Pesudovs, K. (2009). Guttman scale analysis of the distance vision scale. *Investigative Ophthalmology & Visual Science, 50*, 4496–4501.

Guttman, L. (1950). The basis for scalogram analysis. In S. A. Stouffer, L. Guttman, E. A. Suchman, P. Lazarsfeld, S. A. Star, & J. A. Clausen (Eds.), *Measurement and prediction.* Princeton, NJ: Princeton University Press.

Guyatt, G. H., Sullivan, M., Thompson, P., Fallen, E., Pugsley, S., Taylore, D., & Berman, L. (1985). The 6-minute walk: A new measure of exercise capacity in patients with chronic heart failure. *Canadian Medical Association Journal, 132*, 919–923.

Hambleton, R. K., Swaminathan, H., & Rogers, H. J. (1991). *Fundamentals of item response theory.* Newbury Park, CA: Sage.

Handler, J., Zhao, Y., & Egan, B. M. (2012). Impact of the number of blood pressure measurements on blood pressure classification in US adults: NHANES 1999–2008. *Journal of Clinical Hypertension, 14*, 751–759.

Hathaway, S. R., & McKinley, J. C. (1940). A multiphasic personality schedule (Minnesota): I. Construction of the schedule. *Journal of Psychology, 10*, 249–254.

Hays, R. D., Morales, L., & Reise, S. (2000). Item response theory and health outcomes measurement in the 21st century. *Medical Care, 38*(Suppl. 9), II28–II42.

Hickey, A. M., Bury, G., O'Boyle, C., Bradley, F., O'Kelly, F., & Shannon, W. (1996). A new short form individual quality of life measure (SEIQoL-DW). *British Medical Journal, 313*, 29–33.

Holmes, T. H., & Rahe, R. (1967). The Social Readjustment Rating Scale. *Journal of Psychosomatic Research, 11*, 213–218.

Kopec, J. A., Sayre, E., Davis, A., Badley, E., Abrahamowicz, M. Pouchot, J., . . . Esdaile, J. M. (2013). Development of a paper-and-pencil semi-adaptive questionnaire for 5 domains of health-related quality of life (PAT-5D-QOL). *Quality of Life Research, 22,* 2829–2842.

Long, J. S. (1983). *Confirmatory factor analysis.* Beverly Hills, CA: Sage.

Lord, F. M., & Novick, M. R. (1968). *Statistical theory of mental test scores.* Reading, MA: Addison-Wesley.

Migliore-Norweg, A., Whiteson, J., Demetis, S., & Rey, M. (2006). A new functional status outcome measure of dyspnea and anxiety for adults with lung disease: The Dyspnea Management Questionnaire. *Journal of Cardiopulmonary Rehabilitation, 26,* 395–404.

Nunnally, J., & Bernstein, I. H. (1994). *Psychometric theory* (3rd ed.). New York, NY: McGraw-Hill.

O'Boyle, C., McGee, H., Hickey, A., O'Malley, K., & Joyce, C. (1992). Individual quality of life in patients undergoing hip replacement. *Lancet, 339,* 1088–1091.

Oliver, D., Britton, M., Seed, P., Martin, F. C., & Hopper, A. H. (1997). Development and evaluation of evidence based risk assessment tool (STRATIFY) to predict which elderly inpatients will fall: case-control and cohort studies. *British Medical Journal, 315,* 1049–1053.

Patel, K. K., Veenstra, D. L., & Patrick, D. L. (2003). A review of patient-generated outcome measures and their application in clinical trials. *Value Health, 6,* 595–603.

Radloff, L. S. (1977). The CES-D scale: A self-report depression scale for research in the general population. *Applied Psychological Measurement, 1,* 385–401.

Rorschach, H. (1927). *Rorschach test—Psychodiagnostic plates.* Cambridge, MA: Hogrefe.

Sessler, C. N., Gosnell, M. S., Grap, M. J., Brophy, G. M., O'Neal, P. V., Keane, K. A., . . . Elswick, R. K. (2002). The Richmond Agitation-Sedation Scale: validity and reliability in adult intensive care unit patients. *American Journal of Respiratory & Critical Care Medicine, 15,* 1338–1344.

Streiner, D. L. (2003a). Being inconsistent about consistency: When coefficient alpha does and doesn't matter. *Journal of Personality Assessment, 80,* 217–222.

Streiner, D. L. (2003b). Clinimetrics vs. psychometrics: An unnecessary distinction. *Journal of Clinical Epidemiology, 56,* 1142–1145.

Streiner, D. L., & Norman, G. R. (2008). *Health measurement scales: A practical guide to their development and use* (4th ed.). Oxford: Oxford University Press.

Sunderland, R., Hill, J., Mellow, A., Lawlor, B., Gundersheimer, J., Newhouse, P., & Grafman, J. (1989). Clock drawing in Alzheimer's disease: A novel measure of dementia severity. *Journal of the American Geriatric Society, 37,* 725–729.

Üstün, T., Chatterji, S., Kostanjsek, S., Rehm, J., Kennedy, C., Epping-Jordan, J., . . . Pull, C. (2010). Developing the World Health Organization Disability Assessment Schedule 2.0. *Bulletin of the World Health Organization, 88,* 815–823.

Van der Linden, W., & Glas, C. A. (2010). *Computerized adaptive testing: Theory and practice.* Dordrecht, The Netherlands: Kluwer Academic.

Van der Ven, N. C. W., Weinger, K., Yi, J., Pouwer, F., Ader, H., Ploeg, H. M., & Van Der Snoek, F. J. (2003). The confidence in diabetes self-care scale: psychometric properties of a new measure of diabetes-specific self-efficacy in Dutch and US patients with type 1 diabetes. *Diabetes Care, 26,* 713–718.

Varni, J. W., Burwinkle, T., Jacobs, J., Gottschalk, M., Kaufman, F., & Jones, K. (2003). The PedsQL in type 1 and type 2 diabetes: Reliability and validity of the Pediatric Quality of Life Inventory Generic Core Scales and Type 1 Diabetes Module. *Diabetes Care, 26,* 631–637.

Varni, J. W., Magnus, B., Stucky, B., Lin, Y., Quinn, H., Thissen, D., . . . DeWalt, D. A. (2014). Psychometric properties of the PROMIS® pediatric scales: Precision, stability, and comparison of different scoring and administration options. *Quality of Life Research, 23,* 1233–1243.

Varni, J. W., Seid, M., Smith Knight, T., Burwinkle, T., Brown, J., & Szer, I. S. (2002). The PedsQL in pediatric rheumatology: Reliability, validity, and responsiveness of the Pediatric Quality of Life Inventory Generic Core Scales and Rheumatology Module. *Arthritis and Rheumatism, 46,* 714–725.

Ware, J. E., & Sherbourne, C. D. (1992). The MOS 36-item Short Form Health Survey (SF-36). *Medical Care, 30,* 473–483.

Wyatt, G., Sikorski, A., & Wills, C. E. (2013). Development and initial validation of a Complementary and Alternative Medicine (CAM) Knowledge Instrument. *Journal of Nursing Measurement, 21,* 55–63.

Measurement Properties: An Overview

Chapter Outline

Scales and other measures can be assessed in terms of certain measurement properties. A **measurement property** is a characteristic reflecting a distinct aspect of the measure's quality. This chapter provides an overview of properties that are important to those who develop instruments for measurement, select measures to use in research or clinical applications, or evaluate the quality of research evidence as a basis for making clinical practice decisions.

3.1 An Introduction to Measurement Properties

One might think that it would be straightforward to identify the properties that are desirable in a measurement tool, but this has proved not to be the case. Disagreement about measurement properties has arisen between psychometricians who work primarily in psychology and education on the one hand and biomedical/epidemiologic researchers who have concerns regarding clinically relevant outcomes on the other hand. Psychometricians have primarily focused on two measurement properties: *reliability* and *validity* (e.g., DeVellis, 2012; Nunnally & Bernstein, 1994; Streiner & Norman, 2008). Those in health fields have taken a broader view.

To complicate things, the definitions of measurement properties such as reliability and validity are not always consistent. An additional problem is that there is confusion about terminology. For example, the property referred to as *reliability* has been called by such terms as accuracy, agreement, consistency, concordance, dependability, objectivity, precision, repeatability, reproducibility, and stability (DeVet, Terwee, Mokkink, & Knol, 2011; Streiner & Norman, 2008).

3.1.a COSMIN

A study spearheaded by a clinimetrics working group in the Netherlands sought to address problems relating to measurement terminology and definition. Using a Delphi-type approach to achieve consensus among an international panel of measurement experts, the group sought to (1) identify key measurement properties; (2) develop a measurement taxonomy; (3) define the terms in the taxonomy; and (4) develop formal standards for evaluating instruments. The result was the creation of COSMIN, the **Co**nsensus-based **S**tandards for the selection of health **M**easurement **In**struments (Mokkink et al., 2010a, 2010b; Terwee et al., 2012).

For those in health care fields, COSMIN is an important initiative for bringing order to the measurement chaos that has characterized the instrument development literature in the past few decades. Thus, in this book, we follow COSMIN in most respects, and we hope that others will adopt COSMIN's (or our) terms and definitions so that there is greater clarity and cohesiveness in future measurement work.

3.1.b A Measurement Property Taxonomy

The COSMIN group developed a graphic depiction of their measurement taxonomy.[1] While giving full credit for the group's important conceptualization, we have made some small modifications to their taxonomy to more clearly incorporate a time perspective. Our version is presented in Figure 3.1. The taxonomy is the basis for the materials presented in Chapters 8 through 19 (Parts III through V) of this book. As this figure shows, there are two measurement properties that relate to point-in-time (cross-sectional) measurements and two others that relate to longitudinal measurement—that is, the measurement of change.

In brief, the key measurement domains in the taxonomy are reliability, validity, reliability of change, and responsiveness. Each property has multiple aspects, and each is linked to **measurement parameters** that quantify the property so that conclusions can be drawn about an instrument's quality. Additionally, the taxonomy incorporates the issue of interpretability of both point-in-time scores and change scores. Unlike COSMIN, this taxonomy considers the reliability of change scores as a separate domain (i.e., the COSMIN taxonomy has three domains: reliability, validity, and responsiveness).

It may be recalled that in Chapter 1, we posed six measurement assessment questions about scores using as an example the World Health Organization Disability Assessment Schedule (Üstün et al., 2010). In our illustration, the administration of the scale to patients with spinal cord injury resulted in a score of 80 at baseline and 75 at a 3-month follow-up for patient one. These six questions correspond to the key measurement domains in the taxonomy:

1. *Reliability*: Is the score of 80 at baseline the right score value for this patient?
2. *Validity*: Is the scale truly measuring the construct functional ability, or is it measuring something else?
3. *Interpretation of a score*: What does a score of 80 *mean*? Is it high or low for patients with spinal cord injury?
4. *Reliability of change*: Is the change from 80 to 75 a real change, or does it merely reflect random fluctuations in measurement?
5. *Responsiveness*: Does the change from 80 to 75 correspond to a commensurate improvement in the patient's degree of functional ability?
6. *Interpretation of a change score*: What does a 5-point improvement *mean*? Is the improvement large enough to be considered clinically significant?

---

[1]The COSMIN measurement taxonomy is available on the COSMIN website: http://www.cosmin.nl.

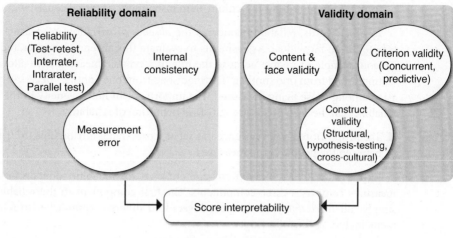

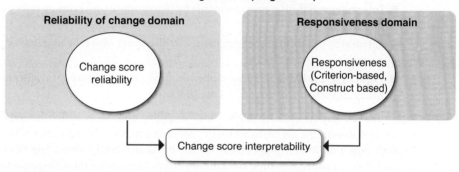

Figure 3.1

A taxonomy of measurement properties for an instrument's scores and change scores.

The remainder of this chapter provides an overview of the taxonomy shown in Figure 3.1, together with some definitions of key measurement terms.

3.2 Reliability

Broadly speaking, **reliability** can be defined as the extent to which a measurement is free from measurement error (Mokkink et al., 2010b). This definition is consistent with classical test theory (CTT), which conceptualizes any obtained score on a measure as the true score, plus or minus any measurement error (Chapter 2). So, according to this definition, if errors of measurement are absent or minimized, the measure would be reliable.

As attractive as this broad definition appears, it is not useful from an operational point of view because there is no way of establishing a person's true score. Reliability must be estimated by examining variation in people's scores. Fortunately, variation is the norm in human attributes. Scores on a measure vary from one person to the next, and they also vary or fluctuate across several measurements of the same person, even when the attribute has not changed. COSMIN offered an extended definition of reliability (Mokkink et al., 2010b), which we have adapted slightly:

■ Reliability is the extent to which scores for people *who have not changed* are the same for repeated measurements, under several situations, including repetition on different occasions, by different persons, or on different versions of a measure, or repetition in the form of different items on a multi-item instrument (internal consistency).

In other words, reliability concerns the *absence* of variation in measuring a stable attribute for an individual. Assessments to evaluate this absence, however, require a heterogeneous sample of people because the role of a reliable measure is to allow people to be distinguished from one another. "Distinguished from one another" necessarily implies variation among those being measured. The importance of heterogeneity in the assessment of reliability can be seen in a more statistical definition of reliability:

■ The proportion of total variance in a set of scores that is attributable to "true" differences between the people being measured

In both the COSMIN taxonomy and our own, the reliability domain for point-in-time measures comprises three components. The first component in the reliability domain is simply called *reliability*. This aspect covers four different approaches to reliability assessment, including the following:

■ **Test–retest reliability:** administration of the same measure to the same people at least twice
■ **Interrater reliability:** measurements by two or more observers or raters using the same instrument
■ **Intrarater reliability:** measurements by the same observer or rater on two or more occasions
■ **Parallel test reliability:** measurements of the same attribute using alternate versions of the same instrument with the same people

The second component within the reliability domain is called **internal consistency**, which concerns the degree to which the items on a multi-item scale covary. When a reflective scale taps a unidimensional construct, the items are ideally measuring the same attribute, so that when added together, any random errors (e.g., errors reflecting a particular wording on an item) cancel each other out. The vast majority of multi-item scales are assessed for internal consistency—although, as pointed out in Chapter 2, it is not appropriate to evaluate internal consistency for formative indexes. Internal consistency, in contrast to the four previously mentioned forms of reliability, can be evaluated through a single administration of the instrument.

The third component of the reliability domain for point-in-time measurement is measurement error. Paraphrasing slightly from COSMIN, **measurement error** is the error in a person's score, including both systematic and random error, that is not attributable to the true value of the construct. **Random errors** are the result of simple and usually small fluctuations that occur by chance in any measurement. A **systematic error** typically reflects biases that distort measurements. Some major types of bias that can affect health measurements are discussed in Chapter 4. Psychometricians have not traditionally treated measurement error as a major measurement property, and so the vast majority of instrument development papers do not present estimates of measurement error. However, measurement error is a key issue in change scores, and COSMIN encourages increased attention to this aspect of reliability. Moreover, measurement error is an important aspect of item evaluation in item response theory. All health care instruments should be assessed for reliability and measurement error within the population of interest.

3.3   Validity

Validity in a measurement context is defined as the degree to which an instrument is measuring the construct it purports to measure. When researchers develop a scale to measure *resilience*, they need to be sure that the resulting scores validly reflect this construct and not something else, such as self-efficacy, mental stamina, or perseverance. Assessing the validity of abstract constructs requires a careful conceptualization of the construct as well as a conceptualization of what the construct is *not*. The construct of interest needs to be carefully differentiated from other closely related constructs. Moreover, a valid measure of the construct should be one whose values are commensurate with the amount of the construct present, for constructs measured on a continuum.

The validity domain, like the reliability domain, encompasses several aspects. As shown in Figure 3.1, one aspect concerns content validity and face validity, which rely on subjective evaluations. **Content validity** is the degree to which the instrument has an appropriate set of items that reflect the full content of the construct domain being measured. Content validity can be enhanced during the development of a scale or index and can be assessed through consultation with experts in the construct domain. The "experts" most often are clinicians, theorists, researchers, or patients. Content validity is important in all multicomponent measures but is especially important in formative indexes because the items essentially define the construct. **Face validity** is the extent to which an instrument *looks* as though it is a measure of the target construct. Face validity is typically not considered a critical measurement property, but it can be important if patients' resistance to being measured reflects the view that the scale is not relevant to their problems or situations. Clinimetricians tend to value face validity more than psychometricians.

Another component in the validity domain is **criterion validity**, which is the extent to which the scores on a measure are an adequate reflection of (or predictor of) a criterion or "gold standard." For example, a new self-report sleep quality scale would have good criterion validity if its scores correlated highly with values from polysomnography. Sometimes, people distinguish two types of criterion validity, depending on whether the instrument is measured at the same time as the criterion (*concurrent validity*) or the criterion is assessed at a later point in time (*predictive validity*).

An especially important but challenging aspect of validity is called *construct validity*. Using language from the landmark work of social scientists Thomas Cook and Donald Campbell (e.g., Cook & Campbell, 1979; Shadish, Cook, & Campbell, 2002), we define **construct validity** as the degree to which evidence about a measure's scores in relation to other scores supports the inference that the construct has been appropriately represented. In a nutshell, construct validity concerns the question: What is *really* being measured?

Construct validity is complex and encompasses multiple aspects. Following COSMIN, one component is structural validity, which is applicable only to multi-item reflective scales that could potentially measure multiple dimensions of a complex construct. **Structural validity** refers to the extent to which an instrument adequately captures the dimensionality of the broad construct through subscales as necessary if the measure is multidimensional.

Efforts to assess construct validity rely heavily on the testing of hypotheses. **Hypothesis-testing validity** refers to the extent to which it is possible to corroborate hypotheses regarding how scores on a measure function in relation to other variables. *If*, for example, my nausea scale is a valid measure of nausea, then I predict higher scores among patients with gastroparesis (delayed gastric emptying) than among patients without this disorder. Evidence confirming such a hypothesis lends support to a claim that the nausea scale is a valid measure of nausea. The more supporting evidence that can be brought to bear on the validity question, the stronger the validity claim.

Many scales undergo translation or adaptation for a particular cultural or language group. In particular, many instruments created in English are adapted for use in non–English-speaking countries, which may differ both culturally and linguistically. **Cross-cultural validity**, as defined by COSMIN, is the degree to which the performance of the items on a translated or culturally adapted instrument adequately reflects the performance of the items on the original instrument (Mokkink et al., 2010b).

As these various aspects suggest, assessing validity and building validity into a new instrument are complex endeavors.

3.4   Reliability of Change

As the title of this book suggests, we are also concerned with measurement parameters relating to change scores. Those who intend to use instruments longitudinally to measure change (e.g., to monitor the course of a disease or to evaluate the benefits of treatment) should also be concerned with the reliability of change scores. All scores have a certain amount of unreliability, to a greater or lesser degree. Errors of measurement can be compounded when an unreliable score at one point in time is subtracted from an unreliable score at another point in time to yield a change score. Thus, an important measurement issue concerns distinguishing a true change from measurement error. We have included the reliability of a change score as a separate domain in our taxonomy.[2]

3.5   Responsiveness

Responsiveness is a measurement property that has stirred controversy and that has led to considerable confusion among those who have defined it. COSMIN defined **responsiveness** as the ability of a measure to detect changes over time in the construct being measured. We elaborate on their definition by noting that changes in a responsive measure should be commensurate with changes in the construct.

Psychometricians have not traditionally considered responsiveness as a measurement property. The term is found nowhere in the writings of prominent psychometricians (e.g., Nunnally & Bernstein, 1994) nor in psychometric guides to scale construction (e.g., DeVellis, 2012). Streiner and Norman (2008), psychometricians who have worked in health measurement, have refuted the idea that responsiveness is a distinctive property, preferring instead to think of it as longitudinal construct validity.

We acknowledge that there is strong conceptual overlap between responsiveness and construct validity, but we agree with the COSMIN group (DeVet et al., 2011) in believing that responsiveness merits independent consideration. Health care professionals are profoundly concerned with the measurement of change—change is what professionals in health fields hope to achieve through intervention with clients. Before the concept of responsiveness was developed, little attention was paid to the issue of longitudinal construct validity. We think it is useful to use a separate label to identify a property of great importance to health care practitioners because it reminds scale developers to incorporate the assessment of change score validity into their development plans.

We also follow COSMIN in distinguishing the *validity* of change scores (responsiveness) and the *interpretation* of change scores. Many writers have confounded interpretation and validity, giving rise to some turmoil about what responsiveness is and how to test it. For example, in an often cited paper, Liang (2000) defined responsiveness as "the ability of an instrument to measure a meaningful or clinically important change in a clinical state" (p. 85). We think that having a measure that can detect a true and commensurate change in a construct of interest (our definition of responsiveness) is different from having a score change that is substantial enough to be clinically meaningful. Of course, responsiveness (and reliability of a change score) are preconditions for clinically important change.

---

[2]In the COSMIN taxonomy, the reliability of change scores was considered an aspect of interpretability of change scores.

3.6   Interpretability and Measurement

Interpretability is not a measurement property, but interpretation plays a key role in the usefulness of any measure. As shown in Figure 3.1, the issue of interpretability is important for understanding any single score or set of scores. COSMIN defines **interpretability** as the degree to which it is possible to assign qualitative meaning to an instrument's scores or change scores. Among clinicians, interpretability concerns the issue of having score values that can be meaningfully applied to clinical situations.

Measures of many physical phenomena are widely understood because people have learned the measurement rules. Even most laypeople know that a body temperature of 102° F is high, for example. Raw scores on most PROs or observational scales, however, do not have direct meaning. Instrument developers can take various steps to enhance the interpretability of scores. For example, they can develop **norms**, which are standards of "normal" or typical values on the scale for a specified population—sometimes for a general population, and sometimes for a population of patients with a particular disease or diagnosis. Interpretability in single scores is discussed in Chapter 16.

Interpretability of change scores is more complex. The central concern is having a method of assessing whether a change in a score is sufficiently large to be *clinically meaningful*. Much has been written on this topic, but there has yet to be devised any easy, widely accepted, or totally satisfactory approach. We delve into this topic in Chapter 19, but recognize that many developments in the interpretation of change scores are likely to emerge in the near future.

3.7   Measurement Quality as an Evidence-Building Enterprise

Developing a new instrument should be undertaken only after careful soul searching about the need for a new measure and an honest assessment of the methodologic skills of a research team. Developing and testing a new instrument with excellent measurement properties requires considerable expertise, a long investment of time, and access to large samples of people for whom the instrument is intended. If item response theory is used in the development of a scale, then specialized software and statistical sophistication are also necessary. It typically takes years to create a high-quality instrument. Many people do not take instrument development as seriously as they should, perhaps because they themselves have completed so many poor-quality scales that they think this is standard or perhaps because they think it is easy to piece together a collection of questions. After all, we all ask questions continually, so it may seem simple. It is not.

When instrument developers create a new measure for use by others, they are expected to present evidence that it has adequate measurement properties. At a minimum, the new instrument's reliability and validity must be evaluated, and those properties must be sufficiently high to persuade others of its merit. If the instrument is expected to be used to monitor change in the target construct over time, then developers also should examine and report on responsiveness and the reliability of change scores.

The development work by researchers who create a new measure is just a point of departure for efforts to understand and document the worthiness of the instrument. Just as a single randomized controlled trial (RCT) seldom provides sufficient evidence for making major treatment changes, so, too, a single instrument development paper does not tell the whole story about a new measure. It takes time and ongoing research to ensure that an instrument has been given sufficient scrutiny. Confidence in the worth of a measure relies on the systematic accumulation of evidence.

One important issue to understand is that, at least within CTT, the measurement properties of an instrument are not *fixed*. Measurement properties apply to a particular *application* of an instrument and for a particular group. The reliability of a CTT instrument can vary from population to population. As we discuss later in this book, a CTT scale will be more reliable in a heterogeneous population than in a homogeneous one. A goal of a scale is to discriminate among people with different amounts of an attribute, and discrimination is harder when the people have similar levels of the attribute than when they are diverse.

In selecting an instrument, clinicians and researchers should be guided by existing evidence of the measure's reliability, validity, and responsiveness. The greater the similarity between the development sample and the patients being measured, the greater the level of confidence one can have that the measure will be of high quality for a new group. However, even with a similar sample, it is wise whenever possible to assess an instrument's measurement properties. A reliability parameter such as Cronbach's alpha is *estimated* during scale development, and multiple estimates of any parameter are desirable, just as multiple estimates of an intervention's effect size are crucial for evidence-based practice.

Some measurement parameters are easier for nondevelopers to evaluate than others. In the realm of reliability, internal consistency assessment with estimates of Cronbach's alpha should be assessed (and reported) whenever a scale is used for research purposes. For observational scales, it is crucial to assess interrater or intrarater reliability for virtually all uses of the instrument because the reliability of the observers, as well as the instrument, is important. Other types of reliability, such as test–retest reliability, are unlikely to be assessed by researchers other than the ones who developed the scale, although this type of assessment should be undertaken if the instrument is used with a different population or in a totally different application or if the instrument is modified.

Evidence in support of an instrument's validity and responsiveness is also cumulative, and the burden of evidence building can be shared by all researchers who use the instrument. Each time a reasonable hypothesis about a construct is supported using a previously validated instrument of the construct, further support for an inference of the measure's validity is provided. For example, if researchers studied patients undergoing pulmonary rehabilitation and found a hypothesized correlation between scores on the Chronic Respiratory Questionnaire or CRQ (Guyatt, Berman, Townsend, Pugsley, & Chambers, 1987) on the one hand and other theoretically linked constructs (e.g., spirometry values) on the other, this research would offer a corroboration of the CRQ's construct validity. And, if changes on the CRQ correlated with changes in spirometry values, this would strengthen claims about its responsiveness.

When assessments of instrument quality are viewed as an evidence-building effort, implications for developers and users of instruments become apparent. For the developers, the obligation is to take extraordinary care in creating high-quality instruments and also to diligently report information about measurement properties. This book offers guidance on how measurement properties can be assessed and also includes suggestions for reporting such information. Additional support is available. For example, the Guidelines for Reporting Reliability and Agreement Studies (GRRAS) are useful, especially for instruments requiring interrater and intrarater reliability (Kottner et al., 2011). The COSMIN work group also has created useful checklists and guidelines (Mokkink et al., 2010a).[3] These checklists are especially useful for evaluating the quality of reporting in a measurement paper and for guiding the preparation of such a paper.

Because evidence about instruments accumulates with ongoing use and can be integrated in systematic reviews, researchers who use instruments in their studies should report information they have gleaned about measurement properties. Those who undertake careful systematic reviews of studies on measurement properties using guidelines and standards such as those offered by COSMIN (Terwee et al., 2012) can play an important role in enhancing the scientific integrity of research in which existing instruments are used to measure key health constructs.

---

[3]The COSMIN checklists are available online at: http://www.cosmin.nl.

References

Cook, T. D., & Campbell, D. T. (1979). *Quasi-experimentation: Design and analysis issues for field settings.* Chicago, IL: Rand McNally.

DeVellis, R. F. (2012). *Scale development: Theory and application* (3rd ed.). Thousand Oaks, CA: Sage.

DeVet, H. C. W., Terwee, C., Mokkink, L. B., & Knol, D. L. (2011). *Measurement in medicine: A practical guide.* Cambridge, MA: Cambridge University Press.

Guyatt, G. H., Berman, L. B., Townsend, M., Pugsley, S., & Chambers, L. (1987). A measure of quality of life for clinical trials in chronic lung disease. *Thorax, 42,* 773–778.

Kottner, J., Audige, L., Brorson, S., Donner, A., Gajewski, B., Hrobjartsson, A., . . . Streiner, D. L. (2011). Guidelines for Reporting Reliability and Agreement Studies (GRRAS) were proposed. *Journal of Clinical Epidemiology, 64,* 96–106.

Liang, M. H. (2000). Longitudinal construct validity: Establishment of clinical meaning in patient evaluation instruments. *Medical Care, 38*(Suppl. II), S84–S90.

Mokkink, L. B., Terwee, C., Patrick, D., Alonso, J., Stratford, P., Knol, D. L., . . . de Vet, H. C. W. (2010a). The COSMIN checklist for assessing the methodological quality of studies on measurement properties of health status instruments: An international Delphi study. *Quality of Life Research, 19,* 539–549.

Mokkink, L. B., Terwee, C., Patrick, D., Alonso, J., Stratford, P., Knol, D. L., . . . de Vet, H. C. W. (2010b). The COSMIN study reached international consensus on taxonomy, terminology, and definitions of measurement properties for health-related patient-reported outcomes. *Journal of Clinical Epidemiology, 63,* 737–745.

Nunnally, J., & Bernstein, I. H. (1994). *Psychometric theory* (3rd ed.). New York, NY: McGraw-Hill.

Shadish, W. R., Cook, T. D., & Campbell, D.T. (2002). *Experimental and quasi-experimental designs for generalized causal inference.* Boston, MA: Houghton Mifflin.

Streiner, D. L., & Norman, G. R. (2008). *Health measurement scales: A practical guide to their development and use* (4th ed.). Oxford: Oxford University Press.

Terwee, C. B., Mokkink, L. B., Knol, D. L., Ostelo, R., Bouter, L. M., & DeVet, H. C. W. (2012). Rating the methodological quality in systematic reviews of studies on measurement properties: A scoring system for the COSMIN checklist. *Quality of Life Research, 21,* 651–657.

Üstün, T., Chatterji, S., Kostanjsek, S., Rehm, J., Kennedy, C., Epping-Jordan, J., . . . Pull, C. (2010). Developing the World Health Organization Disability Assessment Schedule 2.0. *Bulletin of the World Health Organization, 88,* 815–823.

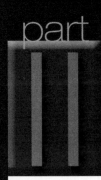

part II

DEVELOPING MULTI-ITEM INSTRUMENTS

chapters

Challenges in Scale Development

Chapter Outline

Scale developers have adopted different approaches to creating multi-item scales. Chapters 5 through 7 present overviews of three approaches that rely on classical test theory (CTT), item response theory (IRT), and clinimetrics, respectively. In this chapter, we review several challenges that are not unique to a particular approach. This chapter aims to make clear that developing a scale from scratch is, if done well, a time-consuming and demanding process. Hopefully, this chapter will also clarify the value of incorporating qualitative research into the instrument development process. It should be noted that this chapter, and the three that follow, focus on structured verbal report measures, such as patient-reported outcomes (PROs), although several issues apply to observational scales as well.

4.1   Conceptualizing the Construct

The importance of a sound, thorough conceptualization of the target construct cannot be overemphasized. It is not possible to quantify an attribute adequately without a thorough understanding of the underlying latent trait. The latent variable is not directly observable, and so appropriate inferences about scores for the variable can be made only if there is an insightful grasp of what the construct is and how it can be made manifest. Scale developers cannot create items to produce the right score, and cannot expect good construct validity, if they are not clear about the construct, its dimensions, and its nuances.

Thus, the initial step in scale development is to become an *expert* on the construct. This means being knowledgeable about theory and research relating to the construct and about any existing (albeit imperfect) instruments. Scale developers usually begin with a thorough review of relevant literature. Developers also benefit from engaging in in-depth discussions (i.e., conducting qualitative interviews) with patients about the attribute to be measured.

Most complex constructs have a number of different facets or dimensions, and it is important to identify and understand each one. In part, this is a content validity consideration: For the overall scale to be content valid, there must be items representing all facets of the construct. Identifying dimensions also has methodologic implications. Scales, or subscales of a broader measure, need to be unidimensional and internally homogeneous, and so an adequate number of items for each dimension needs to be developed. Chapter 11, which focuses on content validity, offers some guidance on developing a conceptual framework of a construct for instrument development purposes.

A full conceptualization of the construct should lead to conclusions about whether the scale will be reflective or formative. In most cases, this is straightforward. However, there are some broad constructs—such as quality of life—that can cause confusion about the nature of the relationship between the construct and the items.[1] Reflective scales, which are most common, involve a conceptualization in which the latent trait is viewed as the *cause* of responses to scale items. When items themselves *define* a construct, the index is formative and, as noted in Chapter 2, the specific items on a formative index are of paramount importance. If there is ambiguity, it may be productive to undertake a "thought experiment" in which you query yourself about the reasonableness of a causal inference. For instance, the 5-item Apgar index to assess newborn health status is an example of a formative index. Is it reasonable to envision a newborn's health status as a *cause* of the infant's respiratory rate? It makes more sense to see respiratory rate as one of several indicators that contribute to the definition of the construct—newborn health status. Chapter 7 discusses the construction of certain types of formative indexes.

During the early conceptualization, scale developers should also think about related constructs that should be differentiated from the target construct. If you are measuring, say, self-efficacy, you have to be sure you can differentiate it from similar but distinct constructs, such as self-confidence. In thinking about the dimensions of the target construct, you should be sure that they are truly aspects of the target construct and not a different construct altogether.

Before getting underway, scale developers should also have an explicit conceptualization of the population for whom the scale is intended. In some cases, this will mean making a decision about whether to create a generic or specific instrument. Understanding the target population for a scale is critical for developing good items. For instruments that are being developed for use by others, it is often advisable to establish an expert panel to review domain specifications in an upfront effort to enhance the scale's content validity (American Educational Research Association, American Psychological Association, & National Council on Measurement in Education Joint Committee, 2014). An iterative, Delphi survey-type approach with opportunities for refinement of the construct specifications by the experts can be useful.

---

[1]Some quality of life measures contain both causal indicators and effect indicators (i.e., they have some elements that are reflective and others that are formative). A *MIMIC model* (Multiple Indicator, Multiple Causes Model) is sometimes used to model relationships in such measures, using structural equation modeling.

4.2 Developing Items for a Scale

Once the construct has been fully conceptualized, the next step is to develop the items. Typically, one starts with a large pool of items from which the best candidates are selected for inclusion in the scale. The method by which the item pool is evaluated and reduced depends of which approach to scale development is being used (Chapters 5 to 7), but all approaches begin with the creation of potential scale items.

4.2.a Sources for Creating the Item Pool

Collectively, items constitute the **operational definition** of the construct. Thus, they need to be carefully crafted to reflect the latent variable they are designed to measure. This is often easier to do as a team effort because different people articulate an idea in diverse ways. Here are some possible sources of scale items for generating an **item pool**:

1. *The literature.* Ideas for item content often come from a thorough understanding of the literature. For those who have become "experts" on the construct, the literature is an obvious source of ideas for items.

2. *Existing instruments.* Sometimes it is possible to adapt an existing instrument rather than starting from scratch. Adaptations often involve adding new items and deleting old ones but may involve item revisions—for example, to make them more culturally appropriate or better suited to a population with low reading skills. It is advisable to obtain permission from the author of the original scale because published scales are often copyright protected.

3. *In-depth qualitative research.* An in-depth inquiry relating to the key construct is a particularly rich source for scale items. A qualitative study involves asking questions about a phenomenon (construct) in a probing and conversational manner, with a sample of people who have experienced the phenomenon. Qualitative studies typically rely on in-depth interviews with a small sample of participants, and one useful sampling strategy is a purposive strategy called *maximum variation sampling.* In this approach, researchers seek out people with variation on dimensions of importance, such as different clinical or demographic profiles. A qualitative study can help you to understand the dimensions of a phenomenon and can also give you actual words for items. For example, Angle and colleagues (2010) conducted in-depth interviews with childbearing women as a preliminary step in developing a scale to measure the quality of neuraxial labor analgesia. Beck and Gable (2001) and Gilgun (2004) offer guidance on using qualitative research to enhance the validity of a new scale. If you are unable to undertake an in-depth study, you should pay careful attention to the verbatim quotes in published qualitative reports about your construct—quotes that perhaps can be used directly as items.

4. *Clinical observations.* Watching patients in clinical settings often provides an excellent resource for scale developers. Ideas for items may come from direct observation of patients' behaviors in relevant situations, from listening to their comments and conversations, from interactions with family members, or from discussions with clinical staff who care for the patients.

4.2.b Decisions About Item Features

In preparing to write items, decisions must be made about such issues as the number of items to develop, the number and form of the response options, whether to include positively and negatively worded items, and how to deal with time.

Number of Items

There is no magic formula for the number of items that should be developed for a scale, but it is a good idea to generate a large pool of items for each dimension of the construct. As you proceed, many items will be discarded. Longer scales tend to be more internally consistent than shorter ones, but long scales are burdensome and run a greater risk of noncompletion than shorter ones. Longer scales also run the risk of being considered inappropriate in clinical settings. Nevertheless, starting with a large number of items is advantageous. DeVellis (2012) recommends starting with 3 to 4 times as many items as you think you will have in your final scale (e.g., 30 to 40 items for a 10-item scale), but at a minimum, there should be 50% more (e.g., 15 items for an anticipated 10-item scale). In scales developed through IRT, a fairly small number of final items is typically needed to achieve adequate reliability, but nevertheless creating and evaluating many items increases the likelihood that the final items will span a good range of difficulty or severity on the latent trait.

Number of Response Options

Scale items for PROs have both **stems** (questions or declarative statements) and **response options**. Traditional Likert scales use response options on a continuum of agreement, but other continua are possible, such as frequency (never/always) or importance (very important/totally unimportant). There is no simple answer to the question of how many response options there should be, but keep in mind that the goal of a scale is to array people on a continuum. Thus, variability is essential. Variability can be enhanced by including many items or by offering numerous response options. However, there is little merit in creating the illusion of precision when it does not exist. With response options on a 0 to 100 scale, for example, the difference between a 96 and a 98 is unlikely to be meaningful. Also, it has been found that too many response options can be confusing to people with limited education. Most Likert scales have five to seven options,[2] with verbal descriptors attached to each option and, often, numbers associated with the options to facilitate coding and to further help people find the right place on the continuum. Note that in IRT, variability can be enhanced by including items at different locations on the attribute continuum, but even in IRT, polytomous response options have been found to yield better discriminatory information than dichotomous ones. In general, it is preferable to use the same number of response options across items in a scale.

Odd Versus Even Response Options

When questions are not dichotomous, developers make a decision about having an odd or even number of response options. An odd number gives people an opportunity to be neutral or ambivalent—that is, to choose a midpoint. Some scale developers prefer an even number (e.g., four or six) to avoid "fence-sitting." However, some respondents may actually *be* neutral or ambivalent, so a midpoint option allows them to express it. The midpoint can be labeled with such phrases as "neither agree nor disagree," "undecided," "neutral," or simply "?". Box 4.1 presents some frequently used response options, without midpoints.

Positive and Negative Stems

A generation ago, psychometricians advised scale developers to include both positively and negatively worded items and to reverse-score the negative ones. As an example, consider two items for a depression scale: "I frequently feel depressed," and "I don't feel sad very often." A key objective of including both types of items was to minimize a bias called *acquiescence*—the tendency to agree with statements regardless of their content. Many experts currently advise against including negative and positive items on a scale because some people are confused by reversing polarities—especially if there are negative words in the

---

[2]George Miller (1956), a cognitive psychologist, wrote an influential and widely cited paper that claimed that seven is a "magic number" in terms of the number of distinctions that are psychologically meaningful to humans. Also, Preston and Colman (2000) found that the number of response options can affect reliability and internal consistency. In their study, both parameters were lowest for 2- and 3-category response options and were highest for response options with 7 to 9 categories; 100 categories (i.e., 0 to 100) resulted in lower reliability.

Box 4.1	Frequently Used Response Options (midpoint term not listed)

- Strongly disagree, disagree, agree, strongly agree
- Disagree strongly, disagree moderately, disagree slightly, agree slightly, agree moderately, agree strongly
- Never, almost never (or rarely), sometimes (or occasionally), often (or frequently), almost always (or always)
- Never, once, twice, 3–4 times, 5 or more times
- None of the time, a little of the time, some of the time, a good bit of the time, most of the time, all of the time
- Very important, important, somewhat important, of little importance, unimportant, totally unimportant
- Definitely not, probably not, possibly, probably, very probably, definitely
- Not at all, slightly, moderately, quite a bit, extremely
- None, very mild, mild, moderate, severe, very severe
- With no trouble, with a little trouble, with some trouble, with a lot of trouble, not able to do

response options (e.g., *never*). There is ample evidence that the inclusion of both types of items on a scale can result in seemingly spurious "dimensions" (*methods factors*) in a factor analysis, even when a scale is really unidimensional (e.g., Hankins, 2008; Marsh, 1996; Motl & DiStefano, 2002).[3] Answering negative item stems appears to be an especially difficult cognitive task for younger respondents. In general, negatively worded items should be avoided.

Item Time Frames

Some items make an explicit reference to a time frame (e.g., "In the past few days, I have had trouble falling asleep"), but others do not (e.g., "I have trouble falling asleep"). Sometimes instructions to a scale can designate a temporal frame of reference: "In answering the following questions, please indicate how you have felt in the past week." Yet other scales ask respondents to respond in terms of a time frame: "In the past week, I have had trouble falling asleep: Every day, 5 to 6 days . . . Never." A time frame should not emerge as a *consequence* of item development. You should decide in advance, based on your conceptual understanding of the construct and the needs for which the scale is being constructed, how to deal with time. (Initial views regarding the time frame could be verified by an expert panel, such as a content validity panel, or by respondents during a pretest.) Also, if the item involves respondents' recall, there should be a sound rationale for the recall period. Items with a short recall period, or that ask for information about a current status, are generally better than ones requiring memory over a long period. There is some evidence from the psychological literature that stability of item responses across time (e.g., in a test–retest situation) may be lower with response options that require a time estimate, such as frequency of occurrence in the past week, than with response options requiring agreement or disagreement (Watson, 2004).

4.2.c Wording of the Items

Items should be worded in a manner that enhances the likelihood that every respondent is answering the same question. Some tips are as follows:

1. *Clarity*. Scale developers should strive for items that are clear and unambiguous. Words should be carefully chosen with the educational and reading level of the target population

---

[3]Some cognitive psychologists have argued that negativity and positivity do not constitute end points of a bipolar dimension but are in fact separate concepts (e.g., Cacioppo & Bernston, 1994; Cacioppo, Gardner, & Berntson, 1999).

in mind. Even beyond concerns about reading levels, you should strive to select words that everyone understands and to have everyone reach the same conclusion about what the words mean.

2. *Jargon.* Jargon should be avoided. Be especially cautious about using terms that might be well-known in health care circles (e.g., lesion, edema) but not familiar to the average person.

3. *Length.* Avoid long sentences or phrases. Simple sentences are the easiest to comprehend. In particular, eliminate unnecessary words. For example, "By and large I do not get a sufficient number of hours of sleep," could be more simply worded as, "I usually do not get enough sleep."

4. *Double negatives.* It is preferable to word things affirmatively ("I am usually happy" than negatively ("I am not usually sad"), but double negatives should always be avoided ("I am *not* usually *un*happy").

5. *Double-barreled items.* Avoid putting two or more ideas in a single item. For example, "I am afraid of insects and snakes" is a bad item because a person who is afraid of insects but not snakes (or vice versa) would not know how to respond. Be on the lookout for use of the word "and" in items.

6. *Bias.* Questions should ideally be worded in a manner that minimizes the possibility of response bias, a topic discussed later in this chapter. Items should not suggest a "right" answer (i.e., a hoped for or socially desirable response).

Special care should be given to item wording when a translation of the scale into another language is planned or anticipated. For example, many health-related scales developed in the United States are translated into Spanish. Wagner and colleagues (1998), who were involved with a project called IQOLA that focused on translating the SF-36 into multiple languages, made some recommendations for easily translatable instruments. They suggested creating items that had simple sentences, that used nouns rather than pronouns, that avoided the subjunctive, and that were written in the active rather than passive voice. Words with a Latin root are advantageous for translation into Romance languages such as Spanish or French. Idiomatic expressions and metaphors are often especially challenging for translators. Additional advice relating to translated instruments is provided in Chapter 15.

The importance of developing a pool of carefully worded items cannot be overstated. Further guidance in wording scale items can be found in Streiner and Norman (2008) and in the classic books by Bradburn, Sudman, and Wansink (2004) and Fowler (1995).

4.3 Early Evaluation of Scale Items

It is challenging to create items that are clear, succinct, and capable of tapping the latent trait adequately. Careful review of items in the initial pool is essential. A review by the research team should focus on several issues, such as the following:

■ Does each item embody the construct?

■ Do the items, taken together, adequately capture the full dimensionality of the construct?

■ In IRT, do the items, taken together, span a wide range of difficulty (severity) level on each dimension of the construct?

■ Are the items grammatical?

■ Are the stems structurally comparable (e.g., do some have gerunds and others have nouns)?

■ Do all of the stems correspond to the response options? (And are the same response options compatible across all stems?)

The latter issue is frequently ignored but can lead to confusion about how to respond. A widely used measure of patient satisfaction with outpatient services provides an example of noncorrespondence. The question "How easy was it to get an appointment for when you wanted?" does not correspond to the response options of *very poor, poor, fair, good,* or *very good.* Some of the items on the patient satisfaction scale can be answered on a *very poor* to *very good* continuum, but others cannot.

The review should also pay careful attention to the issue of the items' understandability.

4.3.a Readability

Unless the scale is intended for a population with known high literacy (e.g., college graduates), it is crucial to assess the scale's **readability**. It is generally recommended that, for a general population, the reading level be at the 6th to 7th grade level or lower. Even some high school graduates may have difficulty reading at a higher level.

Several approaches for assessing the reading level of written documents have been devised, but many methods are inappropriate for evaluating scale items—either because the methods are too time consuming or because they require several hundred words of text.

Many word processing programs provide some information about readability. Microsoft Word, for example, offers two readability statistics, based on the work of Flesch (1948). The first statistic is called the *Flesch–Kincaid grade level,* and the second is the *Flesch reading ease score.* Reading ease scores rate text on a 100-point scale, with higher values associated with greater ease, using a formula that considers average sentence length and average number of syllables. Reading ease scores should usually be at least 65 to 70.

As an example, consider the following two sets of items designed to assess levels of fatigue, which we typed into a Word document:

Set A	**Set B**
I am habitually exhausted.	I am often tired.
I invariably get inadequate sleep.	I do not get enough sleep.

According to the Word software, the two items in Set A have a Flesch–Kincaid grade level of 13.6 and a Flesch reading ease score of 4.8, meaning they are most appropriate for college-educated people. Set B, by contrast, has a grade level of 0.5 and a reading ease score of 100.0. Even though it is advisable to interpret readability statistics from word processing programs cautiously (Streiner & Norman, 2008), it is clear from this analysis that the items in Set B would be superior for a target population that includes people with low reading ability. Two general principles are to avoid long sentences and words with four or more syllables.

As an example of a readability assessment, Olsen, Smith, Oei, and Douglas (2010) computed Flesch scores during the development of a scale to measure cues to starting continuous positive airway pressure (CPAP) in obstructive sleep apnea, the Cues to CPAP Use Questionnaire (CCUQ). They found that the Flesch reading ease score of the CCUQ was 66.1, with the Flesch grade level at 7th grade. It is useful to report readability statistics in papers describing the final instrument.

4.3.b Items and Measurement Properties

A scale's measurement properties are seldom assessed until the full scale has been constructed, but it is sensible to review potential items with an eye toward how they might undermine or contribute to measurement excellence. For example, to achieve high internal consistency in a CTT scale, there needs to be a sufficient number of items to tap each dimension of the construct, and the items need to be measuring the same underlying construct.

Internal consistency is often easy to bear in mind at the stage of item creation and review, but other measurement properties should be considered as well. In particular, researchers can make an effort to anticipate challenges relating to test–retest reliability and responsiveness.

Test–retest reliability involves administering an instrument on two occasions, at an interval in which true change in the construct is not expected to have occurred (Chapter 8). Thus, with the interval for the retest administration in mind, developers can examine each item for its potential stability in the short term. Even better, if a retest administration is completed before the scale is finalized, each item can be evaluated for its stability over the designated interval and this information can contribute to final item selection. Although scrutiny of item performance from a test–retest perspective has been suggested as a means of selecting items (e.g., Nevo, 1977), this is seldom done by health researchers, although there are some exceptions. For example, Ashford, Turner-Stokes, Siegert, and Slade (2013) developed the Arm Activity Measure, which is a patient-reported measure of active and passive function in the paretic upper limb. In finalizing their scale, they examined consistency of responses for each item in a 1-day test–retest analysis, and their results supported the retention of all items. As might be expected, item stability has been found to be predictive of scale stability (Nevo, 1977; Jones & Goldberg, 1967), and so item-level retest analyses, coupled with preestablished standards for item retention, could be a useful strategy for enhancing a scale's retest reliability.

If it is anticipated that an instrument will be used as an outcome measure to evaluate the effect of an intervention, it is useful to consider whether items are capable of reflecting true change when it does occur, which relates to the measure's responsiveness (see Chapter 18). In other words, items should be amenable to change when a true change in the underlying construct has occurred. As an example, an item such as "I have tried cocaine at least once" might be a potential item for a drug use scale. Such an item would be inappropriate if the scale were used to assess the effects of a drug rehabilitation program. No matter how effective the treatment, a person who answered affirmatively before treatment would answer affirmatively after the intervention, barring deception.

4.3.c Pretesting the Scale

There are several approaches to pretesting a new scale. Using multiple methods is an excellent idea, and using at least one method is essential.

The standard pretest method is to try out the scale with a small sample. In preparing for the pretest, care should be taken to write clear instructions for completing the instrument. The instructions should be reviewed by several members of the development team, and a readability assessment of the instructions should be undertaken. The instructions should make clear to respondents exactly what is expected of them. For example, if the points along a response option continuum are not explicitly labeled, guidance to facilitate understanding the end points should be provided.

In a conventional pretest of a new instrument, a small sample of people (25 to 50 or so) representing the target population is invited to complete the items. Respondents might be asked if any of the items were problematic, but conventional pretesting focuses primarily on the assessment of response patterns. For example, analysts look for items with high rates of nonresponse, items with limited variability, or items with numerous midpoint responses (fence-sitting). Such problems signal items that are candidates for deletion or revision.

Pretest respondents can also be asked to provide direct feedback about the clarity of the items. For example, as part of the project to develop and refine physical function items for the PROMIS® databank, 100 subjects initially evaluated the items for clarity on a 4-point scale: *totally clear, somewhat clear, not very clear*, and *not clear at all* (Bruce et al., 2009). As a test of the validity of the responses, the investigators included a few items that were deliberately ambiguous.

Another approach to pretesting involves convening two or three **focus groups**. Focus group interviews are carefully planned discussions that capitalize on group dynamics for accessing in-depth information in a cost-effective manner. In a focus group, a moderator asks a series of open-ended questions, usually with a group of about 5 to 10 people from the target population. For instrument development, the moderator would present items and then ask participants if they are relevant, understandable, culturally sensitive, linguistically appropriate, and perhaps inoffensive.

4.3.d Cognitive Questioning

Developments in cognitive science over the past 25 years have paved the way for a different approach to pretesting, often used to supplement standard pretests.[4] Several models of cognitive processing of questions have been proposed. One such model (Tourangeau, Lance, & Rasinski, 2000) portrays response selection as a four-step process in which a person has to comprehend, retrieve, judge, and select from response options. In **cognitive interviews**, people are asked to reflect upon their interpretation of the items and their answers so that the underlying process of response selection is better understood.

There are two basic approaches to cognitive interviewing. One is called the **think-aloud method**, wherein respondents are asked to explain step-by-step how they processed the question and arrived at an answer. This approach may be especially useful when a question requires recall (e.g., number of times in the past month a medication was missed). A second approach, and one that is gaining favor, is to conduct an interview in which the interviewer uses a series of targeted verbal **probes** that encourage reflection about underlying cognitive processes. Table 4.1 provides examples of possible probes for an item relating to sleeping problems. Such in-depth questioning can be useful in identifying problematic items and in suggesting modifications as well as in offering content validity information (Chapter 11).

As an example of cognitive interviewing during instrument development, Franciosi and colleagues (2012) used cognitive interviews with 17 children and 27 parents in the development of a module for the Pediatric Quality of Life Inventory specific to children with eosinophilic esophagitis. The goal of the cognitive questioning was to obtain patient perspectives on the meaning and clarity of all aspects of the module. Examples of questions relating to specific items include "In your own words, what do you think this question is asking?", "How would you change the words to make it more clear?", and "How did you choose your answer?"

When a large set of items is under consideration for inclusion in a scale, it may be necessary to limit cognitive questioning to a subset of items to minimize respondent burden. One alternative is to question different samples about different item subsets. Another alternative is to focus the cognitive questioning on items most at risk of being problematic. For example, in the previously mentioned project to evaluate items for the PROMIS® databank, the items for the cognitive questioning were ones in which more than 5% of the pretest respondents rated the item as "not clear," or fewer than 70% said the item was "totally clear" (Bruce et al., 2009).

Nápoles-Springer, Santoyo-Olsson, O'Brien, and Stewart (2006) have described a *behavior coding* approach to analyzing responses to cognitive interviews. Transcripts of the cognitive interviews are coded for the incidence of "problematic behaviors," and software for qualitative analysis is used to compute frequency information. Examples of problematic behaviors on the part of respondents include the following: Respondent gives an answer but uses a different response scale than that provided; respondent asks to have the question repeated; respondent asks for clarification of question; and respondent implies that the question asked is repetitive or similar to a previous question (e.g., "You just asked me that"). Such an approach can help to identify items that are repeatedly problematic and may also help to suggest ways to fix the problem.

One final point is that a person's interpretation of a question and the response options may evolve over time if he or she is undergoing health changes. This phenomenon, known as *response shift*, is discussed in Chapters 17 and 19. If researchers are developing an instrument that will measure a health construct over time (e.g., before and after chemotherapy), then it is prudent to undertake cognitive questioning with people at different points in an illness trajectory.

---

[4]One of the earliest "cognitive laboratories" for testing questions for national surveys was developed within the National Center for Health Statistics in 1985, and developments in the application of cognitive science to questionnaire development are continuously unfolding (Presser et al., 2004; Willis, 2005). A useful paper prepared by Gordon Willis called "Cognitive interviewing: A 'how to' guide" can be accessed online at http://appliedresearch.cancer.gov/archive/cognitive/interview.pdf.

Table 4.1	Examples of Cognitive Questioning Using Verbal Probes

Question Example: How often in the past week have you had trouble falling asleep:

1. Much more than usual
2. Somewhat more than usual
3. About the same as usual
4. Somewhat less than usual
5. Much less than usual

Cognitive Questioning Probe Possibilities, by Category:

General probes:
■ What do you think this question means? What does this question mean to you?
■ Was this question easy or hard to answer?
■ Did this question make you uncomfortable in any way? Was it offensive or disturbing?
■ I noticed you hesitated in answering this question. What were you thinking about?
■ I noticed you hesitated in answering this question. On a written questionnaire, might you consider leaving this question blank?

Comprehension probes:
■ Are there any words in the question that are unclear or confusing?
■ Could you explain in your own words what you think the term "trouble" means?

Interpretation probes:
■ When you were asked to compare trouble you are having sleeping in the past week with what is "usual," what did you think of as "usual"? Why did you use that frame of reference?
■ Tell me how you went about calculating the answer you gave for relative frequency of having trouble falling asleep.

Paraphrasing probe:
■ Can you tell me what my question was, in your own words?

Recall probe:
■ Did you easily remember your sleeping troubles for the entire previous week? When you were thinking of "the past week," when did that week start?

Confidence probes:
■ In thinking about your answer, how sure are you that your answer really reflects how much trouble you had with sleeping?
■ Do you think that people will answer this question honestly?

Content probes:
■ Is this question relevant for telling us about your current sleeping problems?

4.4 Bias

A particularly challenging problem confronting developers—and users—of multi-item scales is the risk of biases that can distort scores on an instrument. It is beyond the scope of this book to fully describe the many biases that can occur with multi-item scales, but it is important to consider a few of the more prevalent ones. Here we discuss biases that can emerge in PROs and observational measures. (Recall bias, a bias that is especially relevant to the measurement of change, is discussed in Chapter 17.)

4.4.a Response Biases

Verbal reports are susceptible to numerous biases. A **response bias** is an influence that leads a person to select a response option that does not correspond to his or her true level on the underlying latent trait. Sometimes a bias stems from a particular environment or situation (e.g., which particular person is administering the scale). Sometimes the manner of administration (e.g., orally or in writing) can alter responses. And sometimes *expectation biases* can influence patients' responses, which is why blinding is so important in clinical trials and also in measurement studies when retest reliability or interrater reliability is being evaluated.

Our primary concern in this section is response bias that results from people's reaction to actual scale items. One way to minimize bias is carefully wording questions so that they do not suggest a "right answer" (i.e., avoiding "leading questions"). Other ways to reduce the risk of bias were suggested in our advice about question wording, such as constructing clear, short items with good readability and avoiding double negatives.

Survey researchers have identified several biases that they call **response set biases** because the bias *systematically* influences an entire set of responses in a consistent direction, regardless of the content of the question. Such biases can dampen a scale's validity because the scale is then "measuring" both the focal construct and the bias. Among the more prevalent response set biases are the following:

1. **Social desirability response bias** refers to the tendency of some people to distort their scores by giving answers that are congruent with prevailing social values or congruent with what they believe their health care providers want to hear. Social desirability does not necessarily reflect a desire to deceive but may represent efforts to preserve a positive self-image. This very common bias can undermine the interpretation of average score values; it can also restrict variation, which in turn can reduce group differences as well as estimates of effect size and reliability (Chapter 8). The problem is most acute for the measurement of certain types of constructs, such as socially problematic behaviors (e.g., excessive alcohol consumption, multiple sex partners); feelings of low self-esteem or self-efficacy; illegal acts (e.g., drug use, acts of violence); compliance with medical regimens; and health behavior intentions (e.g., intention to exercise, intention to undergo screening). A particularly worrisome aspect of this bias is that it can distort scores in different directions for different subgroups. For example, men might exaggerate sexual activities, whereas women might underreport them—phenomena described as "*faking bad*" and "*faking good*"[5] when the distortion is deliberate. Although there is no way to eliminate social desirability bias, there are ways to address it. Anonymity is perhaps the single best method of encouraging candor, and written responses rather than oral ones give respondents a greater sense of privacy. When scale developers are measuring sensitive constructs such as those mentioned, they may wish to formally assess a person's tendency to give socially desirable responses. Several social desirability scales have been developed, including the 33-item Marlowe-Crowne Social Desirability Scale (Crowne & Marlow, 1960), shortened versions of that scale (e.g., Strahan, 2007), and the 40-item Paulhus Deception Scale (Paulhus, 2004), which was rigorously constructed. Scale developers can use such scales during development to draw conclusions about the extent to which social desirability is correlated with scores on their new scale or to delete items that seem especially susceptible to this bias. In some cases, it may be beneficial to adjust scores on the target scale statistically based on scores on a social desirability measure. This approach is used in scoring responses to some psychological tests such as the Minnesota Multiphasic Personality Inventory (MMPI), which has a "lie" scale embedded in it. Streiner and Norman (2008) offer additional advice on dealing with social desirability bias.

---

[5]A technique called *differential item functioning* (DIF) can be used to evaluate whether an item is functioning differently for specified subgroups. DIF is discussed in Chapter 6 in connection with IRT, and also in Chapter 15 on cross-cultural validity.

2. **Extreme response bias** is a bias resulting in consistent selection of extreme alternatives (e.g., *strongly agree* or *strongly disagree*) to scale items. These extreme responses distort scores because they do not always signify the most intense feelings about the phenomenon under study but rather reflect a characteristic of the respondent. The opposite tendency to prefer midrange responses, regardless of an item's content, has been called a **moderacy bias** and also a *midpoint* or *end-aversion bias*. Such response set biases are typically viewed as reflecting a stable personality trait (e.g., Weijters, Geuens, & Schilewaert, 2010), and so there may not be much a scale developer can do to counteract it. One possibility is to tinker with the response options. For example, to address a moderacy bias, it may be useful to exclude response options that are extreme (e.g., using *almost always* rather than *always*). The need for such wording might be detected in cognitive interviews or by looking at response patterns in a pretest sample. When a scale is used to reach conclusions about a broad population, or when scales are used to draw comparisons across different cultures or subgroups, it can be useful to model the bias and correct for it. For example, Elliott, Haviland, Kanouse, Hambarsoomian, and Hays (2009) modeled extreme response tendencies and then adjusted for it in a study of consumers' ratings of health care. Concern about extreme response set is especially acute in cross-cultural research because cultures differ in the prevalence of this tendency (Chapter 15).

3. The **acquiescence response set bias** (also called the **yea-sayers bias**) is a tendency to agree with statements (or give positive responses like *true* or *often*), regardless of the item's content. A less common problem is **disacquiescence bias**, which is the opposite tendency for some people (**naysayers**) to disagree with statements independently of question content. Previous advice for combatting these biases was to include both negatively and positively worded items on a scale, but such advice has been discredited. Of course, all items can be worded positively and yet tap opposite directions of the construct, with reverse scoring for relevant items. For example, a scale for depression might include such items as "I frequently feel sad," and "I am happy most of the time." Some scale development experts recommend consistent directionality of item wording (e.g., DeVellis, 2012), whereas other researchers have found evidence for the benefits of reverse-scored items (e.g., Weijters, Geuens, & Schilewaert, 2009). Because there is no firm consensus on this point, if a scale includes item reversals, pretests and cognitive interviews should be used to explore potential problems. Some research suggests that acquiescence can be minimized by putting the most positive response options (e.g., *strongly agree*) at the end of the list rather than at the beginning.

4. A **proximity effect** is a tendency to be influenced in responding to an item by the response to the previous item (Knowles, 1988). This effect can result in overestimates of internal consistency, and so thought should be given to this problem in making decisions about how to order the items. One approach might be to order items randomly. If the scale is designed to measure multiple related dimensions, an alternative approach is to systematically alternate items that are expected to be scored into different subscales or to intersperse scale items with other questions on an instrument (e.g., demographic questions). Based on a careful analysis of data from cognitive interviews and a survey of over 3,000 people, Weijters and colleagues (2009) recommended dispersing items that measure the same construct across a questionnaire.

It is not possible to create scales and indexes that are free from response biases, but scale developers should be aware of the risks of bias as they make decisions about wording items and arranging them on the scale. Some biases can be minimized with subtle or delicately worded questions. It is also important to create scale instructions that reflect open-mindedness and that encourage frankness. Sometimes social desirability bias can be minimized by stating that there are no right or wrong answers, by acknowledging that there are many different opinions and viewpoints about the topic, or by suggesting that

Box 4.2	Instructions for an Index to Measure Academic Integrity[a]

Most students work hard and do their own work. However, we know that students nowadays are under a lot of pressure, and many find it necessary to cut a few corners to get through their coursework.

Example of an item on the index:

How often have you engaged in the following behaviors in your online courses:

Made up or falsified data or results for a project (for example, lab data, research data, time logs)? Options: Never, Once, 2–3 times, 4 or more times

[a]The Academic Integrity Scale for Online Students (AI-SOS), administered anonymously through online surveys (Morgan, Hart, & Polit, 2013)

many people engage in socially risky acts. As an example of the latter, Box 4.2 shows instructions used with an index to assess cheating in online academic courses, which suggests that students face pressures that can lead to cutting some corners. When risk for certain biases seem high (e.g., in a scale to measure socially deviant views or behaviors), it is wise to assess the extent to which biases have influenced scores.

4.4.b Observational Biases

Although this section of the book focuses primarily on the development of verbal report scales (i.e., PROs) rather than observational measures, we note that the risk of bias in observational measures can be high. As with verbal reports, observational biases can influence the reliability and validity of scores. Bias sometimes can be reduced in observational scales by omitting items with a large inferential burden. For example, it is easier to obtain accurate, unbiased information when the observer is recording such behavior as "Patient complained about hospital noise" than "Patient was distressed." Of course, the construct of interest may require the inclusion of behaviors that do require interpretation. When this is the case, the scale developer must take pains to construct a meticulous observational manual that explains each category on the scale in detail so that observers have relatively clear-cut criteria for identifying the occurrence of a specified phenomenon.

Just as response biases often reflect traits of respondents rather than flaws of a verbal report scale, so, too, do observational biases frequently stem from characteristics of observers. For example, the **error of leniency** is the tendency for an observer to rate things too positively, and the **error of severity** is the contrasting tendency to rate too harshly. The **halo effect** is the tendency of an observer to be influenced by one characteristic in judging other, unrelated characteristics. For example, if we formed a positive general impression of a person, we might rate that person as competent, healthy, and energetic simply because these traits are positively valued.

Another observational bias is the **enhancement of contrast effect**, in which an observer distorts observations in the direction of dividing content into clear-cut entities. The opposite effect—a bias toward **central tendency**—occurs when extreme events are distorted toward a middle ground. With **assimilatory biases**, an observer distorts observations in the direction of identity with previous inputs. This bias would have the effect of miscategorizing information in the direction of regularity and orderliness.

The careful construction and pretesting of observational checklists, rating scales, classification/staging systems, and scoring protocols play an important role in minimizing biases. The proper selection, training, and preparation of observers is also crucial. To become good "instruments" for collecting observational data, observers must be carefully screened and trained. The setting during the trial period should resemble as closely as possible the settings that will be the focus of actual observations. Both during the development of an observational system or instrument, and during its use in new settings, it is essential to assess interrater reliability (see Chapter 8).

4.5 Floor and Ceiling Effects

Floor and ceiling effects occur on scales or performance tests when the variability in scores on an attribute is restricted either at the lower end of a continuum (**floor effects**) or at the upper end (**ceiling effects**). Such effects, because they hinder the expression of true variability, can negatively affect estimates of reliability and validity. This is problematic when a large number of people have scores at the upper or lower end and when their "true" score would be higher (lower) except for constraints of the scale or scale items.

Occasionally, floor or ceiling effects might result from efforts to minimize response biases. For example, in a scale to measure alcohol consumption, an item might ask how often a person had five or more drinks on a single occasion. The scale developer might worry that if another item asked about drinking *10* or more drinks on a single occasion, a social desirability bias might induce people to conceal such extreme behavior. However, this decision means that the scale will not be capable of distinguishing between people who drink 5 drinks and people who drink 10 drinks on a single occasion. Such distinctions may not be important, but the item wording should be the result of a conscious decision. Scale developers should pretest items that have such phrases as "…*or more*" or "…*or less*" in them or any phrase suggesting nondifferentiated extremes.

Avoiding floor and ceiling effects also requires careful thought about how and with whom the scale will be used. A scale may have no ceiling effects when administered to adults, for example, and yet be too "difficult" for adolescents. Thus, the scale developer should be clear about the target population and should caution scale users about the absence of information on floor or ceiling effects with a different group. The issue of floor and ceiling effects has been an impetus for the development of specific rather than generic scales (see Chapter 2). For example, a scale to measure activities of daily living (ADL) in a general population is not likely to discriminate sufficiently among patients recovering from a stroke. Several investigators have shown that the SF-36 generic health status scale from the Medical Outcomes Study has floor effects for various clinical populations (e.g., Holmes, Bix, & Shea, 1996; Jacoby, Baker, Steen, & Buck, 1999; Lai, Perera, Duncan, & Bode, 2003).

Another important consideration for scale developers is whether the scale will be used to monitor change over time. If a major purpose of an instrument is to evaluate change, then it must be capable of detecting variability at the extremes at both the posttest and at baseline. Clearly, a person with a score of 1 (on a 25-point scale) at baseline could not deteriorate any further over time, and a person with a score of 25 at baseline could not improve.

Detection of floor and ceiling effects is addressed differently by those using a CTT or IRT approach. We touch on these methods in the next two chapters. However, the issue should be kept in mind during the construction of individual items and during the assemblage of items intended to form the scale. Information about floor and ceiling effects should be included in papers or reports on scale development. For example, Crémers, Phan, Delvaux, and Garraux (2012) developed and evaluated the Dynamic Parkinson Gait Scale and reported that the scale had good internal consistency, reliability, and validity and that floor and ceiling effects were not observed.

4.6 The Challenge of Missing Values

Missing values, the problem that arises when some people fail to answer all items on a scale, is an inevitable challenge for scale developers and scale users. Missing answers could signal problems of interpretation or comprehension, discomfort with the question, inapplicability of the item, and so on and there is no way to know for sure which of these situations is relevant or what the value would be were it not missing. When item scores are added together to form a total scale score, something must be done about missing values or the total score will be wrong.

The first line of defense is to take steps to reduce the risk of missing values. Efforts should be made during the pretest stage to detect problems—for example, by looking at the frequency of missing values for each item and by using cognitive interviews to identify why people might struggle with their answers to certain questions. Even if the finalized items have low rates of missingness in a pretest, guidelines for handling missing values need to be formulated, especially for CTT scales. In particular, scale developers need to establish the maximum number of missing items allowed on a scale before declaring the total score for a person missing. There are no strict rules for what that number is, but it has been suggested that the maximum number of missing items for a given case should not exceed 20% (e.g., Downey & King, 1998).[6] For example, if only 7 items on a 10-item scale were answered, the total score would be coded as missing using this guideline.

The next issue concerns how best to deal with small amounts of missing data when the goal is to preserve the case with CTT scales (As we will see in Chapter 6, missing values can be accommodated with IRT scaling). A wide variety of both simple and sophisticated statistical approaches have been used to impute (estimate and replace) missing item values. (For brief overviews, see Donders, Van der Heijden, Stijnen, & Moons, 2006; Fox-Wasylyshyn & El-Masri, 2005; Haukoos & Newgard, 2007). For example, one could substitute the mean item score of the sample for the missing value. *Mean substitutions* could be done either unconditionally (everyone gets the same imputation) or conditionally, based on some other variable (e.g., separate item means for males and females). Other imputation techniques include regression, expectation maximization, and the "gold standard" imputation technique called **multiple imputation** (MI), all of which are available in widely used statistical software such as SPSS.

One relatively simple approach is to use **case–mean imputation**, which involves using information from the case itself (rather than sample's distribution) to impute a replacement value. For example, on a 10-item unidimensional scale, if Alex missed one item, his missing value would be replaced with the mean of the nine items he completed. The case–mean substitution is analogous to using a total score that is the *mean* of completed items rather than the *sum* of all items. In one simulation study, Roth, Switzer, and Switzer (1999) found that case–mean imputation was robust with up to 20% missing for both random and systematic patterns of missingness. In another simulation study, Shrive, Stuart, Quan, and Ghali (2006) concluded that with only 10% missing, five different imputation methods were about equally satisfactory, but with 20% and 30% missing case–mean substitution worked nearly as well as MI, and it is much simpler to do and easier to communicate to scale users. Decisions about imputations should be made carefully and conservatively. With extensive imputation, the scale's internal consistency is likely to be overestimated.

Methods of handling missing data should be reported in instrument development papers. In the evaluation checklists created by the COSMIN group, there is an explicit item about missing data in the reliability (and other) checklists: "Was there a description of how missing items were handled?" (DeVet, Terwee, Mokkink, & Knol, 2011, p. 289).

4.7   Assessment Challenges

Even in the early stages of scale development, researchers can benefit by anticipating some of the challenges they will face in subjecting their scale to psychometric assessment.

---

[6]A higher percentage of missing might be tolerated in situations in which the missing values are **missing completely at random** (**MCAR**). Rarely, however, would individual scale items be MCAR unless the problem arose because of formatting issues or data entry errors. A participant's decision to leave a question blank is seldom random, which emphasizes the importance of careful pretesting.

One challenge, for example, might be to identify an appropriate "gold standard" if the scale will undergo criterion validity evaluation (see Chapter 12). It is not always easy to identify a gold standard for PRO scales, but creative solutions are sometimes possible and such solutions are desirable because criterion validation can yield very useful information (e.g., diagnostic accuracy statistics such as specificity and sensitivity).

Scales are usually evaluated for test–retest reliability, and a major challenge for such assessments is to decide on the retest interval—that is, the time between the initial test and the retest. As described in Chapter 8, the interval should be short enough to minimize the possibility that the attribute has actually changed but long enough to avoid other biasing carry-over effects. Work undertaken in the early stages of instrument development can inform decisions about a suitable retest interval. For example, during the development of a conceptual model of the construct, researchers should attempt to understand factors that affect the construct's stability and how much short-term stability can be expected. Experts invited to contribute to or comment on the conceptual framework could be asked to estimate the time period within which stability could be expected in the absence of any intervention. During cognitive interviews, patients could be asked how responses to questions might vary over time (e.g., "How might your answer vary from day to day?"). Another strategy is to administer a **health transition scale** to a sample of people from the target population several times to learn about the trajectory of change for the focal attribute. Health transition scales (also called *global rating scales*) are used in many ways in measurement studies (see Chapters 17 to 19). A health transition scale is a single item, often on a 7-point scale, that asks people to rate the extent to which they have improved, deteriorated (e.g., slightly, moderately, greatly), or stayed the same with regard to the attribute. If administered multiple times (e.g., weekly for 4 to 6 weeks), researchers might be better able to identify an appropriate retest interval.

4.8   Practical Challenges

Developing a new instrument in a rigorous manner is an extremely challenging enterprise. To create a scale that has sound measurement properties, years of effort are typically required and, if responsiveness is a property of interest, the work takes even longer to complete. Instrument development requires many diverse skills, which suggests the desirability of a varied and perhaps multidisciplinary development team composed of content experts, psychometricians, statisticians, qualitative research experts, and clinicians from a range of relevant professions. To marshal strong evidence about a scale's measurement properties, developers also need access to a large pool of people from the target population, especially if a factor analysis will be undertaken and if the measure is developed within an IRT framework. This typically means the availability of resources and high levels of institutional support and cooperation.

Careful planning, and having a schedule that allows sufficient time for thoughtful reflection and external review, are essential. Table 4.2 lists key steps in scale development, and additional activities may be required in connection with the approaches discussed in the next three chapters. Many of the steps in this list would involve months of activity. For example, a formal content validity effort might require such activities as preparing a questionnaire, recruiting a panel of experts, gathering and analyzing data, and perhaps doing a second round of expert review (see Chapter 11).[7] Thus, it is wise to think very carefully about the sizeable investment of time that is needed to develop a high-quality scale to measure health constructs.

---

[7]If we had organized this book in a linear fashion according to sequence of tasks, the chapter on content validity would probably have been next. However, to maintain an organization relating to different measurement domains, as described in the taxonomy in Figure 3.1, we have placed the chapter on content validation in Part IV on validity.

Table 4.2	Typical Steps in Rigorous Instrument Development

1. Becoming an expert (e.g., careful review of the literature, analysis of existing instruments, in-depth or focus group interviews with members of the target population, in-depth clinical observations)
2. Elaborating the construct and its dimensionality, preparing a conceptual model and conceptual definitions, getting expert feedback to refine the model
3. Deciding on the type of instrument and the instrument development approach (e.g., CTT, IRT, clinimetric)
4. Developing the item pool
5. Assessing readability, refining items
6. Pretesting the items, undertaking cognitive interviews
7. Reviewing and revising items based on pretest
8. Obtaining expert opinion to evaluate content (and/or face) validity
9. Revising, adding, deleting items based on content validation
10. Undertaking a field test to finalize items and obtain preliminary estimates of scale quality (e.g., in CTT undertaking item analysis and an exploratory factor analysis)
11. Undertaking further developmental testing to gather information about the final scale's reliability, validity, and responsiveness
12. Preparing and publishing instrument development reports

References

American Educational Research Association, American Psychological Association, & National Council on Measurement in Education Joint Committee. (2014). *Standards for educational and psychological testing.* Washington, DC: American Psychological Association.

Angle, P., Landy, C., Charles, C., Yee, J., Watson, J., Kung, R., . . . Streiner, D. (2010). Phase 1 development of an index to measure the quality of neuraxial labour analgesia: Exploring the perspectives of childbearing women. *Canadian Journal of Anesthesia, 57,* 468–478.

Ashford, S., Turner-Stokes, L., Siegert, R., & Slade, M. (2013). Initial psychometric evaluation of the Arm Activity Measure (ArmA): A measure of activity in the hemiparetic arm. *Clinical Rehabilitation, 27,* 728–740.

Beck, C. T., & Gable, R. K. (2001). Ensuring content validity: An illustration of the process. *Journal of Nursing Measurement, 9,* 201–215.

Bradburn, N. M., Sudman, S., & Wansink, B. (2004). *Asking questions: The definitive guide to questionnaire design* (Rev. ed.). San Francisco, CA: Jossey Bass.

Bruce, B., Fries, J., Ambrosini, D., Lingala, B., Gandek, B., Rose, M., & Ware, J. (2009). Better assessment of physical function: Item improvement is neglected but essential. *Arthritis Research & Therapy, 11,* R191.

Cacioppo, J. T., & Berntson, G. G. (1994). Relationship between attitudes and evaluative space: A critical review, with emphasis on the separability of positive and negative substrates. *Psychological Bulletin, 115,* 401–423.

Cacioppo, J. T., Gardner, W. L., & Berntson, G. G. (1999) The affect system has parallel and integrative processing components: Form follows function. *Journal of Personality and Social Psychology, 76,* 839–855.

Crémers, J., Phan, B. R., Delvaux, V., & Garraux, G. (2012). Construction and validation of the Dynamic Parkinson Gait Scale (DYPAGS). *Parkinsonism & Related Disorders, 18,* 759–764.

Crowne, D. P., & Marlowe, D. (1960). A new scale of social desirability independent of psychopathology. *Journal of Consulting Psychology, 24,* 349–354.

DeVellis, R. F. (2012). *Scale development: Theory and application* (3rd ed.). Thousand Oaks, CA: Sage.

DeVet, H. C. W., Terwee, C., Mokkink, L. B., & Knol, D. L. (2011). *Measurement in medicine: A practical guide.* Cambridge, MA: Cambridge University Press.

Donders, A. R., Van der Heijden, G., Stijnen, T., & Moons, K. (2006). Review: A gentle introduction to imputation of missing values. *Journal of Clinical Epidemiology, 59,* 1087–1091.

Downey, R. G., & King, C. (1998). Missing data in Likert ratings: A comparison of replacement methods. *Journal of General Psychology, 125,* 175–191.

Elliott, M. N., Haviland, A., Kanouse, D., Hambarsoomian, K., & Hays, R. (2009). Adjusting for subgroup differences in extreme response tendency in ratings of healthcare: Impact on disparity estimates. *Health Services Research, 44,* 542–561.

Flesch, R. (1948). New readability yardstick. *Journal of Applied Psychology, 32,* 221–223.

Fowler, F. J. (1995). *Improving survey questions.* Thousand Oaks, CA: Sage.

Fox-Wasylyshyn, S. M., & El-Masri, M. M. (2005). Handling missing data in self-report measures. *Research in Nursing & Health, 28,* 488–495.

Franciosi, J., Hommel, K., Greenberg, A., DeBrosse, C., Greenier, A., Abonia, J., . . . Varni, J. W. (2012). Development of the Pediatric Quality of Life Inventory Eosinophilic Esophagitis Module items: Qualitative methods. *BMC Gastroenterology, 12,* 135.

Gilgun, J. F. (2004). Qualitative methods and the development of clinical assessment tools. *Qualitative Health Research, 14,* 1008–1019.

Hankins, M. (2008). The reliability of the twelve-item General Health Questionnaire (GHQ-12) under realistic assumptions. *BMC Public Health, 8,* 355.

Haukoos, J. S., & Newgard, C. (2006). Missing data in clinical research—Part 1: An introduction and conceptual framework. *Academic Emergency Medicine, 14,* 662–668.

Holmes, W., Bix, B., & Shea, J. (1996). SF-20 and item distributions in a human immunodeficiency virus-seropositive sample. *Medical Care, 34,* 562–569.

Jacoby, A., Baker, G., Steen, N., & Buck, D. (1999). The SF-36 as a health status measure for epilepsy: A psychometric assessment. *Quality of Life Research, 8,* 351–364.

Jones, R. R., & Goldberg, L. R. (1967). Interrelationships among personality scale parameters: Item response stability and scale reliability. *Educational & Psychological Measurement, 27,* 323–333.

Knowles, E. S. (1988). Item context effects on personality scales: Measuring changes in the measure. *Journal of Personality and Social Psychology, 55,* 312–320.

Lai, S., Perera, S., Duncan, P., & Bode, R. (2003). Physical and social functioning after stroke: Comparison of the Stroke Impact Scale and the Short Form-36. *Stroke, 34,* 488–493.

Marsh, H. (1996). Positive and negative global self-esteem: A substantively meaningful distinction or artifacts? *Journal of Personality and Social Psychology, 70,* 810–819.

Miller, G. A. (1956). The magic number seven plus or minus two: Some limits on our capacity for processing information. *Psychological Review, 63,* 81–97.

Morgan, L., Hart, L., & Polit, D. F. (2013). Content validity for the Academic Integrity Scale for Online Students (AI-SOS). Saratoga Springs, NY: Humanalysis, Inc.

Motl, R. W., & DiStefano, C. (2002). Longitudinal invariance of self-esteem and method effects associated with negatively worded items. *Structural Equation Modeling, 9,* 562–578.

Nápoles-Springer, A. M., Santoyo-Olsson, J., O'Brien, H., & Stewart, A. L. (2006). Using cognitive interviews to develop surveys in diverse populations. *Medical Care, 44*(Suppl. 3), S21–S30.

Nevo, B. (1977). Using item test-retest stability (ITRS) as a criterion for item selection. *Educational & Psychological Measurement, 37,* 847–852.

Olsen, S., Smith, S., Oei, T., & Douglas, J. (2010). Cues to starting CPAP in obstructive sleep apnea: Development and validation of the Cues to CPAP Use Questionnaire. *Journal of Clinical Sleep Medicine, 6,* 229–237.

Paulhus, D. L. (2004). *Paulhus Deception Scales.* Toronto, CA: Multi-Health Systems.

Presser, S., Rothger, J., Couper, M., Lessler, J., Martin, E., Martin, J., & Singer, E. (2004). *Methods for testing and evaluating survey questionnaires.* Hoboken, NJ: John Wiley & Sons.

Preston, C. C., & Colman, A. M. (2000). Optimal number of response categories in rating scales: Reliability, validity, discriminating power, and respondent preferences. *Acta Psychologica, 104,* 1–15.

Roth, P. L., Switzer, F., & Switzer, D. (1999). Missing data in multiple item scales: A Monte Carlo analysis of missing data techniques. *Organizational Research Methods, 1,* 211–212.

Shrive, F. M., Stuart, H., Quan, H., & Ghali, W. (2006). Dealing with missing data in a multi-question depression scale: A comparison of imputation methods. *BMC Medical Research Methodology, 6,* 57.

Strahan, R. F. (2007). Regarding some short forms of the Marlowe-Crowne Social Desirability Scale. *Psychological Reports, 100,* 483–488.

Streiner, D. L., & Norman, G. R. (2008). *Health measurement scales: A practical guide to their development and use* (4th ed.). Oxford: Oxford University Press.

Tourangeau, R., Lance, J. R., & Rasinski, K. (2000). *The psychology of survey response.* Cambridge, United Kingdom: Cambridge University Press.

Wagner, A. K., Gandek, B., Aaronson, N., Axquadro, C., Alonso, J., Apolone, G., . . . Ware, J. E. (1998). Cross-cultural comparisons of the content of SF-36 translations across 10 countries: Results from the IQOLA project. *Journal of Clinical Epidemiology, 51,* 925–932.

Watson, D. (2004). Stability versus change, dependability versus error: Issues in the assessment of personality over time. *Journal of Research in Personality, 38,* 319–350.

Weijters, B., Geuens, M., & Schilewaert, N. (2009). The proximity effect: The role of inter-item distance on reverse-item bias. *International Journal of Research in Marketing, 26,* 2–12.

Weijters, B., Geuens, M., & Schilewaert, N. (2010). The stability of individual response styles. *Psychological Methods, 15,* 96–110.

Willis, G. B. (2005). *Cognitive interviewing.* Thousand Oaks, CA: Sage.

5 Scale Development: Classical Test Theory

Chapter Outline

Many books and papers about scale development state that classical test theory (CTT) is a "traditional" method that is becoming outmoded and being replaced by more complex, sophisticated methods, namely, those associated with item response theory (IRT). Nevertheless, the majority of health-related scales being created today rely on CTT methods for selecting items from an item pool and creating a final scale, although that situation may well change in the not-too-distant future. This chapter presents some background information about CTT as a supplement to our overview in Chapter 2 and then reviews techniques typically used to finalize scales.

5.1   Classical Test Theory: Some Background

CTT provides a framework for thinking about measurements of various kinds, but it is most often discussed in connection with the development of multi-item scales. In CTT, scale developers create items that are presumed to be roughly comparable indicators of the underlying construct. The items gain strength in approximating a hypothetical true score through their aggregation. Traditional Likert scales, then, rely on items that are deliberately redundant (DeVellis, 2012) in the hope that multiple indicators of the construct will converge on the true score and balance out error. Responses to items on such scales are conceptualized as the effects of the construct, hence the scales that we discuss in this chapter are reflective (Chapter 2).

In the CTT framework, a **domain sampling model** is assumed, which theoretically involves the random sampling of a homogeneous set of items from a hypothetical universe of items reflective of the construct. Of course, random sampling from a *universe* of all possible items is an unrealistic scenario, but it is a principle that is useful to keep in mind. The idea is to generate a fairly exhaustive set of item possibilities, given the construct's theoretical demands. For a traditional scale, redundancy (except for trivial word substitutions) is a good thing—the goal is to measure the construct of interest with a set of items that capture the central theme in slightly different ways so that irrelevant idiosyncrasies of individual items will cancel each other out.

5.2 Designing a Field Test of a Classical Test Theory Scale

Once an item pool has been developed and the items have been pretested and reviewed both internally (e.g., for readability and grammar) and externally (e.g., for content validity), the next step is to undertake a quantitative assessment of the items. Such an assessment requires that the scale be administered to a fairly large development sample. Testing a new instrument is a full study in itself, and care must be taken to design the study to yield useful evidence about the scale's quality. Important steps include developing sampling and data collection strategies.

5.2.a The Sampling Plan

The sample for testing a new CTT scale ideally should be representative of the population for which the scale has been targeted and should be large enough to support complex analyses. Random sampling is seldom possible in scale development studies, but efforts should nevertheless be made to recruit a diverse sample from the relevant population. For example, a good strategy is to recruit a sample from multiple sites, preferably in different locales, to enhance representativeness and to assess geographic and linguistic variation in interpreting items. Other strategies to enhance representativeness should be sought as well—for example, taking steps to ensure that the sample includes people from different age groups, men and women, people with diverse educational and ethnic backgrounds, people with varying disease severity, and so on, if these characteristics are relevant.

Exploratory factor analysis, which is described later in this chapter, is a standard feature of CTT scale development. Although there is no clear consensus on how many participants are needed in a factor analysis, there is agreement that the sample size should be large. Some psychometricians have suggested that 300 is an adequate number to support a factor analysis (Nunnally & Bernstein, 1994; Tabachnick & Fidell, 2013). Others have offered guidance in terms of a ratio of items to respondents. Recommendations range from 5 people per item to 40 or 50 per item, with 10 per item being the number most often recommended (Costello & Osborne, 2005; Osborne & Costello, 2004). That means that if the scale has 20 items, the sample should probably be at least 200, and a larger sample is even better. Having a sufficiently large sample is essential to ensure stability in item covariation estimates. Having a large sample is also advantageous because it could support dividing the sample in half randomly, conducting analyses with one half-sample, and then cross-validating the results with the second half-sample, as we illustrate later.

5.2.b The Data Collection Plan

Decisions have to be made concerning how to administer the scale (e.g., through mailed questionnaires, the Internet, or in-person administration in a paper-and-pencil or computer format) and what to include in the overall instrument. In terms of the mode of administration, it is best to select an approach that approximates how the scale typically would be administered in real-world applications.

The instrument should include the scale items, basic demographic questions, and questions about relevant clinical attributes. The demographic and clinical questions should be ones that are useful in describing the sample but should also be selected with an eye to creating key subgroups for assessing item performance.

Thought should also be given to including measures of other attributes on the instrument. This would be essential if a *separate* study to evaluate the scale's validity is not planned. (Some suggestions about data collection for validation field tests are offered in Chapter 13.) Depending on the nature of the construct, it may be useful to include measures to assess response biases, especially social desirability (Chapter 4). Also, it may be useful to include other measures when there is a concern about possible floor or ceiling effects on the new scale. As an example, to ensure that the scale has adequate distributional properties for people at different levels of physical functioning, it might be useful to administer a well-validated scale measuring functional ability, such as the Barthel Index (Mahoney & Barthel, 1965).

5.3 Basic Item Analysis

Scale development within CTT is associated with a number of statistical analyses, broadly referred to as **item analysis**. A major purpose of item analysis is to draw conclusions about which items to discard or about the possible need to add items. The goal is to arrive at a parsimonious set of items for each dimension of a construct and for the scale or subscales to have acceptable internal consistency. When reporting on scale development, researchers should be explicit about the criteria they used to eliminate items, including what the threshold of acceptability was for such indicators as percentage missing, floor and ceiling effects, and inter-item correlations.

In this chapter, we illustrate aspects of CTT item reduction using data from a sample of 1,000 low-income women (the sample used here was a random sample of a larger sample of nearly 4,000 women in four urban areas; see Polit, London, & Martinez, 2001). These women completed several health scales, including the 20-item Center for Epidemiologic Studies Depression Scale (CES-D; Radloff, 1977). In the CES-D, people are asked to indicate how frequently in the past 7 days[1] they had certain experiences; response options were scored as follows: 0 = *rarely or never* (*less than 1 day*); 1 = *some or a little* (*1 to 2 days*); 2 = *occasionally or a moderate amount* (*3 to 4 days*); and 3 = *most or all* (*5 to 7 days*). To conserve space, we show data for select CES-D items rather than the full 20 items.

5.3.a Distributional Analyses for Individual Items

The first step in item analysis is to check the descriptive statistics for each item. This includes examining the percentage of responses for each response option, the percentage missing, and measures of central tendency, variability, and skewness.

For a CTT scale, items with means that are close to the center of the range of possible scores are especially desirable—for example, a mean near 4.0 on a 7-point (1 to 7) scale or a mean near 1.5 on 4-point CES-D items scored 0 to 3. Ideally, there would be good variability

---

[1]The revised version of the CES-D, the CESD-R, asks about experiences in the past *2* weeks; responses range from 0 (not at all) to 4 (nearly every day for 2 weeks), but scoring for the total scale often involves converting an item score of 4 to 3, so that total scores for the 20 items still range from 0 to 60 (Van Dam & Earlywine, 2011).

on each item, with a near-normal distribution of responses or at least responses covering the full range of response options.

Floor and ceiling effects can be examined by looking at the percentage of people with the highest or lowest possible scores. At the item level, different cutoff values have been used to establish acceptability. For example, Skirko, Weaver, Perkins, Kinter, and Sie (2012) eliminated items if more than 50% of their sample chose the highest (*always*) or lowest (*never*) option on a quality-of-life scale. Holmes, Bix, and Shea (1996) used a criterion of 75% endorsement of extreme options. Pearson's skewness index can also be inspected. Although skewness criteria have not been established for individual items, an item would be extremely skewed if the absolute value of the skewness statistic was 2.0 or greater.

The percentage of missing responses for each item should also be considered when making decisions about item retention. DeVet, Terwee, Mokkink, and Knol (2011) recommend that items with more than 15% missing should be deleted, revised, or replaced, but we are inclined to recommend a stricter criterion—for example, 5% (Yang et al., 2011).

To illustrate, Table 5.1 presents descriptive statistics (from an SPSS analysis) for 12 of the 20 CES-D items administered to the sample of 1,000 low-income women. For all 12 items, there was a slight negative skew, skewing in the direction of not being depressed, but the full range of response options was used for every item, and the means and standard deviations are acceptable. Among these 12 items, the item that might cause some concern is Item 9 (*I thought my life had been a failure*) because it has the highest rate of missingness (5.5%), the highest skewness (1.02), and the highest percentage of responses saying "never" (54.9%), as shown in the shaded cells in Table 5.1.

Item distributions should always be examined for the sample as a whole, but consideration should also be given to looking at distributional characteristics for key subgroups as well. Subgroups could be created on the basis of demographic characteristics, clinical characteristics, or scores on another scale. For example, we scrutinized item 9 (*I thought my life had been a failure*) in greater depth by examining whether the percentage of women who skipped the question differed from those who answered it in terms of educational attainment, employment status, marital status, being above or below poverty, or being in poor or good health (as measured by scores on the SF-12). No significant differences in missingness were found. However, women whose incomes were above the poverty line had a distribution that was more severely skewed (1.50) than women living in poverty (0.89).

5.3.b Correlational Analyses

Within CTT, scale developers seek items that are highly correlated with the true score of the underlying construct. This cannot be assessed directly, but if each item is a measure of an underlying latent variable, then the items should correlate with each another.

The degree of **inter-item correlation** can be evaluated by examining the correlation matrix of all the items (or, if the instrument is expected to be multidimensional, the items on a hypothesized subscale), typically using standard Pearson product–moment correlation. If there are items that were intentionally developed to be reverse scored, it is a good idea to do the item reversals before inspecting the correlation matrix.[2] After such reversals are done, any negative correlations in the matrix are likely to reflect problematic items. For items on the same subscale, inter-item correlations between 0.30 and 0.70 are preferred. Correlations lower than 0.30 suggest limited congruence with the underlying construct and ones higher than 0.70 suggest overredundancy. However, the assessment of correlation values depends on the number of items in the scale. An *average* inter-item correlation of 0.50 is needed to achieve a coefficient alpha of 0.80 on a 4-item scale, but an average of only

---

[2]To reverse score an item, the value of the item should be subtracted from the maximum item value, plus 1. In our CES-D example, which is on a 4-point scale from 0 to 3, a reversed item would be: REVITEM = 4 − OLDITEM.

Table 5.1	Descriptive Statistics for 12 CES-D Items[a] in Sample of Low-Income Women					
Item Number and Stem	% Missing	% Never	% Most Days	Mean	SD[b]	Skewness Index
1. I was bothered by things that don't usually bother me.	2.2	36.9	12.2	1.04	1.0	0.62
3. I felt I could not shake off the blues.	2.0	47.3	11.7	0.87	1.1	0.72
4. I felt as good as other people (reversed).	2.2	16.3	54.0	0.94	1.2	0.78
5. I had trouble keeping my mind on what I was doing.	3.4	44.1	10.4	0.90	1.0	0.85
6. I felt depressed.	3.5	38.2	14.4	1.08	1.1	0.57
7. I felt everything I did was an effort.	4.6	26.7	26.4	1.49	1.1	0.03
8. I felt hopeful about the future (reversed).	3.6	17.2	43.4	1.11	1.1	0.53
9. I thought my life had been a failure.	5.5	54.9	8.8	0.77	1.0	1.02
11. My sleep was restless.	4.2	38.8	16.0	1.10	1.1	0.55
12. I was happy (reversed).	3.7	11.6	40.7	1.02	1.0	0.59
16. I enjoyed life (reversed).	3.9	11.8	54.9	0.82	1.1	0.95
18. I felt sad.	3.8	43.9	10.5	0.93	1.0	0.76

SD, standard deviation.
[a]Responses to 12 of the original 20 items on the CES-D (Radloff, 1977) for a sample of 1,000 low-income women (Polit et al., 2001). The item numbers shown are the original scale numbers. For items marked "reversed," the original percentages for never/most days are shown, but the mean and skewness values are after reversals.
[b]For all items, the range was 0 to 3 (i.e., the full range of response options).

0.29 is needed to achieve the same internal consistency if the scale has 10 items (DeVellis, 2012). For short scales, even items with relatively low inter-item correlations are likely to increase coefficient alpha. Thus, it is probably wise to retain items with modest positive correlations until further analyses are completed.

Continuing with our illustration, Table 5.2 shows the inter-item correlations for five selected items (3, 4, 6, 8, and 12) on the CES-D, correlated with all 12 items from Table 5.1. The average inter-item correlation for these five items, presented in the next-to-last row, range from 0.12 for Item 8 (*I felt hopeful about the future*) to 0.40 (*I felt depressed*). Items 4 and Item 8 (which are items that require reversals) both have low mean inter-item correlations, as well as some negative correlations, and thus suggest potentially problematic items.

A next step is to compute preliminary total scale or subscale scores and then calculate correlations between the items and the total scores on the scales they are intended to represent. If item scores fail to correlate well with scale scores, the item is likely to be measuring a different construct and its inclusion could lower the internal consistency of the

Table 5.2	Selected Inter-Item Correlations for CES-D Items in Sample of Low-Income Women				
Item	Item 3	Item 4	Item 6	Item 8	Item 12
*1. I was bothered by things that don't usually bother me.	0.46	0.06	0.51	0.04	0.24
*3. I felt I could not shake off the blues.	—	0.06	0.61	0.04	0.31
4. I felt as good as other people (reversed).	0.06	—	0.08	0.31	0.31
*5. I had trouble keeping my mind on what I was doing.	0.48	0.03	0.58	0.03	0.24
*6. I felt depressed.	0.61	0.08	—	.05	0.36
*7. I felt everything I did was an effort.	0.26	−0.14	0.30	−0.23	0.04
8. I felt hopeful about the future (reversed).	0.04	0.31	0.05	—	0.28
9. I thought my life had been a failure.	0.45	0.12	0.50	0.03	0.30
*11. My sleep was restless.	0.47	0.05	0.54	−0.03	0.27
*12. I was happy (reversed).	0.30	0.31	0.36	0.28	—
*16. I enjoyed life (reversed).	0.24	0.29	0.29	0.29	0.56
*18. I felt sad.	0.53	0.09	0.63	0.01	0.33
Mean inter-item correlation	0.35	0.14	0.40	0.12	0.29
Mean corrected item-total correlation	0.62	0.19	0.72	0.13	0.52

Note: Correlations ≥0.08 were statistically significant at $p < 0.05$.
*Items used in subsequent analyses; these are the nine items from the 9-item CES-D short form scale developed by Santor and Coyne (1997).

scale.[3] Two types of **item-scale correlations** can be computed. The first is the correlation between an item and a total score that includes the item under consideration (*uncorrected*). The second *corrected approach* involves the correlation of an individual item with the total scale after removing the item (also called *item-partial total correlation*). The corrected approach is preferable because the inclusion of the item on the scale inflates the correlation coefficients, and the inflation factor increases as the number of items on the scale decreases. In SPSS, corrected item-total correlations are calculated in the reliability procedure; uncorrected item-total correlations can be obtained in the correlations procedure. Advice on a minimum criterion for item-total correlations vary. Streiner and Norman (2008) suggest that items with an item-total correlation lower than 0.20 are candidates for deletion, whereas Nunnally and Bernstein (1994) suggest a minimum of 0.30.

The bottom row of Table 5.2 shows the corrected correlations between the 5 selected items and the total summated scale score for all 12 items. Consistent with the picture that emerged for the inter-item correlations, items 4 and 8 did not perform well in this sample of women—the item-total correlations for both were less than 0.20. All future analyses with

---

[3]An item-total correlation is essentially an item *discrimination* index, reflecting the degree to which the item contributes to measurement precision. As we will discuss in Chapter 6, discrimination is an important concept in Item Response Theory.

the CES-D data in this chapter use only the nine items in Table 5.2 marked with an asterisk. Item 9 was deleted because of problems identified with the distribution, as previously noted, and items 4 and 8 had problematic correlational results. As it turns out, the nine remaining items are the same as those selected by Santor and Coyne (1997) in their version of a short-form CES-D.[4]

For constructs that might be affected by a social desirability bias, correlational analyses at both the item-level and scale level can be undertaken if a measure of social desirability was included on the field test instrument. Items that are especially correlated with social desirability measures might bear further scrutiny. Potential scale users should be alerted to the possibility of bias when the total scale scores have high correlations with social desirability scale scores.

Papers on CTT scale development often present the details of item-analysis work as described here. For example, Tsakos and colleagues (2012) developed the Scale of Oral Health Outcomes for 5-year-old children (SOHO-5). The item-total correlations of the seven items on their scale ranged from 0.30 to 0.60, which they concluded was satisfactory. Their average inter-item correlation was 0.29.

5.3.c Distributional Analyses for Provisional Scales and Subscales

The distributional properties of the preliminary total scores should also be subjected to further scrutiny. Such analyses might suggest the need for further revisions, or the need to generate additional items.

Floor effects and ceiling effects can occur for the entire scale or subscales as well as for individual items. If large percentages of the development sample have the most extreme scale scores, then it might suggest the need to take further steps. One possibility is to redefine an appropriate population by looking at floor and ceiling effects within subgroups of the sample. Another possibility is to add items that allow greater variability for people at the extremes. Several people have suggested that floor and ceiling effects are at an unacceptable level if more than 15% of the sample gets scale scores at the extreme (e.g., Cubo et al., 2010; Terwee et al., 2007), although others have used a 20% criterion (e.g., Holmes et al., 1996). Sometimes a scale is expected to pass a skewness test as well, with skewness values less than -1.0 or greater than 1.0 deemed problematic (e.g., Cubo et al., 2010). For the provisional scale composed of the nine CES-D items (Table 5.2), only 4.0% of the sample had the lowest scores of 0, and only 0.4% had the highest score of 27. The skewness statistic for the scale was an acceptable value, 0.57.

Missing values problems should also be analyzed at the scale level. For example, the percentage of the sample that has a missing scale or subscale score should be computed. Equally important, the distribution of the number of missing items across the sample should be analyzed; that is, what percentage of cases have zero missing items, one missing item, and so on? As noted in Chapter 4, it has been suggested that imputation of item values should not be undertaken if a person has more than 20% of the items missing. If many sample members have more than 20% of items missing, this signals a problem with the scale that needs to be addressed. With our CES-D nine-item "scale," only 7.3% of the sample had any missing items. If we were to impute values for women who had one item missing, the percent with a missing scale value would be reduced to 4.1% of the sample. Only 41 out of 1,000 women omitted responses to two or more items. For subsequent analyses, case means were imputed for the single missing item of 32 women.

Depending on the nature of the scale and the population, it might be useful to look for patterns relating to response bias using the provisional total scores, especially if the construct of interest is attitudinal. For example, item distribution information can be used to create indexes of extreme response bias, moderacy bias, and acquiescence.

---

[4]Numerous short-form CES-D scales have been developed, including 10-item scales by Cole, Rabin, Smith, and Kaufman (2004); Kohout, Berkman, & Evans (1993); and Andresen, Malmgren, Carter, and Patrick (1994).

5.4   Exploratory Factor Analysis

A collection of items does not necessarily result in a scale. Items form a summated scale only if they have a common underlying construct, which typically cannot be verified simply by looking at the items. **Factor analysis** disentangles complex interrelationships among items and identifies items that "go together" as unified concepts based on people's responses to the items during the field test. Thus, a factor analysis is an important statistical tool within CTT for understanding whether items can be put together as a unidimensional scale or whether subscales should be created for distinct dimensions of a construct. For example, we might develop a set of items to measure patients' fatigue. We would want to know whether item responses can be scored together to yield a single measure of fatigue or whether there are different aspects to fatigue, such as affective, cognitive, and sensory components, that require scoring into separate subscales.

There are two broad types of factor analyses and multiple variants within the two. This section discusses the first type known as **exploratory factor analysis** (**EFA**), which is a staple analytic tool within the CTT scale development framework. Another type of factor analysis—*confirmatory factor analysis* (CFA)—is a hypothesis-testing procedure that is used to assess structural validity, as described in Chapter 14. (Although both EFA and CFA are often associated with the development and testing of scales in CTT, they also play a role in testing assumptions for IRT measures, as discussed in the next chapter.)

EFA does not require a priori hypotheses about the dimensionality of a set of items. Of course, dimensions of a construct usually *are* envisioned when the scale is being conceptualized, and preliminary ideas about dimensionality may be corroborated by experts during a content validity activity. Preconceptions about dimensions, however, are not always consistent with the reality of actual responses. A factor analysis is a reasonably objective, empirical method of illuminating the underlying dimensionality of a large set of individual measures.

A factor analysis is complex, and so we can provide only an overview. The books by Pett, Lackey, and Sullivan (2003) and Tabachnick and Fidell (2013) are additional resources for learning more about EFA.

5.4.a   Basic Concepts for an Exploratory Factor Analysis

A factor analysis uncovers the structure of a set of items by analyzing intercorrelations among them. In a factor analysis, the underlying dimensions are called *factors*. A **factor** is a hypothetical trait—a *latent trait*—that is presumed to be the basis for people's responses to the concrete measures administered to them.

Mathematically, a factor is a weighted linear combination of variables in a data matrix. A raw data matrix is composed of scores on k item variables for N subjects. A factor could be defined by the following equation:

$$F_1 = b_1X_1 + b_2X_2 + \ldots b_kX_k$$

where F_1 = a factor score for Factor 1
k = number of original variables (items)
b_1 to b_k = weights for each k variable
X_1 to X_k = raw score values on the k variables

A factor analysis solves for the b weights (which are called **factor loadings**) to yield factor scores for the major dimensions underlying the original measures.

One of the products of a factor analysis is a **factor matrix**, in which the original variables are on one dimension and factors are along the other. There are several types of factor matrix, as we discuss subsequently. The entries in a factor matrix are factor loadings that tell us about the relationship between the original items and the underlying factors.

Table 5.3	**Hypothetical Factor Matrix for Six Pain Items[a]**		
	Factor		**Communality[b]** (h^2)
Items	**I**	**II**	
A	0.81	0.21	0.70
B	0.67	0.20	0.49
C	0.74	0.13	0.56
D	0.17	0.70	0.52
E	0.22	0.80	0.69
F	0.27	0.61	0.45
Eigenvalue	1.81	1.60	3.41
Explained variance	30.2%	26.6%	56.8%

[a]Hypothetical results for a rotated factor matrix for six items on patients' pain; Factor I represents pain intensity and Factor II represents pain interference.
[b]Common factor variance.

Table 5.3 shows a hypothetical example of a factor matrix. In this example, suppose that the variables A through F in the first column are six items tapping patients' pain. Factors I and II are empirically derived factors that might represent pain intensity (Factor I) and pain interference (Factor II). Except as we discuss later, factors loadings can be interpreted much like correlation coefficients. The first entry in the matrix (0.81) indicates a strong positive correlation between Item A and Factor I. Items A, B, and C have high loadings on Factor I, whereas all the loadings for Items C, D, and E on Factor I are less than 0.30. Conversely, the first three items have modest loadings on Factor II, but the last three items have loadings of 0.61 or greater on this factor. We would interpret the factors by trying to conceptualize what Items A, B, and C have in common and what they do *not* have in common with Items D, E, and F.

Table 5.3 has two other types of useful information. The **communality** is a measure of a variable's *shared* variance (sometimes called *common factor variance* and sometimes labeled h^2). The communalities of the original items are equal to the sums of squares of the factor loadings for those items. Thus, for Item A, the communality is $(0.81)^2 + (0.21)^2 = 0.70$. The common factor variance of each item indicates the variance that it shares in common with other items. The variability of each item in Table 5.3 can be expressed as follows:

$$\sigma^2_{Total} = \sigma^2_{CommonFactor} + \sigma^2_{Specific} + \sigma^2_{Error}$$

where σ^2_{Total} = Total variance
$\sigma^2_{CommonFactor}$ = Common factor variance (h^2)
$\sigma^2_{Specific}$ = Variance specific to the item
σ^2_{Error} = Error variance

Using Item A to illustrate, the total variance in patients' scores on Item A consists of (1) variance that Item A has in common with the other five items, plus (2) variance that is specific to Item A, plus (3) error variance (e.g., unreliability). Across the two factors, 70% of the variance in Item A is common factor variance; the remaining 30% is **unique variance**, which is partly item-specific variance and partly error variance. Table 5.3 indicates that Item A has the highest proportion of common factor variance (0.70), whereas Item F has the lowest (0.45). A factor analysis allocates the total common factor variance of items (h^2) to the different factors.

A row near the bottom of Table 5.3 is labeled eigenvalue. An **eigenvalue** is the sum of the squared item loadings for a specific factor. For Factor I, the eigenvalue is $(0.81)^2 + (0.67)^2 + (0.74)^2 + (0.17)^2 + (0.22)^2 + (0.27)^2 = 1.81$. An eigenvalue indicates how much variance is explained by a given factor. Each item is standardized to have a variance of 1.0, so the total amount of variance in the analysis is the number of items times 1.0, here 6.0. In this example, the eigenvalues for both factors are similar (1.81 and 1.60), indicating that both pain intensity and pain interference account for a comparable percentage of variance in the six item scores. The amount of variance is shown in the bottom row: 30.2% for Factor I and 26.6% for Factor II. Together, the two factors account for 56.8% of the total variance in the six items (the combined eigenvalue of 3.41, divided by 6.0).

Inasmuch as a factor analysis uses a correlation matrix as its starting point, the assumptions underlying the correlational analysis should be kept in mind. The variables in a factor analysis are generally measured on a scale that is interval or ratio or on an ordinal scale that approximates interval properties (such as individual Likert-type items). Each pair of variables in the correlation matrix should be linearly correlated; curvilinear relationships degrade the analysis. Normally distributed variables enhance the factor analytic solution.

5.4.b Phases in an Exploratory Factor Analysis

A factor analysis typically involves several phases, each with iterations and feedback loops. The first step involves transforming the raw data matrix into a correlation matrix and undertaking some preliminary analyses to assess whether, in fact, a factor analysis makes sense. In other words, an initial task is to assess whether the correlation matrix is *factorable*.

In EFA, underlying constructs are assumed to be responsible for correlations among the items, consistent with the model for a reflective scale (Chapter 2). Ideally, the factor solution will reveal a small number of interpretable and meaningful dimensions of a construct that are substantively interesting. The phase called **factor extraction** is used to assess how many factors are needed to adequately capture the variance in the items. Different approaches to factor extraction are available, and different criteria can be applied to draw conclusions about the appropriate number of factors. The product from this phase of analysis is an **unrotated factor matrix**.

The goal of factor extraction is to maximize variance. An unrotated factor matrix, however, does not yield readily understandable results. In the next phase of a factor analysis, **factor rotation**, the original factors are transformed so that the results are more interpretable. As with factor extraction, there are alternative methods of factor rotation. The result of this phase of the analysis is a **rotated factor matrix**. Table 5.3 presented a fictitious rotated factor matrix.

The next phase of a factor analysis typically involves interpreting, evaluating, and refining the factors. Interpretation is a key activity in a factor analysis, and interpretation can sometimes be aided by testing alternatives to see if different analytic decisions result in a better and more interpretable solution. Thus, EFA is widely used and valued, but its many options for key decisions, the absence of clear-cut criteria for decision making, and the importance of interpretation make it different from standard hypothesis-testing statistical procedures.

5.4.c Evaluation of Factorability

A first step in drawing conclusions about whether a correlation matrix is factorable concerns the size of the sample, which should be large enough to rule out spurious intercorrelations. Having a large overall sample does not necessarily provide a sufficient basis for factor analysis if there are large amounts of missing data. As we illustrated earlier, case mean substitution can be used to impute small amounts of missing data, and even more sophisticated options such as multiple imputation are available. If the analysis is done in SPSS or other widely used multipurpose statistical software, it is best not to use the *missing values option* within the factor analysis procedure because this will replace missing values with item means for the entire sample and will replace all missing values without considering the percentage of items skipped per case. (Under no circumstances should the *pairwise deletion* option be used in a factor analysis, which yields a nonrectangular matrix of correlation coefficients based on a varying number of cases.) If missing values are extensive, a factor analysis may not be appropriate.

To be factorable, a correlation matrix should have a number of sizeable correlations between items. When inter-item correlations are low, the items are unlikely to be capturing a common underlying construct. Thus, if the correlation matrix consists mainly of coefficients with an absolute value less than 0.30, there is probably nothing to factor analyze. On the other hand, if correlations are too high, problems with multicollinearity may occur. If there are items with intercorrelations greater than 0.80, some should be dropped because they are likely to be redundant and also because they can result in an unstable solution.

Factor analysis software typically offers diagnostic tools for evaluating factorability in terms of item intercorrelations and *sampling adequacy*, which refers to the adequacy of sampling *items*. One such tool is **Bartlett's test of sphericity**, which tests the null hypothesis that the correlation matrix is an *identity matrix*—one in which correlations among the variables are zero. If this null hypothesis cannot be rejected, factor analysis is inappropriate. If Bartlett's test is significant, further evaluation of the factorability of the data is warranted. However, the test is almost significant because it is influenced by sample size, which is usually large.

A more important tool is the **Kaiser-Meyer-Olkin (KMO) test**, a measure of sampling adequacy that compares the magnitude of correlation coefficients to the sizes of partial correlation coefficients (i.e., correlations after controlling for the effects of all other variables). In a factorable set of data, partial correlations should be small in relation to observed correlation coefficients. The KMO index of sampling adequacy can range from 0 to 1, and the closer the value is to 1, the better the prospects for factor analysis. KMO values of 0.80 or higher are considered good, and those in the 0.70s are fair. Anything below 0.60 is considered questionable for a factor analysis (Tabachnick & Fidell, 2013). KMOs can be computed for all items combined as well as for each item individually.

For several parts of our discussion, we will be describing a factor analysis of the nine CES-D items discussed earlier in connection with basic item analyses, with analyses performed in SPSS. Because our sample size was large, we randomly divided the sample in half, so that the results in the first half-sample could be cross-validated with the other half-sample (about 500 women in each sample). Table 5.4 presents the results for Bartlett's test and the

Table 5.4	**Results From an Analysis of Factorability for Nine CES-D Items, Sample 1 of Low-Income Women ($N = 481$)**	
Kaiser-Meyer-Olkin and Bartlett's Test		
Kaiser-Meyer-Olkin Measure of Sampling Adequacy		**0.873**
Bartlett's Test of Sphericity	Approximate Chi-Square	1450.9
	df	36
	Sig.	0.000

overall KMO test for these data for the first half-sample. As this figure shows, Bartlett's test is significant (p <0.001) and the KMO value (0.873) is very good.

KMO values for individual items (called *measures of sampling adequacy* or *MSA*) can be found on the diagonal of the *anti-image correlation matrix*. Although not shown here because of its size, the anti-image matrix for our example showed KMO values ranging from a low of 0.749 for one item to a high of 0.940 for another. These values further support a decision to proceed with a factor analysis.

5.4.d Factor Extraction in Exploratory Factor Analysis

In factor extraction, the computer program seeks clusters of intercorrelated items in the correlation matrix and extracts as much variance as possible. Different models and statistical criteria can be used to extract factors; most factor analysis programs offer several alternatives.

A frequently used method of factor extraction is called principal components. **Principal components analysis (PCA)** differs from other factor analytic methods in that it analyzes *all* variance in the item scores, not just common factor variance. The key issue concerns the value placed on the diagonal of the correlation matrix prior to matrix operations because the variance subjected to analysis is the sum of values on the positive diagonal. With PCA, all diagonal values are 1.00, representing total item variance. Thus, there is as much variance to be analyzed in a PCA as there are items. All variance in the original items are distributed to the factors, including each item's unique variance and its error variance.

PCA creates successive linear combinations of the items in the analysis. The first factor, or *principal component*, is a linear combination that accounts for the most variance, using a least-squares criterion. The second component, formed from residual correlations, accounts for the second largest amount of variance that is uncorrelated with the first component. Successive components account for smaller and smaller proportions of total variance in the data, and all are orthogonal to (uncorrelated with) previously extracted components. The extracted factors (components)[5] thus represent independent sources of variation.

In PCA, there are as many factors as there are variables, but with factorable data only the first few account for a sizeable proportion of variance. Table 5.5 presents a summary table from a PCA factor extraction of the nine CES-D items. In this analysis, nine factors were extracted. The amount of variance explained by each factor is shown in column 2 (Total), which represents initial eigenvalues for each factor. All of the variance in the nine CES-D items is accounted for by the nine factors in PCA: Summing the eigenvalues in column 2 yields a total of 9.0 and cumulatively, the nine factors account for 100% of the variance in the original items. To compute the proportion of variance explained by a factor, the eigenvalue associated with the factor is divided by 9.0. For the first factor in this example, $3.95 \div 9.0 = 0.4389$. In other words, 43.89% of the variance in the nine items is accounted for by the first factor. Subsequent factors account for declining percentages of variance (e.g., 14.74% for factor 2). The final column shows the cumulative percentage of variance explained by the factor for that row, plus all preceding factors. Thus, the first two factors account for about 59% of the variance in the nine variables. As a general rule of thumb, 60% or more of variance explained by the key factors is considered good.

In other methods of factor extraction, only common factor variance is analyzed and unique variance is excluded. The most popular common factor extraction method is called the **principal factors** (PF) method (or *principal-axis* factoring method). The PF method

---

[5]Some writers do not call PCA a factor analysis. For simplicity, we refer to components as factors even when PCA was performed.

Table 5.5	Total Variance Explained, Principal Components Analysis for Nine CES-D Items, Sample 1 of Low-Income Women ($N = 481$)		
Component (Factor)	Initial Eigenvalues		
	Total Value	% of Variance	Cumulative %
1	3.95	43.89	43.89
2	1.33	14.74	58.63
3	0.82	9.10	67.73
4	0.63	6.99	74.72
5	0.58	6.48	81.21
6	0.54	6.02	87.23
7	0.41	4.57	91.80
8	0.40	4.45	96.25
9	0.34	3.75	100.0
Total	9.0	100.0	

puts estimates of item communalities, rather than 1s, on the diagonal of the correlation matrix. The initial communality estimates are the squared multiple correlation coefficients for the specified item, with all other items as predictors. As an index of shared variance, R^2 is a reasonable proxy for common factor variance. The communalities are repeatedly and iteratively reestimated from the factor loadings until there are only negligible changes in the communality estimates. As with PCA, the goal of a PF extraction is to extract the largest possible amount of variance with successive factors.

Other methods of factor extraction include the *alpha method, maximum likelihood extraction, image factoring, and generalized least squares factoring*. There may be sound substantive or methodologic reasons for preferring one method over another, but when there are a fairly large number of items and a large sample of participants, differences in factor extraction solutions tend to be small.

5.4.e Number of Factors to Extract in Exploratory Factor Analysis

In doing a factor analysis, researchers must decide how many factors to extract and rotate. There are two competing goals in making the decision. The first is to maximize explained variance. The larger the number of factors, the greater the percentage of variance explained. Table 5.5 shows that we can account for 100% of the variance in the nine CES-D items by using nine factors, but this would defeat the purpose of a factor analysis. The competing objective is parsimony: The fewer the number of factors, the more parsimonious is the solution in characterizing the dimensionality of the set of items. Yet, if too few factors are extracted, the proportion of explained variance might be insufficient, and important dimensions of the broader construct might go unidentified. If we used only the first factor in Table 5.5, for example, we would account for only about 44% of the variance in the items. The aim, then, is to balance the two goals by using as few factors as is adequate in explaining a high proportion of variance.

Researchers can use various criteria in deciding how many factors to rotate. The simplest method is to inspect eigenvalues from an initial run with PCA. A component with an eigenvalue less than 1 can usually be discounted. In PCA, an eigenvalue lower than 1.0 is less important in accounting for variance in a factor than an original item. According to this criterion, we would conclude from Table 5.5 that the CES-D items encompass two key factors because only the first two factors have eigenvalues greater than 1.0. In SPSS, this criterion is used as the default.

A second approach is a **scree test**, in which successive factors and their eigenvalues are plotted. Figure 5.1 shows a scree plot in which the nine factors from Table 5.5 are graphed along the X axis and their eigenvalues are plotted on the Y axis. What one looks for in a scree plot is a sharp discontinuity in the plot's slope that separates larger, more important factors from smaller, less reliable ones. In other words, one looks for the point in the plot where a line drawn through the points sharply changes slope. In this example, an argument could be made that a break in the slope occurs between factors 2 and 3, which is consistent with the criterion based on eigenvalues.

Other criteria for deciding on the number of factors have been proposed, such as examining communalities, the proportion of variance accounted for by a factor, and values in the residual correlation matrix. These and other decision-making strategies are described in Tabachnick and Fidell (2013).

The decision about the number of factors to retain and rotate is usually more critical than the decision about which factor extraction method to use. Yet, the decision is not always straightforward because different criteria can lead to different conclusions. If the number of important factors is not clear cut, it is advantageous to inspect more than one rotated factor matrix to assess which solution is most theoretically sensible. It is usually better to begin with too many rather than too few factors and to cut back if necessary.

5.4.f Factor Rotation in Exploratory Factor Analysis

The factor matrix resulting from factor extraction decisions is usually difficult to interpret. Factor rotation helps researchers to better understand the meaning of underlying factors by maximizing high item loadings on those factors that have been deemed important,

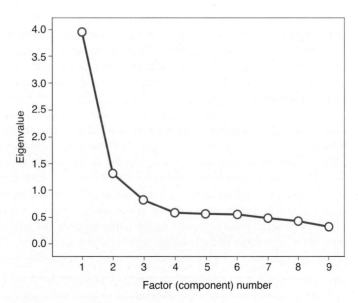

Figure 5.1
Scree plot for nine CES-D items, sample 1.

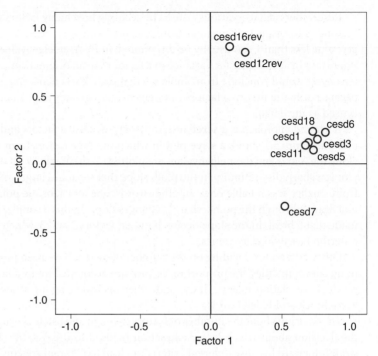

Figure 5.2

Rotated plot for nine CES-D items, two-factor solution, sample 1.

according to criteria described in the previous section. Rotated factors are equivalent to unrotated ones mathematically. Factor loadings change after rotation because the axes are altered, but the communalities and the total percentage of variance explained by the rotated factors do not change. Readers interested in a more complete explanation of factor rotation, together with graphic illustrations of the rotation process can consult DeVellis (2012) or Pett and colleagues (2003).

The objective of rotation is to align items more clearly along axes and thus derive factors that are as "pure" as possible. An ideal rotation solution results in items with high loadings on one and only one factor. Also, a good solution yields loadings as close to 1.00 (or −1.00) as possible for items aligned with a factor and loadings as close to zero as possible for items not aligned with that factor. In the real world, ideal factor solutions are seldom achieved.

Multiple methods of factor rotation have been developed, and so factor analysts must make additional decisions. Rotation methods fall into two major groupings: orthogonal rotation and oblique rotation. **Orthogonal rotation** results in factors that are uncorrelated with one another. During factor extraction, the factors are always orthogonal because each new linear combination is uncorrelated with previously created factors. Orthogonal factors are at right angles and are independent of one another. Several techniques that use different statistical criteria can be used for orthogonal rotation. *Varimax rotation* is the most widely used type of orthogonal rotation.[6] As the name suggests, the goal of varimax rotation is to maximize the variance of the loadings within factors, across items. Figure 5.2 presents a plot of the two retained CES-D factors after varimax rotation. The horizontal axis passes close

---

[6]Another orthogonal method, *quartimax rotation*, emphasizes the simplification of items rather than factors. Quartimax rotation aims to increase the dispersion of the loadings within the items, across factors. A third orthogonal method, *equimax rotation*, attempts to combine the goals of quartimax and varimax rotations by aiming to simplify factors and items simultaneously.

to a cluster of six items, and the vertical axis is most clearly aligned with two items. Rotated factor loadings from this plot are discussed in the next section.

Oblique rotation results in correlated factors. Oblique rotation allows the axes in the rotated factor space to depart from a 90-degree angle, thereby allowing items to be more closely associated with factors. When oblique rotation is used, the method is usually one called *direct oblimin*. With direct oblimin rotation, users specify a value for *delta*, which is an index that affects the allowable amount of correlation between factors. The default for delta in SPSS is zero, which allows solutions with moderately correlated factors. Negative delta values result in nearly orthogonal rotations, whereas delta values near +1 allows high correlations among rotated factors.

Oblique rotations result in two matrices, a **pattern matrix** and a **structure matrix**. The pattern matrix shows partial regression coefficients between items and factors, whereas the structure matrix indicates factor-item correlations. (With orthogonal rotation, the correlations and regression coefficients are identical, so only one factor matrix is needed to display the results.) Oblique rotation also yields a **factor correlation matrix**, which shows the correlation coefficients for each factor with every other factor, like a correlation matrix. With the CES-D example, using oblimin rotation and delta = 0, the correlation between factors 1 and 2 was a modest 0.18.

Not everyone agrees on which rotation approach is preferable. People who favor orthogonal rotation claim that it leads to greater theoretical clarity. Orthogonal rotation also makes it easier to compare factor structures across studies and simplifies reporting. Advocates of oblique rotation note that, in reality, the dimensions of a construct usually *are* correlated. For example, people high on pain intensity are likely to be higher than average on pain interference as well. Oblique rotation can, however, result in peculiarities that are difficult to interpret. A useful approach might be to apply oblique rotation first and then examine the factor correlation matrix. Orthogonal rotation might be contraindicated if the factor correlations are sizeable. If, however, the correlations among factors are modest (for example, all 0.30 or less), then orthogonal rotation probably can be justified. With a strong, factorable data matrix, results at the item level are often similar regardless of which rotation method is used.

5.4.g Interpreting Factors

The rotated factor loadings from an orthogonal rotation are correlations between the items and the factors. Squared loadings, as noted earlier, indicate the amount of variance in an item that is explained by the factor (i.e., the latent trait). Thus, variables with high factor loadings should be examined to help identify the underlying dimension corresponding to the factor. By looking at the group of items with high loadings, one can conceptualize and *name* the underlying dimension.

The higher an item loads on a factor, the better it is at capturing the essence of the factor. Loadings in excess of 0.70 (indicating at least 50% overlapping variance between the item and the factor) are especially desirable for interpretive purposes. Different criteria have been proposed as minimum loadings. Tabachnick and Fidell (2013) recommend that loadings should have an absolute value of 0.32 or greater, but 0.40 is sometimes suggested as the cutoff value. Ideally, there will be at least one **marker variable** in each factor. A marker variable is one that is highly correlated with one and only one factor and hence helps to define the nature of the factor and suggests how to label it. Marker variables tend to be robust; that is, they tend to load on a factor regardless of which method was used to extract and rotate factors.

The process is similar for oblique rotation. Interpretation is based on inspection of the pattern matrix. Although the coefficients in the structure matrix represent correlations between items and factors, their values are inflated by the overlap between factors. For this reason, the pattern matrix tends to be more interpretable than the structure matrix.

To illustrate the interpretive process, let us consider the factor analysis of the nine CES-D items. Table 5.6 presents the orthogonally rotated factor matrix for a two-factor solution. In this table, the items are listed in descending order of magnitude for the factor loadings; loadings of 0.32 or greater are bolded. Even though the CES-D is a widely used scale that has been factor analyzed many times, the results in Table 5.6 are not ideal. The first seven items have loadings on Factor 1 of 0.52 or higher, suggesting a strong first factor. The highest loading (0.82) was for Item 6 (*I felt depressed*), which can be considered a marker variable. Consistent with others who have factor analyzed the CES-D, we will call this factor *Depressed Affect*.

Factor 2 has two items with loadings above 0.80—the two reverse-scored items dealing with happiness and enjoyment of life. Others have called this factor (lack of) *Positive Affect* or, more clinically, *Anhedonia*.

Difficulties arise in connection with Item 7 (*I felt everything I did was an effort*), which had relatively high loadings both on Factor 1 (.52) and Factor 2 (−0.32). Inspecting the rotated plot of the two factors in Figure 5.2, it can readily be seen that Item 7 is an outlier that is not clearly aligned with either factor, nor with the two clusters of items. Women who said that everything was an effort for them on most days in the previous week tended to have higher scores on the other six depressed affect items but also tended to say they were happy or enjoyed life, a seemingly contradictory response pattern. When an item loads highly on two factors, researchers must make a decision about what to do. One option is to drop the item. Another rule of thumb is that if the difference in loadings is at least 0.20, then the item is assigned to the factor with the higher loading. In this example, this would mean assigning Item 7 to Factor 1, which is how this item typically is scored. In fact, Item 7 has been a valued item, having been retained in several short forms of the CES-D (Cole et al., 2004; Kohout et al., 1993; Santor & Coyne, 1997).

If we were developing this scale from scratch, however, we might consider dropping or revising Item 7 because the response pattern suggests confusion or ambiguity in this

Table 5.6	Rotated Factor Matrix for Nine CES-D Items, Sample 1 of Low-Income Women (*N* = 481)[a]		
		Factor	
Items		**1**	**2**
6. I felt depressed.		**0.82**	0.19
3. I couldn't shake off blues.		**0.78**	0.17
18. I felt sad.		**0.74**	0.24
5. I had trouble keeping my mind on things.		**0.73**	0.11
1. I was more bothered by things than usual.		**0.68**	0.13
11. My sleep was restless.		**0.63**	0.20
7. I felt everything I did was an effort.		**0.52**	**−0.32**
16. I enjoyed life (reversed).		0.13	**0.86**
12. I was happy (reversed).		0.26	**0.81**

[a]Extraction method: principal components; extraction criterion: eigenvalue ≥1.0; rotation method: varimax; rotation converged in three iterations.

Table 5.7	Summary of Cross-Validated Results From Factor Analysis of Nine CES-D Items, for Two Random Half-Samples of Low-Income Women		
		Random Half-Samples	
Results		**Sample 1**	**Sample 2**
Kaiser-Meyer-Olkin Measure of Sampling Adequacy		0.873	0.875
Factor 1 eigenvalue (% of variance explained)		3.95 (43.9)	3.99 (44.3)
Factor 2 eigenvalue (% of variance explained)		1.33 (14.7)	1.32 (14.6)
Factor 3 eigenvalue (% of variance explained)		0.82 (9.1)	0.82 (9.1)
Item 6 factor loading, Factor 1 (felt depressed)		0.82	0.82
Item 6 factor loading, Factor 2		0.19	0.23
Item 7 factor loading, Factor 1 (required effort)		0.52	0.53
Item 7 factor loading, Factor 2		−0.32	−0.30
N		481	480

population of low-income women.[7] At a minimum, the results shown in Table 5.6 and Figure 5.2 suggest the desirability of further exploration, a procedure that is common in doing a factor analysis with unexpected results. For example, we might take a closer look at an oblique rotation, or we might adjust the value of delta. In this example, when we used a direct oblimin rotation with delta set at 0.75, the problem was exacerbated: The loadings for Item 7 were 0.65 on Factor 1 and −0.46 on Factor 2. We might explore what happens when a different number of factors is extracted. When three rather than two factors were rotated, Item 7 had a loading of 0.97 on the third factor and loadings of 0.20 or less on the first two factors, confirming that this item was in a realm of its own in this sample. Further inspection of this item seems warranted. When we looked more closely at frequency distributions, for example, we found that a higher percentage of women said that this item applied to them most days of the previous week (26.4%) than any other item and that, unlike other items, responses were about equally dispersed across the four response options. When we reran the PCA with varimax rotation with eight rather than nine items (i.e., removing Item 7 from the analysis), two strong factors emerged, and these two factors accounted for a higher percentage of variance (64%) than in the original analysis (59%).

Finally, we completely reran all the factor analysis with the second half-sample to see if the results for Item 7 were spurious or could be cross-validated. The results, shown in Table 5.7, confirm that the two-factor solution for the nine CES-D items was robust, and that Item 7 was problematic in both samples.

---

[7]In previous work with the CES-D in low-income populations, Polit has repeatedly found that Item 7 performed poorly. She has speculated that some of the women interpret the item as a positive attribute, perhaps reading into it something like, "I put effort into the things that I did" (Polit et al., 2001). Another team of researchers (Canady, Stommel, & Holzman, 2009) reported similar problems with Item 7 in a sample of African American and Caucasian pregnant women, and others have noted that the item may inflate estimates of depression for elderly or chronic pain populations (e.g., Obayon & Schatzberg, 2003).

This example illustrates that a fair amount of "sleuthing" may be necessary in doing a factor analysis. Because of the many decisions that must be made, a team approach to decision making seems advisable.

5.4.h Factor Scores

Researchers can use the results of a factor analysis to create **factor scores**. Most factor analysis software offers alternative methods for creating a composite score on each factor for each person in the analysis. For example, SPSS offers three methods for computing factor scores (*regression*, *Anderson-Rubin*, and *Bartlett*), each of which uses different calculations. However, all three methods involve assigning weights to items, multiplying the weight times the original value on each item in the factor analysis for the particular participant, and then summing to arrive at a composite score. Factor scores for all methods are standardized to have means of zero and standard deviations of 1.0. When PCA is used to extract factors, all three methods yield the same factor scores. The regression approach to calculating factor scores is the most widely used method.

In a more typical scenario for CTT measures, researchers use factor analysis to select items for subscales, summing together item scores for those items with high loadings on the factor. This method results in scales and subscales that can be replicated with other samples. In our example, each person could have two subscale scores for the CES-D, a Depressed Affect score (Items 1, 3, 5, 6, 7, 11, and 18) and a Positive Affect score (Items 12 and 16). However, even though a two-factor solution to CES-D items has been found by many researchers, total CES-D scores are usually computed by adding together all item scores, an issue we discuss further in Chapter 14.

5.5   Conclusions

The CTT techniques described in this chapter remain the most widely used analytic tools for creating verbal report scales (i.e., patient-reported outcomes [PRO]), although it is likely that future researchers will use IRT techniques with greater frequency (see Chapter 6). Productive ways to combine CTT and IRT methods may well be pursued by future scale developers, as noted by DeVellis (2012).

Researchers who adopt the item analysis and EFA methods summarized here to create a CTT measure are most likely to turn next to an analysis of internal consistency before finalizing their scales. Evaluation of internal consistency is described in Chapter 9. It is also likely to be useful to pursue item-level test–retest reliability analyses before finalizing a scale, as discussed in Chapter 8.

The analytic methods associated with CTT are appropriate exclusively for reflective scales. Formative scales are composed of items that are not necessarily highly intercorrelated, and so the items are not typically factorable using EFA.[8] An item analysis and EFA can be productively used with measures other than PROs, however, as long as the scales are reflective. For example, EFA has been used to identify dimensionality (subscales) for observation-based measures and performance tests. As an illustration, Escalante, Haas, and DelRincon (2004) did an EFA (principal components) with several performance-based rheumatology function tests and learned that they all loaded on a single factor that explained more than 70% of the variance in the individual tests, leading them to recommend a global physical function scale with rescaled values.

---

[8]Structural equation modeling (and hence confirmatory factor analysis) does, however, allow models to be fitted with formative indicators (see Brown, 2006).

References

Andresen, E. M., Malmgren, J., Carter, W., & Patrick, D. (1994). Screening for depression in well older adults: Evaluation of a short form of the CES-D. *American Journal of Preventive Medicine, 10,* 77–84.

Brown, T. A. (2006). *Confirmatory factor analysis for applied research.* New York, NY: The Guilford Press.

Canady, R. B., Stommel, M., & Holzman, C. (2009). Measurement properties of the Centers for Epidemiological Studies Depression Scale (CES-D) in a sample of African American and non-Hispanic white pregnant women. *Journal of Nursing Measurement, 17,* 91–104.

Cole, J. C., Rabin, A. S., Smith, T. L., & Kaufman, A. S. (2004). Development and validation of a Rasch-derived CES-D short form. *Psychological Assessment, 16,* 360–372.

Costello, A., & Osborne, J. (2005). Best practices in exploratory factor analysis: Four recommendations for getting the most from your analysis. *Practical Assessment, Research & Evaluation, 10*(7), 1–9.

Cubo, E., Velasco, S., Benito, V., Villaverde, V., Galín, J., Santidrian, A., . . . Leon, J. (2010). Psychometric attributes of the DISC predictive scales. *Clinical Practice & Epidemiology in Mental Health, 6,* 86–93.

DeVellis, R. F. (2012). *Scale development: Theory and application* (3rd ed.). Thousand Oaks, CA: Sage.

DeVet, H. C. W., Terwee, C., Mokkink, L. B., & Knol, D. L. (2011). *Measurement in medicine: A practical guide.* Cambridge, MA: Cambridge University Press.

Escalante, A., Haas, R., & DelRincon, I. (2004). Measurement of global functional performance in patients with rheumatoid arthritis using rheumatology function tests. *Arthritis Research & Therapy, 6,* 315–325.

Holmes, W., Bix, B., & Shea, J. (1996). SF-20 and item distributions in a human immunodeficiency virus-seropositive sample. *Medical Care, 34,* 562–569.

Kohout, F. J., Berkman, L. F., & Evans, D. A. (1993). Two shorter forms of the CES-D depression symptoms index. *Journal of Aging and Health, 5,* 179–193.

Mahoney, F., & Barthel, D. W. (1965). Functional evaluation: The Barthel Index. *Maryland State Medical Journal, 14,* 61–65.

Nunnally, J., & Bernstein, I. H. (1994). *Psychometric theory* (3rd ed.). New York, NY: McGraw-Hill.

Obayon, M. M., & Schatzberg, A. F. (2003). Using chronic pain to predict depressive morbidity in the general population. *Archives of General Psychiatry, 60,* 39–47.

Osborne, J., & Costello, A. (2004). Sample size and subject-to-item ratio in principal components analysis. *Practical Assessment, Research & Evaluation, 9*(11), 8.

Pett, M., Lackey, N., & Sullivan, J. (2003). *Making sense of factor analysis: The use of factor analysis for instrument development in health care research.* Thousand Oaks, CA: Sage.

Polit, D. F., London, A., & Martinez, J. (2001). *The health of poor urban women: Findings from the Project on Devolution and Urban Change.* New York, NY: Manpower Demonstration Research.

Radloff, L. S. (1977). The CES-D scale: A self -report depression scale for research in the general population. *Applied Psychological Measurement, 1,* 385–401.

Santor, D. A., & Coyne, J. C. (1997). Shortening the CES-D to improve its ability to detect cases of depression. *Psychological Assessment, 9,* 233–243.

Skirko, J. R., Weaver, E., Perkins, J., Kinter, S., & Sie, K. (2012). Modification and evaluation of a velopharyngeal insufficiency quality-of-life instrument. *Archives of Otolaryngology—Head & Neck Surgery, 138,* 929–935.

Streiner, D. L., & Norman, G. R. (2008). *Health measurement scales: A practical guide to their development and use* (4th ed.). Oxford: Oxford University Press.

Tabachnick, B., & Fidell, L. (2013). *Using multivariate statistics* (6th ed.). Boston, MA: Pearson Education.

Terwee, C., Bot, S., de Boer, M., van der Windt, D., Knol, D., Dekker, J., . . . de Vet, H. C. (2007). Quality criteria were proposed for measurement properties of health status questionnaires. *Journal of Clinical Epidemiology, 60,* 34–42.

Tsakos, G., Blair, Y., Yusuf, H., Wright, W., Watt, R., & MacPherson, L. (2012). Developing a new self-reported scale of oral health outcomes for 5-year-old children (SOHO-5). *Health and Quality of Life Outcomes, 10,* 62.

Van Dam, N. T., & Earlywine, M. (2011). Validation of the Center for Epidemiologic Studies Depression Scale-Revised (CESD-R): Pragmatic depression assessment in the general population. *Psychiatry Research, 186,* 128–132.

Yang, F., Heslin, K., Mehta, K., Yang, C. W., Ocepek-Welikson, K., Kleinman, M., . . . Teresi, J. A. (2011). A comparison of item response theory-based methods for examining differential item functioning in object naming test by language of assessment among older Latinos. *Psychological Test and Assessment Modeling, 53,* 440–460.

6

Scale Development: Item Response Theory

Chapter Outline

Item response theory (IRT) gained attention in the 1970s in standardized educational testing (Lord & Novick, 1969) and has been a major force in psychometrics since the 1980s. IRT has become increasingly attractive as a foundation for developing multi-item health scales because the theory solves many of the measurement challenges found in scale construction under classical test theory (CTT). One example of a measurement challenge is separating the properties of the questions used in a scale from the underlying construct that the scale is intended to measure. In CTT, measurement of the underlying construct is dependent on the questions chosen for the scale, whereas in IRT, the underlying construct is based on the estimation of a model. Under IRT, the properties of both the underlying construct and the test questions are *invariant*. The estimation of the construct will be the same even with different sets of items, and the characteristics of the items are (in theory) independent of the people who respond to them.

In this chapter, we provide a brief overview of IRT, with the goal of introducing readers to basic IRT models, features, methods, and procedures for choosing items for a scale. We illustrate the evaluation of items for a scale using IRT approaches with an analysis of selected items from the Center for Epidemiologic Studies Depression Scale (CES-D) (Radloff, 1977), using data collected from 1,000 low-income women—the same data set used in the previous chapter (Polit, London, & Martinez, 2001). We briefly discuss the future of IRT in scale construction in the health field using the National Institutes of Health (NIH) Patient Reported Outcomes Measurement Information System (PROMIS®) Roadmap Initiative (http://www.nihpromis.org) as an example. Finally, major differences between CTT and IRT are reviewed, including their advantages and disadvantages.

Because the complexity of IRT makes it impossible for us to provide extensive detail, interested readers are urged to consult other sources for more in-depth coverage. Good resources that offer fairly nontechnical overviews of IRT are DeMars (2010) and Embretson and Reise (2000). Other good sources of information on IRT are the books by Hambleton, Swaminathan, and Rogers (1991) and de Ayala (2009). Bond and Fox (2007) and Andrich (1988) provide accessible descriptions of the Rasch family of models.

6.1   The Basics of Item Response Theory

IRT does not refer to a single specific technique but rather to a measurement framework that encompasses multiple models for analyzing item-level data. In essence, IRT analyses involve modeling the probability of people's response to an item as a function of the underlying trait and one or more **item parameters**. In IRT models, every respondent is assumed to have a true location on a continuous latent trait dimension, and the person's location on the continuum is assumed to underlie how he or she responds to an item.

Many terms have been used interchangeably in the IRT literature to refer to the underlying construct of interest. These include *trait* (Zhang & Walker, 2008), *latent trait* (Fraley, Waller, & Brennan 2000; Lord, 1953), *ability* (E. Cole, Wood, & Dunn, 1991), *latent ability* (Lord, 1980; Samejima, 1969), and *theta* (McDonald, 2010; Whittaker, Fitzpatrick, Williams, & Dodd 2003). Several of these terms (e.g., ability) derive from the early popularization of IRT in the field of education. In the context of health measurement, the construct being measured is most often referred to as the "latent trait."[1]

In IRT models, the amount of the latent trait is expressed on a continuum that is much like a standard score, with a mean of zero and an *SD* of 1. The standardized metric or "ruler" can be used to locate both people, in terms of the amount of the trait they possess, and items, in terms of how "difficult" it is to endorse them. Thus, model-based estimation is used to separate the measurement properties of the person's responses to items on the one hand and the person's underlying level of the trait being measured on the other.

---

[1] An exception in the health field is in the measurement of a patient's cognitive status or cognitive ability (Yang et al., 2012).

IRT methods are most often used to create scales based on self-reports (i.e., patient-reported outcomes [PROs]), but multi-item observational scales (e.g., for assessing patient confusion) can also be developed or refined with IRT methods. Because the person's latent trait is conceptualized as being the "cause" of item responses, IRT scales are always reflective (Chapter 2). In using IRT to construct a scale, an objective is to identify a small set of items (typically fewer than are needed with scales created using CTT methods) that span the range of the latent trait or that span the range that is of greatest interest in terms of the scale's measurement precision and its ability to discriminate among people.

6.1.a Assumptions in Item Response Theory

Several important assumptions underlie the use of IRT. Unlike CTT, which has "soft" assumptions that are often ignored, it is critical to evaluate the extent to which IRT's "hard" assumptions have been met. Four assumptions for parametric IRT models are described here.

■ *Unidimensionality.* A core assumption in IRT is that the latent trait being measured is **unidimensional** (i.e., a single trait or a single facet of a complex trait). In a unidimensional scale, the trait is assumed to account for all of the item intercorrelations. Unidimensionality in a set of items is never perfect, and so one issue is whether any departure from unidimensionality is substantial enough to justify the construction of separate subscales to represent important distinctions with the set of items. The most common method used to evaluate the dimensionality of a set of items is factor analysis. Both exploratory factor analysis (EFA; Chapter 5) and confirmatory factor analysis (CFA; Chapter 14) have been used to evaluate dimensionality in IRT analyses.[2] If a single dimension or factor is found in the data, then the assumption of unidimensionality is met.

■ *Local independence.* A related assumption is **local independence**, which assumes that the trait itself is the sole influence on a person's response to an item other than random error. The assumption of local independence implies that a person's responses to items are not statistically related to each other, after controlling for the latent trait. There are two basic components in local independence. The first component is that only one latent trait is specified (i.e., unidimensionality), and the second is that the response to one question is not contingent upon a response to another question. Local dependence can potentially be jeopardized in some situations—for example, when there is extreme redundancy of item content. Inter-item correlations greater than about .80 should generally be avoided. Changing polarity of items can also result in responses that are dependent on respondents' cognitive ability, as has been found with the four positively worded items on the CES-D for certain populations (Carlson et al., 2011). Local independence can be evaluated by various means, including inspection of the residual matrix in a CFA; excessive covariation among the residuals can be indicative of local dependence. However, outside of educational testing, local dependence is not commonly encountered (Streiner, 2010).

■ *Monotonicity.* In IRT, the probability of endorsing an item is directly related to the person's trait level. **Monotonicity** means that the probability of responding to a given item should increase monotonically with increased levels of the trait.

■ *Invariance.* Another IRT assumption and goal concerns sample, item, and latent trait **invariance**. Under this assumption, the estimation of the item parameters and the latent trait is presumed to be independent of the particular sample used and the particular items in the analysis. For example, if invariance holds, the item parameters for the CES-D question, "I was bothered by things that don't usually bother me," would be similar for different samples of people completing the CES-D, if the items were calibrated with a large sample from a heterogeneous population.

---

[2]Although CTT has no formal assumption regarding the unidimensionality of true scores, the interpretation of scores from scales constructed using CTT methods also requires that a single construct is influencing responses to scale items.

In the case of the CES-D items administered to a sample of low-income women, we already learned in the exploratory factor analysis in Chapter 5 that 12 CES-D items did not form a unidimensional scale. We will find further evidence in Chapter 14 (in a confirmatory factor analysis) that an assumption of unidimensionality is not tenable. Thus, the IRT analyses we use here for illustrative purposes focuses on the seven CES-D items that we used to construct a short "Depressed Affect" subscale.

6.1.b Overview of Item Response Theory Models

IRT models provide a mathematical equation to characterize the relationship between the probability of a person's response to an item and the amount of his or her latent trait. Many IRT models have been developed, only a few of which will be discussed in this chapter. Most models are parametric, but there are nonparametric variants (e.g., *Mokken models*). Nonparametric models may be attractive in some situations because they relax some of the strong assumptions associated with parametric IRT models. Information about such models may be found in Mokken (2010) and Molenaar (2010).

One important way in which IRT models vary concerns how many item parameters are estimated, which is a focus of the next section (6.2) of this chapter. In brief, IRT includes models for one-, two-, three-, and four-item parameters. The one-parameter IRT model (1-PL) is similar to another model, the Rasch model. Differences and similarities between the 1-PL model and the Rasch model will be described in a subsequent section. Three-parameter (3-PL) and four-parameter (4-PL) models are used infrequently in health research, and this chapter focuses primarily on one- and two-parameter IRT models.

Another key way in which IRT models vary concerns whether the items in the analysis are **dichotomous** (binary) or **polytomous** (i.e., three or more response options). The simplest and most basic IRT models are for binary data, in which there are only two response options. In performance or ability tests, the dichotomy is between *correct* and *incorrect* answers (even when the test has multiple choice questions). In health scales, the more typical dichotomies are for responses of *yes* versus *no*, or *true* versus *false*. As an example, a version of the CES-D used in the Health and Retirement Study (Juster & Suzman, 1995) used dichotomous items. On this nine-item scale, people were asked to state whether or not they experienced various feelings much of the time in the previous week. As an example, one item was, "Much of the time during the week, I felt depressed. Would you say yes or no?"

Polytomous IRT models are used with items that have three or more ordered response categories, reflecting intensity or frequency of a symptom, feeling, or condition. Most health scales rely on polytomous items, as in the case of the CES-D. As discussed in Chapter 5, the four CES-D response categories include rarely or none of the time (<1 day), some or a little of the time (1 to 2 days), occasionally or a moderate amount of the time (3 to 4 days), and most or all of the time (5 to 7 days), with these rank-ordered options scored 0, 1, 2, or 3, respectively.

Table 6.1 presents the names of several IRT models that are frequently found in the health literature. The model names are shown for one- and two-parameter models and for items with dichotomous and polytomous response options. Features of the various polytomous IRT models are discussed elsewhere (e.g., Nering & Ostini, 2011; van der Linden & Hambleton, 2010) and will not be described here. In this chapter, our example with the CES-D data will be based on the **graded response model**, which is most often used to estimate IRT models for Likert-type scales (Samejima, 2010).

6.1.c Item Characteristic Curves

A basic feature of an IRT analysis is the **item characteristic curve** (ICC), described briefly in Chapter 2. An ICC is most commonly defined as a logistic (S-shaped) function that models the relationship between people's responses to an item and their level of the latent trait. Figure 6.1 presents an example of an ICC for a single dichotomous item. In this figure, the

Table 6.1	Frequently Used Parametric IRT Models			
	Parameter Name		**Dichotomous Response Options (e.g., Yes/No)**	**Polytomous Response Options (e.g., Likert type)**
Number of Parameters	**Difficulty/ Location**	**Discrimination**		
1	X		Rasch model 1-PL model	Rating scale model Partial credit model Many-faceted model
2	X	X	2-PL model	Graded response model (GRM) Generalized partial credit model

X axis represents the latent trait continuum, labeled theta (θ). The Y axis, sometimes shown as $P(\theta)$, represents the probability of endorsing the item, ranging from 0.0 to 1.0. ICCs are sometimes referred to as *item response functions*, or IRFs.

As an example, let us assume that the latent trait for Figure 6.1 is depression, with negative values corresponding to lower levels of depression and higher positive values corresponding to increasingly more severe levels of depression. Suppose the item is "I am unhappy some of the time," to which people answer *yes* or *no*. For this particular hypothetical item, the probability of endorsing the item is 0.5 for those whose value on the latent depression trait is exactly at the mean of 0.0. For those who are more depressed, the probability of endorsing the item increases. For example, the probability increases to about 0.75 for those

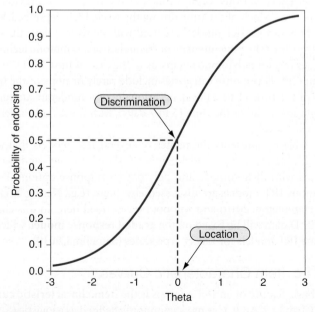

Figure 6.1

Item characteristic curve for a dichotomous item.

with a latent trait value of 1.0. As we shall see in the next section, different parts of an ICC reveal information about the item's parameters. These visual representations of item properties are one of the many attractive features of IRT and provide useful information for selecting items that cover the desired range of the trait.

Theoretically, the continuum for theta ranges from $-\infty$ to $+\infty$. But we know that, for normally distributed traits, 99.9% of values fall between -4 and $+4$ in standard deviation (*SD*) units from the mean. Most ICCs are shown with values on the X axis that range from ± 3 or ± 4 *SD*s from the mean of 0. For traits with a highly skewed distribution, the range may be asymmetric. For example, the theta scale for symptom items to measure *Diagnostic and Statistical Manual of Mental Disorders* 4th edition (*DSM-IV*) conduct disorders ranged from -1.0 to $+5.5$ (Gelhorn et al., 2009).

6.2 Item Parameters in Item Response Theory

Item characteristic curves can differ from one another along four dimensions: their location along the trait continuum theta, the steepness of their slopes, and where they flatten out at the bottom or at the top. These four dimensions correspond to four potential item parameters; only the first two will be discussed at any length in this chapter.

6.2.a Item Difficulty: The Location Parameter

The term **item difficulty** is used in educational testing to describe how difficult an item is along the latent ability trait to achieve a 0.5 probability of a correct response. In testing situations, the more difficult the item, the higher the students' ability must be to have a 50% probability of answering the question correctly. The difficulty of an item indicates where along the trait continuum the item functions best. All IRT models estimate the difficulty parameter of items.

In health fields, the term **item location** is often used in lieu of "difficulty"; *item severity* is sometimes used in the psychiatric literature. However, one can also conceptualize an item for health constructs as being more "difficult" to agree with or endorse among people who do not have high levels of the trait. For example, it is more difficult for people who are slightly depressed to agree to an item such as "Sometimes I think about committing suicide" than to agree to the item "I am unhappy some of the time." In Figure 6.1, using our previous example, the location of the ICC for the dichotomous "unhappy" item centers at the mean theta level of 0. The ICC for the "suicide" item would be located far to the right on the theta continuum. By determining an item's difficulty level (location), researchers can establish how much of the trait is required for a person to have a specified probability of endorsing the item.

In modeling item responses, the item location parameter is noted by b for item i (b_i). In Figure 6.1, $b = 0.0$. With polytomous items, there are multiple location parameters because each rank-ordered response has a different location on the theta continuum. We illustrate this with two CES-D items later in this chapter.

6.2.b Item Discrimination: The Slope Parameter

The **item discrimination** parameter provides information about the degree to which an item can unambiguously differentiate between those whose trait level is below the item location and those whose trait level is above—that is, how well an item can identify patients with different levels of the latent trait. The item discrimination parameter is also called the *slope parameter*, with steeper slopes at a particular theta level offering better discrimination than less steep slopes, as depicted on the item's ICC. With steep slopes, large changes in the probability of endorsing the item can be observed for small changes in the trait level. Flatter

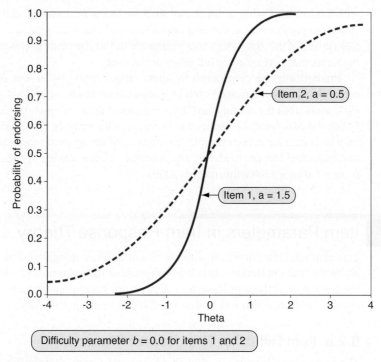

Figure 6.2

Item characteristic curves for two dichotomous items varying in item discrimination.

ICCs are less discriminating across a broad range of the latent trait: The probability of an endorsement at low theta levels is nearly the same as it is at higher levels. In Figure 6.1, the steep slope of the ICC directly above the theta level of 0.0 (at the 0.5 probability point) indicates good discrimination at that level. The discrimination parameter in IRT is similar to an item-total correlation in CTT.

Estimates of the item discrimination parameters are noted by the letter a for each item i (a_i). The range of possible values for a_i are from $-\infty$ to $+\infty$, but negative values are rare and signal a potential problem because they suggest that people with increasing levels of the latent trait are less likely to endorse more severe response options. Under a logistic model, the discrimination parameter typically ranges from 0.5 to 2.0. Higher values for a are associated with items that are better able to discriminate between adjacent trait levels near the inflection point; therefore, high values are generally preferred. All items in an IRT analysis, whether they are dichotomous or polytomous, have a discrimination parameter a, but in some models, a is not estimated (i.e., it is assumed to be a constant).

Figure 6.2 shows ICCs for two dichotomous items that have identical location parameters ($b = 0.0$ for both) but that differ in slope. Item 1 is a better (more discriminating) item, with a steeper slope and $a = 1.5$. The flatter ICC of Item 2 ($a = 0.5$) reflects an item with greater ambiguity. In other words, Item 1 discriminates more effectively than Item 2 between those who endorse or do not endorse the item. This illustrates how the ICCs of items can help scale developers to better understand the strengths and weaknesses of individual items.

6.2.c The Guessing and Carelessness Parameters

In educational tests, students with low ability may guess the correct answer on a multiple-choice question. Such guessing can be modeled with a guessing or *pseudo-chance-level parameter*, designated as c_i for item i. This parameter is determined by the point at which the ICC intersects the Y axis (the lower asymptote). The value of c_i is the probability of getting the item correct by guessing. If a person with the very lowest level of ability still has (say) a 0.20 probability of answering a test question correctly, this is likely accounted for by guessing.

In health fields, c is rarely estimated because items do not typically have right or wrong answers, although there has been some discussion in the psychopathology and personality literature about whether the lower asymptote parameter might reflect a social desirability bias (Reise & Waller, 2003). A more in-depth discussion of the c parameter can be found in Lord (1974).

Another rarely used item parameter in health fields is called the *carelessness parameter* (d_i). IRT models with four-item parameters (4-PL) incorporate an upper asymptote parameter for item-specific carelessness, which can occur on a test when a person with the very highest level of ability gets a question wrong due to negligence. It can also occur on a scale when even those with the highest possible level of the trait resist endorsing an extreme item, such as (for example) an item about suicide ideation on a scale of depression.

In Figure 6.2, we can see that the lower asymptote for both ICCs is at 0.0, and the upper asymptote is at 1.0. Thus, the guessing and carelessness parameters would not be relevant.

6.2.d Scaling Factor: D Constant

In IRT models (but not in Rasch models), there is often a *scaling factor, D*, which is a constant with the value 1.7. This scaling factor makes the ICC for a logistic function equal to that of a normal distribution (normal ogive) function. The logistic function was introduced by Birnbaum (1968) to easily calculate the item parameters and the probability of theta without using more complicated mathematical integration in the normal ogive function (Lord, 1952). Certain software, such as the Mplus program (Muthén & Muthén, 2014) uses this scaling factor.

6.3 | Item Response Theory and Rasch Models

The item parameters described in the previous section are the basic elements of IRT models. In this section we describe three unidimensional IRT models: the one-parameter logistic model, the Rasch model, and the two-parameter logistic model.

6.3.a The One-Parameter Logistic Model

The **one-parameter logistic (1-PL) model** is an IRT model that includes only the item location (b_i) parameter. In a 1-PL model, it is assumed that only the item's location parameter and the underlying latent trait influence a person's response to a question. In a 1-PL model, the slopes of the ICCs—the items' discrimination—are assumed to be the same. That is, it is assumed that the ICCs are parallel and do not cross each other. Figure 6.3 presents two ICCs that have the same discrimination but different locations on the trait continuum—an ideal situation for a 1-PL model.

Two features of the 1-PL model are depicted in the ICCs. One feature is that the probability of endorsing a more severe response for each item increases monotonically with increasing theta. The second feature is that the ICC changes from an accelerating function to a decelerating function curve when the probability of endorsing the response option to an item is at 0.5, which is sometimes called the *threshold level* of the b_i parameter.

6.3.b The Rasch Model

In the literature on IRT, it is not uncommon to see Rasch and 1-PL models discussed as though they were synonymous. The **Rasch model** is similar to the 1-PL IRT model in many

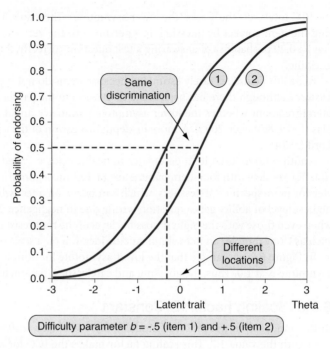

Figure 6.3

Item characteristic curves for two dichotomous items varying in item location.

respects, the most noteworthy being that both models assume that all items being evaluated have the same discrimination. In other words, in both 1-PL and Rasch models, the only item parameter that is estimated is item difficulty/location. Other parameters such as discrimination and guessing are constrained and set to a constant. Both Rasch and 1-PL models, which are mathematically similar, can estimate the location parameter for binary and polytomous items, as shown in Table 6.1. Popular one-parameter models for polytomous items include the *rating scale, partial credit,* and *many-faceted models.*

Although the Rasch and 1-PL models are similar, there are some conceptual differences. In Table 6.2, we summarize some of the more noteworthy distinctions. One major difference concerns the goal of the analysis. In IRT modeling, the objective is to identify a model that best fits a set of data and adequately describes item response patterns. In Rasch analysis, the model itself is paramount, and the intent is to find a set of items that fit a Rasch model. IRT models predominate in the United States, whereas researchers in other parts of the world often prefer Rasch analysis.

6.3.c Two-Parameter Logistic Model

The **two-parameter logistic (2-PL) model** includes both the discrimination (a_i) and location (b_i) parameters. Because discrimination parameters are estimated in the 2-PL model, discrimination for different items can be different from each other and different in their relationship to the latent trait. The ICCs in the 2-PL model can cross each other because each discrimination parameter is freely estimated.

To illustrate an item response function, we offer the following equation for a 2-PL model for dichotomous item *i*:

$$P(X_i = 1)|\theta = \frac{\exp(1.7a_i(\theta - b_i))}{1 + \exp(1.7a_i(\theta - b_i))} \tag{6.1}$$

Table 6.2	Comparison of 1-PL Model and Rasch Model	
Issue/Aspect	**1-PL IRT Model**	**Rasch Model**
Goal	To seek a model to fit the data and explain item response patterns; model is *descriptive* of the data	To develop a measurement system based on Rasch measurement principles; the model is paramount and *prescriptive*
Fit evaluation	Global fit of the model to the data, model accepted or rejected	Local fit of the data to the Rasch model, one parameter (item) at a time
Data–model mismatch	Data misfit leads to consideration of adding parameters, notably discrimination	Items violating model are scrutinized for possible deletion from the model
Parameterization	The person sample is parameterized by a mean and *SD* for item estimation; local origin of the scale is the average person ability: norm referenced	Each individual in the person sample is parameterized for item estimation; local origin of the scale is the average item difficulty (or difficulty of a specified item): criterion referenced
Item discrimination	Item characteristic curves are modeled to be parallel, with a slope of 1.7 (the scaling factor), approximating slope of cumulative normal ogive	Item characteristic curves are modeled to be parallel with a slope of 1.0, the natural logistic ogive

SD, standard deviation.
Note: Entries in this table are based on Andrich (1988), Doucette and Wolf (2009), and Streiner and Norman (2008).

where P is the probability of a response X being an endorsement of (or correct response to) item i, conditional on the latent trait (θ); exp is the exponential function, 1.7 is the scaling factor D, a_i is the discrimination parameter for item i, and b_i is the location parameter for item i. In estimating a person's latent trait using the 2-PL model, items are assigned different weights in accordance with the values of the discrimination parameters. The higher the value of a_i, the more weight is assigned to the item in estimates of the latent trait. Note that if a_i is set to 1 (or another constant) in equation 6.1, the result is the model for a 1-PL.

The equation for a 2-PL model (6.1) is for dichotomous items with one ICC for each item, but the same principles for interpreting the item parameters can be extended to polytomous IRT models. As shown in Table 6.1, two popular 2-PL models for polytomous ordinal items include the *generalized partial credit model* (a generalization of the Rasch model) and the *graded response model* (GRM), which we will use to illustrate an IRT analysis of CES-D items.[3] The GRM (Samejima, 2010) is an extension of the 2-PL model that includes at least two location (b_{ij}) parameters. Within the GRM, a polytomous item is treated as a

---

[3]A model called the *nominal model* can be used to analyze polytomous items that are categorical (nominal) rather than ordinal. This model is used infrequently in health applications.

series of dichotomies, equal to the number of response options, minus one. The GRM estimates the probability of a patient's response (x) at or above a given category threshold (j) on the latent trait level, given one discrimination parameter (a_i), and the corresponding number of location thresholds (b_{ij}). With polytomous items, **category response curves** (CRCs) represent the probability of a person's response in each category, given his or her latent trait. We illustrate CRCs for two CES-D items in section 6.4.c.

6.4   Evaluation of Rasch and Item Response Theory Models

In this section, we briefly review methods of evaluating Rasch and IRT models and items for a scale and also discuss the issue of scoring. We begin with Rasch models but focus mainly on IRT and an illustration using items from the CES-D.

6.4.a Evaluation of Rasch Models

As noted in Table 6.2, Rasch analyses are more focused than IRT analyses on the local fit of each item to the model, and so item fit statistics are provided in Rasch software. *Mean square fit* is an index of item fit and is calculated by averaging the squared residual for each person–item combination—that is, averaging across every person in the sample for a given item. Mean square fit is evaluated for two types of fit. The **infit statistic** is sensitive to response patterns across items; it measures unexpected responses to items with a difficulty level near a person's trait level. The **outfit statistic** is an indicator of respondent outliers—that is, it captures unexpected responses to items that are at the extremes of the trait continuum. Items that are very low or high on the fit statistics are either redundant (*overfit*) or are likely not measuring the construct of interest (*misfit*). Infit and outfit estimates, for items with a good fit, are expected to range between 0.7 and 0.14 (Bond & Fox, 2007). Thus, items with high or low infit and outfit statistics are candidates for deletion. When the misfitting items are omitted, the Rasch analysis needs to be rerun.

Another evaluation step in a Rasch analysis concerns whether the items with a good model fit cover the trait range sufficiently. Rasch software can be used to create a **person–item map**, which shows the distribution of people along the latent trait (often on the left side of a vertical "ruler" for the trait) and the distribution of items (on the right side of the same trait ruler).[4] Figure 6.4 shows an example of such a person–item map from a study that used a Rasch analysis of a 39-item measure of visual performance, the Self-Report Assessment of Functional Vision Performance, or SRAFVP (Velozo et al., 2013). This map shows that the people in the sample spanned a wide range of visual performance ability, ranging from about −3 (in logits) on the trait continuum to nearly +4.0. In this example, each "X" on the left represents a sample member, but with large samples, each "X" might correspond to some multiple (e.g., 5 or 10 people). On the right side, the items are shown at their difficulty location. The most difficult item is the person's *ability to read a telephone directory* (difficulty = 3.55). The least difficult items are *avoiding collisions* and *tripping* (difficulty = −2.82). The map shows that the items cover a broad range of difficulties and that item gaps are not large. The biggest gap is near the trait mean of 0.0. It might be useful to add an item whose difficulty lies between *ability to use an oven to prepare a meal* (difficulty = −0.35) and *ability to address an envelope* (difficulty = +0.35), especially if the desire is to discriminate in the middle range of the trait.

6.4.b Evaluation of Item Response Theory Model Fit

IRT is based on model estimation, so the fit of the model to the data is an important evaluation criterion. This section introduces basic fit statistics used to evaluate IRT models, without the mathematical formulations.

---

[4]Some software uses a horizontal format for the person–item map. In such cases, the items are typically depicted below the horizontal trait continuum and people are represented above it.

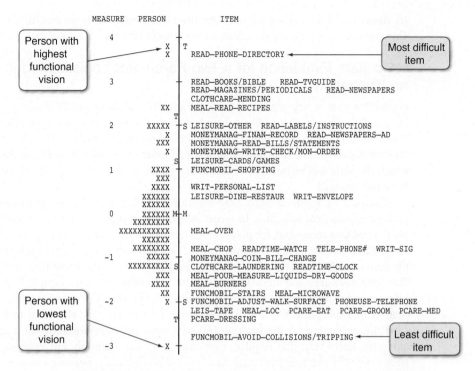

Adapted from Velozo et al. (2013), Fig 4. Each "X" represents a respondent. On the "ruler", M is the mean, S is 1 SD from the mean, and T is two SDs. (See reference for full explanation of each item.)

Figure 6.4

Person–item map on the same trait (logit) scale for the Self-Report Assessment of Functional Vision Performance (SRAFVP).

Many statistics can be used to evaluate the overall fit of IRT models, varying with regard to the items' level of measurement and the software used. Some fit statistics are sensitive to sample size, notably the chi-square (χ^2) goodness of fit statistic (described in greater detail in Chapter 14). Two common fit statistics in IRT analyses are the **root mean square error of approximation** (**RMSEA**) (Browne & Cudeck, 1993) and the **comparative fit index** (**CFI**) (Bentler, 1990). RMSEA provides a measure of discrepancy while considering the degrees of freedom (*df*) in the model. The closer the RMSEA value is to zero, the better the fit of the model to the data. The cutoff values recommended by Browne and Cudek (1993) for the RMSEA is less than or equal to 0.1 for an adequate fit of the model to the data, but Hu and Bentler (1998) suggest a more stringent cutoff value of less than or equal to 0.06. The CFI ranges between zero and one; values of greater than or equal to 0.95 generally indicate adequate fit (Bentler, 1990). Various factors can contribute to poor fit statistics for IRT models, including the violation of assumptions, speededness (when tests are timed), and rates of missingness.

As noted earlier, we used the seven CES-D items that we identified as forming a short "Depressed Affect" subscale (Chapter 5) to illustrate an IRT analysis. The fit statistics for the 1-PL and 2-PL GRM for the seven items are as follows:

■ 1-PL: $\chi^2 = 527(df = 20)\ p < .001$, RMSEA $= 0.16$, CFI $= 0.911$
■ 2-PL: $\chi^2 = 22(df = 14)\ p = .07$, RMSEA $= 0.03$, CFI $= 0.999$

The 1-PL model has a poorer fit to the data; the value of RMSEA for the 1-PL is unacceptably high, and the CFI for the 2-PL is better. (Also, for the chi-square test, nonsignificant values are desired, and the chi square value for the 1-PL model was large and highly significant). Thus, we use the 2-PL model to illustrate IRT output for the CES-D items.

6.4.c Item Evaluation for a Two-Parameter Logistic Model: An Illustration

Even when a set of items is found to have a good overall fit to an IRT model, scale developers use the output from an IRT analysis to evaluate individual items. Typically, the analysis begins with a larger set of items than are needed to reliably measure the latent trait, and so the best items must be selected. What is "best," however, usually depends on the purpose to which the scale will be put. (Of course, when items are deleted or revised, the model needs to be reevaluated).

When a 2-PL model is used, both location and discrimination parameters play an important role in item selection. In terms of location, it is desirable to have items that span the desired trait range and, for polytomous items, to have response options that have a good range across the trait. When examining the ICCs and CRCs, the steeper the slope, the better the item is at discriminating between high and low levels of the latent trait. Items with high discrimination are likely to be very useful for screening tests, for example, in primary care offices when clinicians would like to figure out quickly whether a patient would benefit from referral to a specialist. Yet, low discrimination parameters may also need to be examined carefully, particularly if the location (b_i) parameter offers information for a severity level along the latent trait that requires immediate medical attention. For example, in depression, a suicidal ideation item may have poor discrimination because few people admit to or experience suicidal ideation. Nevertheless, when such an item is found to be endorsed at higher levels of the latent depression trait, it might serve an important diagnostic function.

Item parameter information for the seven CES-D items we used to illustrate an IRT analysis is presented in Table 6.3. This table shows that the discrimination (a) parameter ranges from a low of 0.73 for Item 7 ("I felt everything I did was an effort") to a high of 3.67 for Item 6 ("I felt depressed"). These results are consistent with what we observed using the same data set for the analyses in Chapter 5, which suggested that Item 6 was a "marker" variable in the exploratory factor analysis, and Item 7 had questionable utility.[5] For example, of the 12 items in the factor analysis, Item 6 had the highest factor loading on the Depressed Affect subscale (0.82). Item 7 had the lowest loading (0.52) and also loaded moderately highly on a second factor.

In IRT, an important concept concerns how much *information* an item provides. An item response function can be transformed into an **item information function (IIF)**. Item information is maximized near the item's location, and the amount of information is a direct function of item discrimination. Because item information is closely associated with measurement error in IRT, we postpone a fuller discussion of this topic until Chapter 10, where we illustrate the IIFs of CES-D Items 6 and 7. Suffice it to say here that item information is another important tool for evaluating and selecting items for a scale.

In terms of the location parameters in Table 6.3, we explained earlier that there are as many location parameters (often called *category threshold parameters*) as there are response options, minus 1. Thus, with the four-category response options for CES-D items, there are three category threshold parameters. For example, for the item "I felt depressed," b_1 would correspond to the probability of moving from a response of "none of the time" to "some of the time," b_2 would correspond to the probability of moving from "some of the time" to "a moderate amount of the time," and b_3 would correspond to the probability of moving from "a moderate amount of the time" to "most of the time." Specifically, the category threshold parameters represent the point along the latent trait continuum at which the respondent

---

[5]When we ran an IRT analysis with all 20 CES-D items, Item 4 ("I felt I was just as good as other people") had the lowest discrimination value ($a = 0.35$). This is consistent with the fact that the item was excluded from further analyses in Chapter 5 due to the poor item-total correlation of .19 (see Table 5.2).

Table 6.3	IRT Item Parameters for Seven-Item CES-D Subscale, Depressed Affect, 2-PL Model (N = 983)				
Items		a	b_1	b_2	b_3
1 I was bothered by things that usually don't bother me.		1.57	−0.52	0.76	1.72
3 I felt that I could not shake off the blues even with help from my family or friends.		2.21	−0.09	0.68	1.53
5 I had trouble keeping my mind on what I was doing.		1.85	−0.22	0.94	1.74
6 I felt depressed.		3.67	−0.34	0.50	1.18
7 I felt that everything I did was an effort.		0.73	−1.46	0.15	1.62
11 My sleep was restless.		1.72	−0.41	0.61	1.40
18 I felt sad.		2.20	−0.22	0.77	1.60

Note: a is the item discrimination parameter; b_1 is the category threshold parameter between a response of 0 (rarely) and 1 (some of the time); b_2 is the category threshold parameter between 1 (some of the time) and 2 (occasionally); and b_3 is the category threshold parameter between 2 (occasionally) and 3 (most of the time)

has a 0.50 probability of responding above that threshold. For Item 6 (I felt depressed), a person with a depression trait level of −0.34 has a 0.50 probability of responding "none of the time" versus any response indicating greater frequency. A person with a trait level of +1.18 (b_3) has a 0.50 probability of answering "occasionally" versus "most of the time."

Graphic depictions also help in the evaluation of items. Figure 6.5 (panel A) presents the CRCs for Item 6 of the CES-D. These functions suggest a good spread across the latent trait, and good differentiation across response categories. This figure shows that the probability of a person answering in a particular response category is conditional on the latent trait (Depressed Affect). At any point along the X axis, the sum of probabilities is 1.0 because respondents have selected one of the four response options. The item location parameters (the bs) are where the curves intersect. For example, the CRC for response category 0 (*none of the time*) crosses the CRC for response category 1 (*some of the time*) at −0.34. This is the same value shown as b_1 for Item 6 in Table 6.3. By contrast, the CRCs for Item 7 (panel B of Figure 6.5) clearly suggest that the item does not do a good job of discriminating across different categories, consistent with the low value of a for this item. As we concluded in the previous chapter, Item 7 would probably be dropped if we were developing a Depressed Affect subscale from scratch, at least for use in a population of low-income women.

The items for this CES-D subscale appear to work best near the middle of the latent trait, which seems appropriate for an instrument used to measure depressed affect in a general population. For clinical purposes, some items with location parameters (bs) of 2.0 and higher would be desirable. Scales other than the CES-D have been created for such purposes. In fact, Olino and colleagues (2012) used IRT methods to calibrate the CES-D, the Beck Depression Inventory (BDI), and another depression scale in a sample of adolescents. Their findings were that the BDI provided more information at higher severity levels of depression, consistent with the widely held view that the CES-D is useful in epidemiologic studies, whereas the BDI is better suited for clinical samples.

Yang and colleagues (2013) offer a detailed example of selecting items based on IRT. The scale in question, a measure of delirium, included a mixture of self-report items and items based on observation.

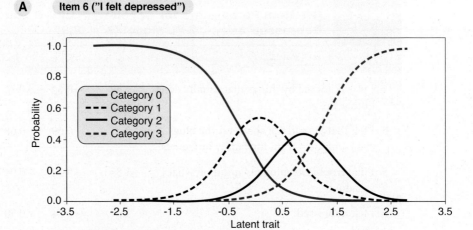

A   Item 6 ("I felt depressed")

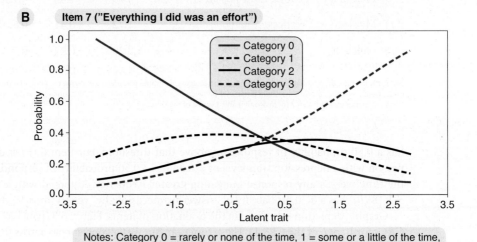

B   Item 7 ("Everything I did was an effort")

Notes: Category 0 = rarely or none of the time, 1 = some or a little of the time, 2 = occasionally, 3 = most or all of the time.

Figure 6.5
Category response curves for two CES-D items.

6.4.d Scoring for Item Response Theory Scales

In IRT and Rasch scaling, the item responses from a set of items with known item response functions are used to estimate a person's position on the latent trait continuum. With a Rasch model, the observed raw scores for a set of items comprising a scale are sufficient for estimating latent trait scores, using a nonlinear transformation. The summated scores from Rasch models are based on maximum likelihood estimations (MLEs) that calculate the latent trait level (θ) for each respondent. This is done by summing the likelihood or logits of each estimated item response, which are independent and uncorrelated with each other, controlling for θ. The maximum of the likelihood function, which is defined by the software, is the assigned Rasch score. Limitations of MLE are that it cannot estimate θ for patients who have either missing responses or have chosen the same response for every question.

In 2-PL models, raw scores are not sufficient for estimating trait scores because the discrimination parameter needs to be taken into account. Item scores are weighted by the discrimination score, such that people who have higher item response scores on discriminating items are assigned higher theta estimates. As a result, people with the same unit-weighted total raw score may obtain different theta values, depending on the response pattern on specific items. Indeed, a virtue of the 2-PL model is that the weighted item sums provide more information (and less measurement error) than unweighted item sums (Reise & Henson, 2003).

The specific scoring methods for IRT scoring are complex and are not described in detail here. Scoring is based on the estimator that is used in the IRT software program for the particular model used. For a 2-PL GRM, which we used in the analysis of the CES-D items, a person's responses can be scored using the *maximum a posteriori* (MAP) and the *expected a posteriori* (EAP) estimation methods, both of which are based on a Bayesian model. The MAP is a Bayes model estimation based on an iterative scoring process that identifies the mode of the posterior distribution of theta. The posterior distribution of theta is based on prior information of IRT parameters and the observed log-likelihood function. The EAP is based on the mean of the posterior distribution for all possible response patterns, which includes missing or intentionally omitted responses. A detailed discussion regarding these two scoring processes is found in Embretson and Reise (2000).

For the seven-item CES-D Depressed Affect subscale, IRT-based latent trait scores for each of the 983 women who answered at least one of the seven questions were estimated using the EAP. The IRT scores ranged from −1.59 (for women who answered all questions with "Rarely or none of the time") to +2.41 (for those who responded to all the questions with "Most or all of the time"). The corresponding CTT summated scores ranged from zero to 21 points. As this illustrates, IRT-derived scores are more immediately interpretable than summated raw scores.

6.5 Designing a Field Test of an Item Response Theory–Based Scale

The initial phases of an IRT-based scale development project are much the same as for the development of a CTT-based scale. That is, an item pool needs to be developed, and the items under consideration are reviewed for readability, comprehensibility, construct relevance, and so on. Pretests and cognitive interviews are also used to refine or prune items. After preliminary work, the next step is a formal field test with a fairly large development sample (i.e., the sample used to estimate item parameters). In this section, we discuss two specific issues relating to study design: the sampling plan and the selection of IRT software.

6.5.a The Sampling Plan

When a field test is undertaken to calibrate item parameters for an IRT-based scale, care needs to be taken to recruit a sample that is representative of the population for which the scale is targeted. The sample should be heterogeneous with respect to the latent trait to ensure stability of parameter estimates at all levels of the trait. In particular, the sample should contain a sufficient number of respondents at the extremes of the trait continuum to reduce measurement errors at those levels. Also, for polytomous items, there needs to be an adequate distribution of responses in each response category. If differential item functioning (DIF) will be assessed for key subgroups of respondents, then the sample must contain a sufficient number of respondents in each subgroup (DIF is explained in a later section).

With respect to sample size, large samples are preferred for IRT analyses. For example, Tsutakawa and Johnson (1990) recommended a sample size of 500 for accurate estimation of parameters. In a Monte Carlo simulation study, Reise and Yu (1990) found that for a GRM with response options ranging from zero to four, a sample size of 500 produced estimated item parameters closest to the predicted model item parameters. Cella and Chang (2000) suggested that as many as 1,000 cases may be needed for estimating a 2-PL model.

Recruiting such large samples is often challenging in health fields. However, sample size requirements vary depending on several factors. For example, the purpose of the field test needs to be considered because different levels of precision may be acceptable in different circumstances. If the items are being calibrated for a scale that would be widely used to derive accurate individual scores, or if item parameters are being calibrated for an item bank, then large samples are needed. Smaller samples might be acceptable for a scale with more limited use or for evaluating item properties of an existing or adapted scale.

The scale purpose can also affect sample size needs. For example, for a scale used to describe a general population (rather than, say, make a clinical evaluation of individual patients), smaller sample sizes may be needed because high precision at the extremes might not be necessary.

In general, sample size requirements increase with the complexity of the model. This means that larger samples are needed for 2-PL compared to 1-PL models, for models of polytomous items rather than dichotomous items, and for models with a greater number of items. It has also been found that the better the data meet the assumption of unidimensionality, the smaller the sample needs to be (Edelen & Reeve, 2007).

Smaller sample sizes have been reported as adequate for Rasch compared to IRT models. For example, Linacre (1994) claimed that sample sizes as small as 100 to 150 are adequate for stable estimates of Rasch parameters. He demonstrated that with 150 cases, there is 99% confidence that item calibrations are within 0.5 logits of their expected value.

6.5.b Item Response Theory Software

Data management and IRT analysis software are not currently integrated into a single statistical package. Although certain statistical packages, such as Stata, can "run" other IRT packages through customized macros, IRT software still needs to be purchased separately.

More than a dozen software programs have been developed to analyze items with IRT and Rasch methods, and some are more versatile than others. For the IRT analyses performed with the seven CES-D items in this chapter, the program Mplus was used (Muthén & Muthén, 2014). Mplus can be used to estimate unidimensional and more complex IRT models and is appropriate for 1-PL, 2-PL, and GRMs. (It is also widely used for structural equations modeling). Other popular software for IRT models includes PARSCALE and MULTILOG. IRTPRO is a single program that integrates four widely used IRT programs, including PARSCALE and MULTILOG (Cai, Thissen, & du Toit, 2011). IRTPRO can be used for 1-PL, 2-PL, and 3-PL models; GRM; and generalized partial credit models. IRTPRO is commercially available through Scientific Software International.

For Rasch models, one popular program is WINMIRA 2001, which can also be used for the partial credit model and the rating scale model. WINMIRA can read and write data directly in Statistical Package for the Social Sciences (SPSS) file format, and person-fit statistics can be appended directly to an SPSS data file. WINSTEPS (an earlier version was called *BIGSTEPS*) is another program designed for analyses using the Rasch model. Commercial versions of these two programs are available from Assess.com and Winsteps.com, respectively.

There is not much guidance on which IRT/Rasch software to select, and the selection may depend mainly on what is available in a given institution or on what software has been used by colleagues. Yang and colleagues (2011) compared several different programs in a DIF analysis of the Spanish and English Neurological Assessment Scales (SENAS). The researchers found that, overall, there was moderate to near perfect agreement across methods and programs.

6.6   The Application and Future Use of Item Response Theory in Health Measurement

In this chapter we have shown how IRT methods can be used to develop a multi-item scale. Among the many advantages of IRT is the fact that it has several applications beyond scale construction. In this section, we briefly review a few major applications and discuss the role of IRT in the future of health measurement.

6.6.a Item and Scale Improvement

IRT methods can be used to improve the psychometric adequacy of an existing scale. Many CTT scales were developed without giving much consideration to item difficulty, and indeed, in a typical CTT scale, item difficulty for most items is similar. In a CTT scale, score variability in a population is expected to result from differences in degree of endorsement of items of moderate difficulty or severity. Unfortunately, this often results in a measure that is not able to discriminate well across all levels of the trait or across the trait levels where discrimination is more desired. Using IRT methods (assuming model assumptions have been met), researchers can analyze data from an existing scale and more carefully evaluate the performance of each item. For example, IRT models can help to identify *disordered thresholds* (i.e., a transition between response categories that is not consistent with an increase in the underlying trait). Most importantly, IRT methods can identify *item gaps* (locations on the trait continuum where more items are needed) as well as item redundancies (locations on the trait continuum where there is an abundance of items). For example, Court and colleagues (2014) used a Rasch analysis to analyze data from a sample of patients with bipolar disorder who had completed the Hypomania Checklist (HCL-32), a measure that is used widely to screen for hypomania. Based on their analysis of model fit and item characteristics, the researchers recommended removal of four items on the HCL-32.

6.6.b Creation of Short Forms

In CTT, there is an inevitable tension between the desire to create a scale with high internal consistency on the one hand and to minimize respondent burden on the other. To improve internal consistency, one need only add items, but lengthening the scale makes it more burdensome to patients and sometimes more costly to those administering it. Brief scales have an additional advantage of being amenable to adoption in busy clinical settings. IRT methods allow researchers to create short forms from existing scales and at the same time achieve a comparable (or improved) level of precision. Moreover, IRT methods can maximize precision along the entire range of interest on the latent trait continuum. Edelen and Reeve (2007) provide a particularly good description of their process of developing a 10-item short form to measure depression in adolescents. The 19-item Feelings Scale, with many items identical to items on the CES-D, was administered to more than 6,500 adolescents in the National Longitudinal Study of Adolescent Health, and responses were analyzed with a GRM. The researchers selected 10 items that had high information levels, balanced content, and minimal content overlap. For example, the item "I felt depressed" was retained in the short form but "I felt sad" was not. The 10-item scale had only marginally higher measurement error than the full 19-item scale.

6.6.c Confirmation of Psychometric Properties and Linearization

Psychometric evidence from IRT analyses is sometimes used to offer corroborating evidence of an existing scale's measurement properties. In particular, IRT model fitting is used to further support a claim of the scale's unidimensionality (and hence, structural validity), measurement precision, and the justification for summing item scores. Another reason for applying an IRT model to data from an existing scale is to linearize the total score. For example, the widely used Oswestry Disability Index (ODI) was originally developed using CTT methods more than 30 years ago (Fairbank, Couper, Davies, & O'Brien, 1980) and has been found to have good reliability, validity, and responsiveness. There have been several IRT analyses of the ODI designed to examine and confirm the soundness of its psychometric properties using modern measurement theory. Lu and coresearchers (2013), for example, used a Rasch analysis with ODI data from a sample of 408 patients with back pain in Taiwan. In this study, all 10 of the ODI items had a good fit with the model, and the analysis further revealed that there were no major gaps in the items nor significant floor or ceiling effects. The overall precision of the test was high, with the most precise estimation of functional limitations in the range of -2.3 to $+2.3$ logits. The match between item difficulty and person ability was high. Many researchers are now combining IRT and CTT methods to provide a comprehensive assessment of a scale's psychometric properties and to derive scoring on a scale that has interval-level properties.

6.6.d Differential Item Functioning

A question that arose in the context of standardized testing is whether some items function differently for different subgroups, for example, whether subgroups of people (e.g., males vs. females) respond differently to an item, despite having the same trait level. Items that exhibit **differential item functioning (DIF)** can bias trait scores for subgroups and are therefore candidates for deletion, revision, or cautious interpretation.

In health fields, interest in DIF has focused primarily on differences for key demographic characteristics, such as sex, age, race, and ethnicity.[6] The phrasing of a question could, for example, involve words that are more culturally familiar to one group than to another. For example, "blues" in a depression item might not be interpreted by all cultural groups as implying a feeling or emotion. A good example of DIF for gender subgroups is the CES-D item "I had crying spells," for which there are numerous reports of DIF. Even when controlling for level of depression, females are more likely than males to endorse the "crying" item, which results in artificially inflated depression scores for women (e.g., Carleton et al., 2013; S. R. Cole, Kawachi, Maller, & Berkman 2000; Yang & Jones, 2007).

Yang and Jones (2008) have shown that DIF in the CES-D could also be attributable to chronic or other health differences. For depressive symptoms, especially among older adults, attention needs to be paid to comorbid conditions, such as cardiovascular diseases and risk factors that might inflate depression scores. For example, illnesses can affect somatic symptoms (e.g., restless sleep, poor appetite), without being caused by depression.

There are many approaches to studying whether items function in a comparable fashion across respondent subgroups, as we discuss in more detail in Chapter 15 on cross-cultural validity. In some cases, the different DIF approaches lead to similar conclusions (e.g., Yang & Jones, 2007), but in other cases, as described in Chapter 15, results vary considerably. There is no consensus regarding which of the many DIF methods is preferable, but IRT is considered a particularly elegant framework for empirically assessing DIF (Yang et al., 2011; Yang & Jones, 2007), although DIF analysis requires a larger sample for IRT methods than for other methods. When 2-PL models are used, subgroups can exhibit DIF in terms of item discrimination and item location (as well as in the separation between response alternatives for polytomous items), and this information can be useful in coming to conclusion about how to proceed with an item. Some researchers prefer IRT to other procedures, notably the Mantel–Haenszel method, because of evidence that IRT provides better estimates of *nonuniform DIF* (i.e., DIF that occurs only at certain levels of the trait) (Hambleton & Rogers, 1989). For example, using an IRT approach, Carleton and colleagues (2013) found that men and women answered the "crying" item on the CES-D similarly when depression levels were low, but gender DIF was detected at higher levels of depression.

6.6.e Computerized Adaptive Testing and PROMIS®

Computerized adaptive testing (CAT) is a popular application of IRT. With CAT, a computer algorithm is used to select a subset of highly discriminating items from a carefully calibrated *item bank* (a set of items, with known item parameters, for a particular latent trait). Items are selected to optimize measurement precision for each respondent. Typically, a

---

[6]DIF is also used to explore differential responses to items based on how the scale is administered. For example, Chan, Orlando, Ghosh-Dastidar, Duan, and Sherbourne (2004) found that for 12 CES-D items, a telephone interview mode resulted in more extreme responses than when the items were answered in a mailed survey.

person begins by answering an item of moderate difficulty (i.e., near the middle of the latent trait continuum). The response to that item provides a preliminary estimate of the latent trait level, and the computer then selects another item from the item bank that would improve the estimate. For example, those not endorsing an item would be given an "easier" item, whereas those endorsing it would be given a more "difficult" item. This iterative process continues until a good trait estimate is obtained, usually when a prespecified and low amount of measurement error is achieved. Through this process, it is typically possible to get a good trait estimate with relatively few items.

In health fields, measures of numerous patient-reported outcomes are available for CAT administration through NIH's PROMIS® initiative (Cella et al., 2010; Cella et al., 2007). PROMIS® includes items from the public domain that have undergone rigorous selection, refinement, and IRT calibration. Examples of constructs (traits) for which there are PROMIS measures for adults include ones in the physical health domain (e.g., physical function, pain intensity, fatigue, sleep disturbance), in the mental health domain (e.g., depression, anxiety, anger), and in the social health domain (e.g., satisfaction with participation in social roles, social support). Measures are available for both adult and pediatric populations, and the pediatric scales are available both as self-report and parental proxy. Details regarding the methodology for the PROMIS® item banks are found at http://www.nihpromis.org.

PROMIS® measures are available for CAT administration to researchers and clinicians online or for offline computers or tablets. Static long and short forms that can be administered in paper-and-pencil (or interview) format are also available. Items selected from the item bank for the short forms (typically 4 to 10 items) are those contributing the highest information to the latent trait. CAT-administered measures tend to yield more precise scores and typically involve only 3 to 7 items. CAT-based measurement is advantageous because of high precision, because scoring is in real time, and because the questions are more relevant to patients (i.e., they are targeted to their trait level). Because questioning is brief and relevant, CAT administration can decrease patients' fatigue, boredom, and frustration, especially when multiple traits are being assessed. Most PROMIS® instruments are available through the PROMIS® Assessment Center (https://www.assessmentcenter.net).

As an example, the PROMIS® item bank for the measurement of depression includes 28 items, 8 of which make up the static short form. The items ask people to indicate, on a 5-point scale ranging from "never" to "always," how often in the past 7 days they experienced certain feelings (e.g., I felt worthless, I felt depressed, I felt unhappy). Figure 6.6 shows how one CAT item from the PROMIS® item bank for depression would appear on a computer screen. Figure 6.7 shows how scoring information can be presented to the person completing the depression scale.

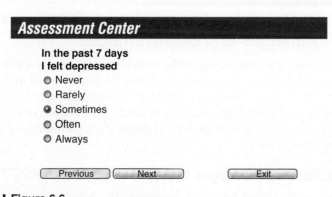

Figure 6.6

Example of a CAT-administered depression item from PROMIS®.

Your scores for the CATs you completed are shown below.

The diamond ◆ is placed where we think your score lies. This diamond is placed on your T-Score, which is a standardized score that is based on an average score of 50, based on responses to the same questions in the United States general population. The T-score also has a standard deviation of 10 points, so a score of 40 or 60 represents a score that is one standard deviation away from the average score of the general US population.

The Standard Error (SE) is a statistical measure of variance and represents the possible range of your score. The lines on either side of the diamond in your profile report show the possible range of your actual score around this estimated score. It is very likely that your score is in the range of these lines.

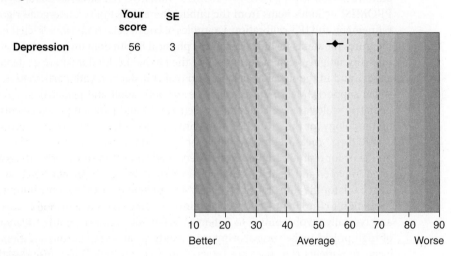

Figure 6.7
Example of scoring information on depression scale from PROMIS® CAT administration.

PROMIS® illustrates a state-of-the-art application of IRT. The questions can be self-administered on a computer or tablet, which decreases data entry errors that may occur when an interviewer or data clerk transfers answers to the computer. Responses can be saved immediately on a password protected database. With more than a dozen countries linked to PROMIS and several language translations, PROMIS® is a growing clinical and research measurement tool for assessing patient health outcomes.

6.7 Item Response Theory Versus Classical Test Theory: Advantages and Disadvantages

CTT approaches to scale construction have been used to create health-related scales for many decades, and most scale developers have been trained in this psychometric tradition. Yet, the use of IRT in the construction of health scales is becoming increasingly popular as its great advantages become more apparent. This section reviews the major benefits of IRT relative to CTT, as well the disadvantages. We begin with disadvantages because there are far fewer of them.

6.7.a Disadvantages of Item Response Theory

The single biggest barrier to developing IRT-based scales is that the models themselves are complex, and both statistical and measurement sophistication are required to estimate them. Moreover, none of the software for IRT analyses is particularly user friendly, and the software is usually expensive. Documentation for the software is often highly technical and error messages are sometimes difficult to comprehend. Another factor is that IRT analysis requires very large samples to yield stable item parameter estimates along a trait continuum, and large samples may be beyond what is available in most health settings.

Another impediment is that in clinical settings, unit-weighted summated scoring is simple to calculate, whereas IRT-based scoring is not. The widespread availability of computer tablets and other handheld technology, however, will likely overcome this problem as IRT-based scales become available for instantaneous online scoring.

Reluctance to pursue a more arduous and complex scale development process is likely nurtured by the considerable evidence indicating a high correlation between IRT-based scale scores and CTT-based raw scores using the same items. For example, Reise and Henson (2003) noted that they routinely observe correlations of .98 or higher. Yet, as they pointed out, optimal scaling via IRT can in some cases alter substantive conclusions.

6.7.b Advantages of Item Response Theory

It should be obvious from our description of IRT that this approach offers rich information about individual items that is not available using CTT methods. The graphic tools—such as item characteristic curves, CRCs, and so on—provide powerful visual information about individual items and the population of respondents, allowing for the optimal selection of items for a scale.

A particularly attractive feature of IRT-based scales is that, unlike CTT scales, the measurement of a latent trait is not *test dependent*. In a CTT scale, adding or omitting an item results in a different scale and different scores, but IRT-based scores are not dependent on a particular set of items. In other words, with IRT methods, a person's position on a latent trait continuum does not depend on the specific items that are administered. Such "item-free" scaling of individual differences is possible because IRT includes both item and person parameters into the same model. This seems intuitively desirable; a person's level of a trait (say, depression) is, at any point in time, a given amount, and it is useful to estimate that value regardless of which items are completed. This item-free scaling makes CAT feasible. Also, it means that missing data can be tolerated. A person's trait level can be estimated with a subset of items that have been calibrated in an IRT analysis, even if some questions are left unanswered.

Just as IRT-based trait estimates are invariant to specific items, another advantage is that item characteristics are generally sample independent. When an IRT model fits a population, ICCs should be the same in different samples (within a linear transformation, and aside from sampling error). Item parameters estimated in one sample can often be linearly transformed to be equal to parameters in a different sample, even if the sample means are different. This advantage, however, does not hold true universally. Streiner and Norman (2008) have noted that a number of studies have found sizeable differences in item parameters in different populations, and indeed such differences are what is under study in DIF analyses. Nevertheless, it is true that with CTT scales, scale properties are always sample dependent. With a traditional scale, a percentile rank for a person's score very much depends on who else completed the scale.

A particularly significant difference between CTT and IRT concerns measurement error, which we discuss in greater depth in Chapter 10. In brief, in CTT measures, a single index of measurement error (the *standard error of measurement*, or *SEM*) is computed for a sample, and the *SEM* is the same value for everyone in that particular sample (and the *SEM* is sample dependent). In IRT scales, measurement error is different at different points along the latent trait continuum, and so the degree of precision is person specific.

In traditional scales, internal consistency reliability can be improved simply by adding items. Indeed, CTT scales are often relatively long because of the desire to produce a high coefficient alpha. However, IRT-based scales of the same length as a CTT scale are almost always more precise. In turn, this means that for a desired level of precision, fewer items are needed for IRT scales, especially if items can be targeted to a respondent's trait level, as is the case with CAT. Shorter scales are beneficial because respondent burden is reduced, and this in turn may improve researchers' recruitment and retention efforts (and lower their costs).

A frequently cited advantage of IRT and Rasch scales is that they yield scores that are more truly interval level than CTT scales. Traditional scales yield measurements that are more accurately described as being ordinal level, although this fact is widely ignored in the subsequent analysis of scale scores. Indeed, even CTT items are treated as interval level when in reality the "distance" between "strongly agree" and "agree" (for example) is rarely equivalent to the distance between two other options, and the distance between response categories likely changes from item to item. Yet, when items are added together by unit weighting, equivalent distances between response options are assumed. As Streiner and Norman (2008) have noted, there is no need to play "let's pretend" (p. 324) about the measurement level of IRT-derived scales. In IRT scoring, moving from 0 to +1 logits on the trait continuum is equivalent to moving from +1 to +2 logits. Moreover, the scores from IRT scaling are more directly interpretable than scores from a traditional scale (see Chapter 16).

Interval-level measurement of a trait has beneficial implications for measuring change (see Chapter 17). And, because measurement error in IRT is person dependent, rather than sample dependent, measurement is more sensitive to change at the individual level than with CTT scales. Moreover, the fact that the exact same items do not need to be administered on a second testing in order to derive an estimate of a trait level in IRT means that the risk of carryover effects (e.g., remembering a previous response to an item) is reduced. Also, in measuring improvements or deterioration using IRT-based scales, there is less likely to be a problem with floor or ceiling effects, assuming adequate item coverage across the full range of the trait. IRT analysis provides useful information about where additional items are needed (i.e., their location) to minimize measurement problems at the extremes.

Another advantage of IRT scaling is that it can readily accommodate different response formats. In CTT, it is desirable to combine items with similar variances, which means that the response options are almost always the same for all items. The GRM allows items to have varying numbers of response alternatives (e.g., a five-point agreement continuum for some items, plus a three-point frequency continuum for others). Thus, in IRT the scale developer has more flexibility in phrasing appropriate questions.

Finally, as we have seen, IRT methods lend themselves to important applications, such as CAT and DIF. Another interesting application is that IRT-based linking methods allow the comparison of people who have completed different scales measuring the same construct or different versions of the same scale (Reise & Henson, 2003; Streiner & Norman, 2008).

References

Andrich, D. (1988). *Rasch models for measurement*. Newbury Park, CA: Sage.

Bentler, P. M. (1990). Comparative fit indexes in structural models. *Psychological Bulletin, 107*, 238–246.

Birnbaum, A. (1968). Some latent trait models. In F. Lord & M. Novick (Eds.), *Statistical theories of mental test scores*, (pp. 397–424). Reading, MA: Addison-Wesley.

Bond, T. G., & Fox, C. M. (2007). *Applying the Rasch model: Fundamental measurement in the human sciences*. Mahwah, NJ: Lawrence Erlbaum Associates.

Browne, M., & Cudeck, R. (1993). Alternative ways of assessing model fit. In K. Bollen & J. Long (Eds.), *Testing structural equation models*, (pp. 136–162). Thousand Oaks, CA: Sage.

Cai, L., Thissen, D., & du Toit, S. (2011). *IRTPRO for Windows*. Lincolnwood, IL: Scientific Software International.

Carleton, R. N., Thibodeau, M. A., Teale, M. J. N., Welch, P. G., Abrams, M. P., Robinson, T., & Asmundon, G. J. (2013). The Center for Epidemiologic Studies Depression Scale: A review with a theoretical and empirical examination of item content and factor structure. *PLoS ONE, 8*(3), e58067.

Carlson, M., Wilcox, R., Chou, C.-P., Chang, M., Yang, F., Blanchard, J., . . . Clark, F. (2011). Psychometric properties of reverse-scored items on the CES-D in a sample of ethnically diverse older adults. *Psychological Assessment, 23*, 558–562.

Cella, D., & Chang, C. H. (2000). A discussion of item response theory and its application in health status assessment. *Medical Care, 38*(Suppl. II), II66–II72.

Cella, D., Riley, W., Stone, A., Rothrock, N., Reeve, B., Yount, S., . . . Hays, R. (2010). Initial adult health item banks and first wave testing of the Patient-Reported Outcomes Measurement Information System (PROMIS) network: 2005–2008. *Journal of Clinical Epidemiology, 63*, 1179–1194.

Cella, D., Yount, S., Rothrock, N., Gershon, R., Cook, K., Reeve, B., . . . Rose, M (2007). The Patient-Reported Outcomes Measurement Information System (PROMIS®): Progress of an NIH Roadmap cooperative group during its first two years. *Medical Care, 45*(5, Suppl. 1), S3–S11.

Chan, K. S., Orlando, M., Ghosh-Dastidar, B., Duan, N., & Sherbourne, C. D. (2004). The interview mode effect on the Center for Epidemiological Studies Depression (CES-D) scale: An item response theory analysis. *Medical Care, 42*, 281–289.

Cole, E., Wood, T. M., & Dunn, J. M. (1991). Item response theory: A useful test theory for adapted physical education. *Adapted Physical Activity Quarterly, 8*(4), 317–322.

Cole, S. R., Kawachi, I., Maller, S. J., & Berkman, L. F. (2000). Test of item-response bias in the CES-D scale: Experience from the New Haven EPESE study. *Journal of Clinical Epidemiology, 53*, 285–289.

Court, H., Forty, L., Jones, L., Gordon-Smith, K., Jones, I., Craddock, N., & Smith, D. (2014). Improving the psychometric utility of the Hypomania Checklist (HCL-32): A Rasch analysis approach. *Journal of Affective Disorders, 152–154*, 448–453.

De Ayala, R. J. (2009). *The theory and practice of item response theory.* New York, NY: The Guilford Press.

DeMars, C. (2010). *Item response theory.* New York, NY: Oxford University Press.

Doucette, A., & Wolf, A. W. (2009). Questioning the measurement precision of psychotherapy research. *Psychotherapy Research, 19*, 374–389.

Edelen, M. O., & Reeve, B. B. (2007). Applying item response theory (IRT) modeling to questionnaire development, evaluation, and refinement. *Quality of Life Research, 16*, 5–18.

Embretson, S. E., & Reise, S. P. (2000). *Item response theory for psychologists.* Mahwah, NJ: Lawrence Erlbaum Associates.

Fairbank, J. C., Couper, J., Davies, J. B., & O'Brien, J. P. (1980). The Oswestry low back pain disability questionnaire. *Physiotherapy, 11*, 271–273.

Fraley, R. C., Waller, N. G., & Brennan, K. A. (2000). An item response theory analysis of self-report measures of adult attachment. *Journal of Personality and Social Psychology, 78*, 350–365.

Gelhorn, H., Hartman, C., Sakai, J., Mikulich-Gilbertson, S., Stallings, M., Young, S., . . . Crowley, T. (2009). An item response theory analysis of DSM-IV conduct disorder. *Journal of the American Academy of Child & Adolescent Psychiatry, 48*, 42–50.

Hambleton, R. K., & Rogers, J. (1989). Detecting potentially biased test items: Comparison of IRT area and Mantel-Haenszel methods. *Applied Measurement in Education, 2*, 313–334.

Hambleton, R. K., Swaminathan, H., & Rogers, H. J. (1991). *Fundamentals of item response theory.* Newbury Park, CA: Sage.

Hu, L., & Bentler, P. (1998). Fit indices in covariance structure analysis: Sensitivity to underparameterized model misspecifications. *Psychological Methods, 4*, 424–453.

Juster, F. T., & Suzman, R. (1995). An overview of the Health and Retirement Study. *Journal of Human Resources, 30*, S7–S56.

Linacre, J. M. (1994). Sample size and item calibration stability. *Rasch Measurement Transactions, 7*(4), 328.

Lord, F. M. (1952). *A theory of test scores.* New York, NY: The Psychometric Society.

Lord, F. M. (1953). The relation of test score to the trait underlying the test. *Educational and Psychological Measurement, 13*, 517–549.

Lord, F. M. (1974). Estimation of latent ability and item parameters when there are omitted responses. *Psychometrika, 39*, 247–264.

Lord, F. M. (1980). *Applications of item response theory to practical testing problems.* Hillsdale, NJ: Lawrence Erlbaum Associates.

Lord, F. M., & Novick, M. (1969). *Statistical theories of mental test scores.* Reading, MA: Addison-Wesley.

Lu, Y. M., Wu, Y. Y., Hsieh, C., Lin, C., Hwang, S., Cheng, K., & Lue, Y. (2013). Measurement precision of the disability for back pain scale by applying Rasch analysis. *Health Quality of Life Outcomes, 11*, 119.

McDonald, R. P. (2010). Normal-ogive multidimensional model. In W. J. van der Linden & R. K. Hambleton (Eds.), *Handbook of modern item response theory* (pp. 258–270). New York, NY: Springer-Verlag.

Mokken, R. J. (2010). Nonparametric models for dichotomous responses. In W. J. van der Linden & R. K. Hambleton (Eds.), *Handbook of modern item response theory,* (pp. 351–368). New York, NY: Springer-Verlag.

Molenaar, I. W. (2010). Nonparametric models for polytomous responses. In W. J. van der Linden & R. K. Hambleton (Eds.), *Handbook of modern item response theory* (pp. 369–380). New York, NY: Springer-Verlag.

Muthén, L. K., & Muthén, B. O. (2014). *Mplus version 7.* Los Angeles, CA: Muthén & Muthén.

Nering, M. L., & Ostini, R. (Eds.) (2011). *Handbook of polytomous item response theory models.* New York, NY: Taylor & Francis.

Olino, T. M., Yu, L., Klein, D., Rohde, P., Seeley, J., Pilkonis, P., & Lewinsohn, P. (2012). Measuring depression using item response theory: An examination of three measures of depressive symptomatology. *International Journal of Methods in Psychiatric Research, 21*, 76–85.

Polit, D. F., London, A., & Martinez, J. (2001). *The health of poor urban women: Findings from the Project on Devolution and Urban Change.* New York, NY: Manpower Demonstration Research Corporation.

Radloff, L. S. (1977). The CES-D scale: A self-report depression scale for research in the general population. *Applied Psychological Measurement*, *1*, 385–401.

Reise, S. P. & Henson, J. M. (2003). A discussion of modern versus traditional psychometrics as applied to personality assessment scales. *Journal of Personality Assessment*, *81*, 93–103.

Reise, S. P., & Waller, N. G. (2003). How many IRT parameters does it take to model psychopathology items? *Psychological Methods*, *8*, 164–184.

Reise, S. P., & Yu, J. (1990). Parameter recovery in the graded response model using MULTILOG. *Journal of Educational Measurement*, *27*, 133–144.

Samejima, F. (1969). Estimation of latent ability using a response pattern of graded scores. *Psychometrika Monograph Supplement*, *37*(1, Pt. 2), 68.

Samejima, F. (2010). Graded response model. In W. J. van der Linden & R. K. Hambleton (Eds.), *Handbook of modern item response theory* (pp. 85–100). New York, NY: Springer-Verlag.

Streiner, D. L. (2010). Measure for measure: New developments in measurement and item response theory. *Canadian Journal of Psychiatry*, *55*, 180–186.

Streiner, D. L., & Norman, G. R. (2008). *Health measurement scales: A practical guide to their development and use* (4th ed.). Oxford: Oxford University Press.

Tsutakawa, R. K., & Johnson, J. C. (1990). The effect of uncertainty of item parameter estimation on ability estimates. *Psychometrika*, *55*, 371–390.

Van der Linden, W. J., & Hambleton, R. K. (Eds.). (2010). *Handbook of modern item response theory*. New York, NY: Springer-Verlag.

Velozo, C. A., Warren, M., Hicks, E., & Berger, K. (2013). Generating clinical outputs for self-reports of visual functioning. *Optometry and Vision Science*, *90*, 765–775.

Whittaker, T. A., Fitzpatrick, S. J., Williams, N. J., & Dodd, B. G. (2003). IRTGEN: A SAS macro program to generate known trait scores and item responses for commonly used item response theory models. *Applied Psychological Measurement*, *27*, 299–300.

Yang, F. M., Grigorenko, A., Tommet, D., Farias, S.T., Mungas, D., Bennett, D.A., . . . Crane, P. K (2012). AD pathology and cerebral infarctions are associated with memory and executive functioning one and five years before death. *Journal of Clinical and Experimental Neuropsychology*, *35*, 24–34.

Yang, F. M., Heslin, K. C., Mehta, K. M., Yang, C. W., Ocepek-Welikson, K., Kleinman, M., Mungas, D. (2011). A comparison of item response theory-based methods for examining differential item functioning in object naming test by language of assessment among older Latinos. *Psychological Test and Assessment Modeling*, *53*, 440–460.

Yang, F. M., & Jones, R. N. (2007). Center for Epidemiologic Studies-Depression scale (CES-D) item response bias found with Mantel-Haenszel method was successfully replicated using latent variable modeling. *Journal of Clinical Epidemiology*, *60*, 1195–1200.

Yang, F. M., & Jones, R. N. (2008). Measurement differences in depression: Chronic health-related and sociodemographic effects in older Americans. *Psychosomatic Medicine*, *70*, 993–1004.

Yang, F. M, Jones, R. N., Inouye, S., Tommet, D., Crane, P., Rudolph, J., . . . Marcantonio, E. (2013). Selecting optimal screening items for delirium: An application of item response theory. *BMC Medical Research Methodology*, *13*, 8

Zhang, B., & Walker, C. M. (2008). Impact of missing data on person—Model fit and person trait estimation. *Applied Psychological Measurement*, *32*, 466–479.

7

Developing Clinimetric Measures

Chapter Outline

Alvan Feinstein originated the term **clinimetrics** to designate a domain concerned with indexes, scales, and classification criteria for clinical phenomena. In numerous articles and in his book on clinimetrics, Feinstein (1987) called attention to the need to formalize clinical observations and judgments in a manner that would yield greater uniformity. He was not only critical of the medical community for not formulating coherent methods for clinical classifications and ratings but also critical of psychometric approaches for being clinically naïve (Feinstein, 1982). He wanted clinicians to challenge themselves to "dissect" and specify the components of their clinical judgments so that decisions could be more systematic and generalizable.

Feinstein made a major contribution by bringing increased attention to measurement issues in medicine, especially with regard to the "soft" information that is routinely gathered in clinical work (e.g., symptoms, clinical signs). Clinimetrics has, however, had a rocky history. Some enthusiasts have proposed abandoning traditional psychometric approaches. For example, Fava and Belaise (2005) have written about "the misleading effects of psychometric theory" in psychiatric research. At the other extreme, Streiner (2003b) advocated that the term *clinimetrics* "gracefully fade from use" (p. 1142), seeing it as an unnecessary distinction from psychometrics. More moderate opinions urge researchers to blend aspects of clinimetrics and psychometrics to yield measurements with high clinical relevance while still meeting widely accepted psychometric standards of excellence (e.g., Bech, 2004; DeVet, Terwee, & Bouter 2003; Ribera et al., 2006).

This chapter discusses clinimetric measures, with particular emphasis on how their construction differs from methods discussed in the previous two chapters.

7.1 Basics of Clinimetrics

Before explaining the methods that have been used to create clinimetric measures, we discuss a little background.

7.1.a Early Clinimetric Measures

Clinimetricians often state that one of the earliest examples of a clinimetric measure is the widely used Apgar (1953) score for assessing infants' health status. Feinstein himself used the Apgar score as an example of how clinical observations could be made more systematic through the development of rules for evaluating clinical phenomena. As illustrated in Figure 2.4, the Apgar score combines clinicians' ratings (on a scale from zero to two) of five separate constructs (e.g., pulse, respiration), so that scores can range from 0 to 10.

Another early example of a clinimetric measure cited by Feinstein is the Jones criteria for diagnosing acute rheumatic fever (Jones, 1944). Jones' pioneering idea was to address diagnostic challenges by demarcating clearly defined criteria that enhanced consistency across clinicians. Feinstein (1982) noted that the Jones criteria were not perfect and they have undergone several revisions, but they nevertheless had a profound impact on clinical science. He pointed out that standardizing the process of diagnosing rheumatic fever "has allowed us to investigate it precisely, to treat it effectively and to prevent it" (Feinstein, 1982, p. 1).

These early examples illustrate that clinimetric measures can involve scaled values that yield continuous scores or classification criteria that yield nominal information: a positive or negative diagnosis. Many classification systems and diagnostic criteria that are not specifically called *clinimetric* could qualify for this designation. Indeed, it has been pointed out that the criteria for psychiatric diagnoses in the *Diagnostic and Statistical Manual for Mental Disorders* (*DSM*) are clinimetric in nature (Fava et al., 2004). For the most part, however, the term *clinimetric* is used to indicate a multicomponent measure that provides a continuous score for a clinically relevant outcome. The components of such measures typically involve either clinician ratings (e.g., the Apgar score) or patient reports (e.g., symptom checklists).

7.1.b The Nature of Clinimetric Measures

Some of the tension between clinimetrics and psychometrics is attributable to a fundamental difference that is not always recognized. The phenomena in which psychologists have been interested are primarily constructs that can be measured with reflective scales, as illustrated in Figure 2.3. For such constructs as intelligence, motivation, or self-esteem, one can conceptualize the construct as being the *cause* of people's responses to a set of items. Feinstein recognized this and used the term *homogeneous scales* when referring to *reflective scales*. With a homogeneous scale, the goal is to assemble a set of items that share a common cause—the latent trait that is being measured. When a researcher desires to combine a set of homogeneous items as effect indicators of the underlying trait, it is appropriate to use statistical ("psychometric") methods that are designed to examine and assess homogeneity, such as exploratory factor analysis (Chapter 5) and internal consistency (Chapter 9).

In clinimetric measures, by contrast, a heterogeneous set of signs and symptoms are combined. Feinstein called clinimetric measures *heterogeneous* because they often involve disparate symptoms, signs, and patient functions that are not necessarily correlated. He also preferred the term *index* for clinimetric measures rather than scales. Thus, clinimetric measures are usually *formative indexes* (Chapter 2). For indexes that are formative rather than reflective, classical test theory (CTT) methods such as factor analysis and internal consistency assessment, as well as item response theory (IRT) approaches, are typically not appropriate because there is no requirement that items be intercorrelated (Fayers & Hand, 2002; Streiner, 2003a).

Thus, it is not so much that psychometric approaches are "misleading" for clinical measures. Rather, the two psychometric measurement models (CTT and IRT), as well as certain standard psychometric procedures, are not relevant for the type of measures that some clinicians construct. If symptoms are combined into an index to shed light on the extensiveness of a health problem, there is no expectation that each item is measuring the same thing. Items that "measure the same thing" are characteristic of reflective (homogeneous) scales but not of formative (heterogeneous) indexes. In summarizing differences between the two, Fayers and Hand (2002) observed that the aim of psychometric approaches "might be characterized as attempting to measure a single attribute by using multiple items. In contrast, clinimetric methods attempt to summarize multiple attributes with a single index" (p. 240).

For formative indexes, the approach to reliability assessment is test–retest or interrater methods (Chapter 8) and not internal consistency. Similarly, structural validity (via a factor analysis) is seldom relevant. If the components are heterogeneous, the data would not typically be factorable. Indeed, Fayers and Hand (2002) have noted that when clinimetric scales such as symptom checklists are subjected to factor analysis, it is difficult to get stable results; factor structures tend to vary from study to study.

Validity assessments of clinimetric measures do, however, involve methods from the psychometric arsenal. Content validity is especially important because each component of a composite index should be relevant to the attribute being measured, and the measure should comprehensively include all relevant components. Clinimetricians often pursue what has been called **incremental validity**—that is, that each item or component of a measure contributes something unique to the assessment of an attribute. A content validity assessment can examine the extent to which this has been achieved. Criterion validity and hypothesis-testing construct validity are also used to assess the quality of clinimetric measures. Thus, methods traditionally associated with clinimetrics can profitably be combined with methods originating in psychometrics. No matter how a measure is constructed, its measurement properties need to be assessed, and those properties are not unique to one discipline. One of the biggest problems with clinimetric indexes is that many have been of an ad hoc nature and not subjected to rigorous testing.

7.1.c Clinimetric Domains

Feinstein described four kinds of medical data: demographic (e.g., age), paraclinical (e.g., laboratory tests, biopsies), therapeutic (e.g., drug regimens), and clinical. He categorized the first three as yielding "hard data," meaning information that is precise and reproducible. His clinimetric focus was on clinical information that could be considered "soft data."

Clinimetric measures are sometimes designed for a general purpose (e.g., pain assessment), but many are disease specific. The domains for clinimetric assessment, several of which were identified by Fava, Tomba, and Sonino (2012), include the following:

■ *Symptoms, states, and clinical manifestations.* For example, Castilhos and colleagues (2012) developed the Severity Score System for Progressive Myelopathy, a clinimetric measure to assess symptom severity.

■ *Functional status and functional ability.* For example, Chen et al. (2013) examined the clinimetric properties of the Spinal Alignment and Range of Motion Measure for children with cerebral palsy.

■ *Illness behavior.* For example, the Amyotrophic Lateral Sclerosis Frontotemporal Dementia Questionnaire is a clinimetric measure to assess behavioral disturbances in patients with amyotrophic lateral sclerosis (Raaphorst et al., 2012).

■ *Quality of life.* Ribera and colleagues (2006) evaluated a revised version of the clinimetrically developed Quality of Life after Myocardial Infarction questionnaire (QLMI).

■ *Allostatic load.* Fava, Giusi, Semprini, Tomba, and Sonino (2010) proposed clinimetric criteria for a determination of allostatic load, the cumulative effect of stressful experiences in everyday life.

■ *Lifestyle and behavior.* As an example, the widely used Alcohol Use Disorders Identification Test (AUDIT) for screening for alcohol use disorders in medical settings was developed using clinimetric principles (Bohn, Babor, & Kranzler, 1995).

7.2 Developing Clinimetric Indexes

Wright and Feinstein (1992) stated that clinimetric indexes are typically developed in three steps: (1) developing a preliminary pool of items, (2) selecting items for retention in the index, and (3) combining the information in a manner that gives appropriate emphasis to the retained items. Before items are generated, however, researchers need to be clear about the nature of the proposed measure. In particular, it will be impossible to devise a strong plan for constructing and formally assessing a new measure without knowing whether it will be a reflective scale or a formative index. In some cases, particularly in quality of life measures, formative and reflective subscales may be present in the same multidimensional instrument (Fayers, Hand, Bjordal, & Groenvold, 1997).

7.2.a Item Generation for Clinimetric Indexes

In formative clinimetric indexes, the specific items are extremely important. As "causal" indicators (Chapter 2), each item represents an important facet of the attribute being measured. Breadth of coverage, and thus content validity, is extremely important to an even greater extent than with reflective scales.

As with reflective scales, a first step in developing a clinimetric measure is to construct an overarching conceptualization of the attribute being measured. For example, Marx, Bombadier, Hogg-Johnson, and Wright (1999a) developed an instrument called the DASH—Disabilities of the Arm, Shoulder, and Hand. They sought to have their measure encompass four domains: symptoms, physical disability, social disability, and emotional disability. Their conceptual model and preliminary items were based on a review of the disability literature, inspection of existing scales, and input from experts. Some clinimetricians also derive items from direct observations of patients as well as discussions or in-depth interviews with patients and family members. Content validation efforts (Chapter 11) may contribute ideas for additional items.

Typically, the item pool is large and needs to be reduced. In the Marx et al. (1999a) study, the initial item pool was 821 items, which the researchers subsequently reduced to 30. They began by eliminating redundancies or obviously unsuitable items, then turned to clinimetric strategies.

7.2.b Final Selection of Items: The Clinical Impact Method

Clinimetric indexes are most distinctive from reflective scales in terms of the methods used to select the final items for the scale. Several clinimetric proponents have criticized the statistical and nonclinical approach to final item selection used by psychometricians, such as item analysis and factor analysis. Given that these methods are not even appropriate for formative indexes, their criticism is often justified.

The approach that is often used in developing clinimetric indexes has come to be called the **clinical impact method**. This method involves undertaking a substudy to ascertain which items in the item pool are most relevant and important, usually to patients.

We illustrate the method with a hypothetical index to measure autonomic dysfunction in patients with Parkinson disease (PD). Our example is a broad adaptation of several existing measures, including an index developed using the clinical impact method by Visser, Marinus, Stiggelbout, and van Hilten (2004). After developing our pool of possible items—symptoms of autonomic dysfunction—we would recruit a sample of patients with PD and ask them to answer two questions about each symptom: a frequency question (e.g., How often have you experienced this problem in the past month?) and an importance question

Table 7.1	Clinical Impact Scoring for a Hypothetical Set of Items for an Index of Autonomic Dysfunction in Parkinson Disease		
Symptom: In the past month, have you experienced:	Frequency[a]	Importance[b]	Impact[c]
Difficulty swallowing	4	5	20
Choking	3	5	15
Drooling, saliva dribbling from your mouth	5	4	20
Feeling bloated	2	2	4
Constipation	3	4	12
Diarrhea	2	2	4
Flatulence, feeling gassy	4	2	8
Involuntary loss of urine	4	5	20
Incomplete emptying of bladder	3	3	9
Light-headed feeling upon standing	3	4	12
Fainting or feeling faint	3	3	9
Excessive or unexpected sweating	3	4	12
Difficulty tolerating the cold	3	3	9
Difficulty tolerating the heat	4	2	8
Flaky skin or scalp	1	1	1

Note: Fictitious values are shown for a single patient.
[a]Frequency: In the past month, how often did you experience this problem? 1 = Never; 2 = Rarely; 3 = Occasionally; 4 = Often; 5 = Very often.
[b]Importance: How troubled are you by this problem? 1 = Not at all troubled to 5 = Severely troubled.
[c]Clinical impact = Frequency × Importance.

(e.g., How much does this problem trouble you?). Table 7.1 presents some possible items for this index. Information from these two questions is combined to generate item-level clinical impact scores, as described subsequently. Then the items are rank ordered on the basis of these impact scores, and the items with the greatest impact are selected for inclusion in the index.

There is considerable diversity in how the item impact scores are derived. Sometimes frequency and importance scores are added together, but most often they are multiplied, as in the example in Table 7.1. There is also diversity with regard to how the computations are handled. Sometimes an item impact score is obtained for each subject, as in Table 7.1, and then averaged across all sample members. Other researchers compute an average frequency and importance score across all subjects, and then multiply.

Different measurement scales have been used to measure frequency and importance as well. For example, frequency is sometimes captured dichotomously as present versus absent, but others use a scale of three or more ordinal points, as in our example (never, rarely, occasionally, often, very often). Importance, or the amount of burden, is almost always scaled, sometimes using three points (e.g., not at all, a little bit, a lot) but often scaled for five, seven, or more points. Based on the work of Visser et al. (2004), we would expect that several of the items listed in Table 7.1 would be eliminated (e.g., *Feeling bloated*, *Flaky skin or scalp*) because of low clinical impact rankings.

Researchers differ on how they make decisions about how many items to include. Sometimes there is a number of items that is considered desirable a priori, perhaps for the purposes of minimizing patient burden. For example, Marx and colleagues (1999a) knew in advance that they wanted 30 items for the DASH, so they selected the 30 items with the highest clinical impact rankings. Others use an impact score cut point (e.g., Juniper, Guyatt, Streiner, & King 1997). In our example, item impact scores (using the multiplication method at the subject level) could range from 1 (symptom not experienced, not troubling) to 25 (symptom occurs very often and is severely troubling). A researcher could decide that all items whose mean impact scores were 10.0 or higher (for example) would be included in the index.

Fortunately, Marx and coresearchers (1999b) investigated whether the methods used to derive impact scores affect item selection. They used six different scoring algorithms (e.g., adding frequency and importance, multiplying the two, using different scaling) and found little effect on item rankings. They concluded that the choice of scoring methods is not especially important, but they nevertheless recommended the use of ordinal scales with five or more categories for both frequency and importance.

Thus, a feature that distinguishes most clinimetric indexes from traditional "psychometric" scales is that the former are usually developed with patient input. By design, they embody and standardize what occurs in clinical settings when clinicians seek to learn how their patients are doing and what types of problems patients are experiencing.

Clinimetric measures are not necessarily finalized on the basis of clinical impact rankings alone, however. Often, there is a further review (akin to a content validity evaluation) from a panel of clinical experts. For example, in constructing their DASH index to measure activity limitations, Marx and colleagues (1999a) first selected the 30 items (out of 70 tested) with the highest impact rankings. They then asked experts with experience in upper limb disorders to review the 30 included and the 40 excluded items and to suggest any needed modifications. Clinicians suggested substituting 10 items. For example, the item "Having a frequent feeling of weakness in your arm, shoulder, or hand" was dropped after clinician review, but items such as "Turning a key" and "Pouring from a jug or teapot" were added. A further assessment indicated that the version with clinician input had better measurement properties than the version without the input, so the final scale retained clinician-suggested items.

7.2.c Scoring and Weighting in Clinimetric Indexes

There are many ways to combine information from individual items in clinimetric indexes. The simplest, and perhaps most frequent for multicomponent indexes, is to simply add item scores together, as is the case with Apgar scores. As noted in Wright and Feinstein (1992), other methods of aggregation are also possible. For example, the score could be a count of the number of items with a positive response or the percentage of items with a positive response. When the final score is a classification or staging, Wright and Feinstein suggest a variety of clustering methods or "Boolean unions" (p. 1203).

The issue of weighting is of greater importance in formative indexes than reflective scales. Weighting items before creating a composite score is seldom worth the effort in CTT scales because items are usually comparable. Many commentators have argued, however, that giving differential emphasis to items is appropriate in clinimetric indexes. This makes sense: Given that the items are all different constructs, some are likely to be more important than others in defining the attribute. When weighting is not used, the implicit assumption is that all components merit equal emphasis.

When weighting is used, the weights may be derived from patients' or clinicians' judgments about relative importance, such as using impact scores. Sometimes, if there is a well-accepted criterion or outcome, regression analyses are undertaken to establish weights.

One trouble with weights, however, should be kept in mind. We will point out repeatedly in this book that the measurement properties of a CTT instrument (e.g., reliability, validity) can vary from one population to another or from one application of an instrument to another. Similarly, weights created in one population may not be appropriate for another population or even for another sample from the same population. As with all research, replication is important to understand the generalizability of a measure's properties.

7.3 Other Issues Concerning Clinimetric Measures

This section discusses several issues that are relevant to clinimetrics, including assessment criteria, comparisons with psychometric scales, and reporting on clinimetric measure development.

7.3.a Clinimetrics and "Sensibility"

Clinimetrically developed instruments should meet standards of measurement excellence, to the same degree as any other measures. In terms of the taxonomy developed by the Consensus-based Standards for the selection of health Measurement Instruments (COSMIN) (and refined by us in Figure 3.1), the key measurement properties are reliability (test–retest and interrater or intrarater reliability), measurement error, content and face validity, criterion validity, hypothesis-testing construct validity, change score reliability, and responsiveness. In translated indexes, cross-cultural validity may be relevant. These properties and relevant parameters are all described in Parts III and IV of this book.

Feinstein (1987) used the term **sensibility** as the overall quality criterion for evaluating clinimetric indexes. Sensibility covers several properties that are considered important in psychometrics (e.g., content validity) and others that concern prudent instrument development, such as having clear instructions (what Feinstein referred to as *replicability*) and item clarity (*comprehensibility*).

Feinstein was an early advocate of creating measures that are *sensitive to treatment*—the characteristic called *responsiveness* in many measurement papers. Several clinimetricians have expressed doubt that homogenous scales are sufficiently sensitive to capture expected change (e.g., Fava & Belaise, 2005; Wright & Feinstein, 1992). Developers of traditional reflective scales do not specifically select items based on responsiveness. Moreover, psychometricians have resisted acknowledging responsiveness as a separate measurement property (e.g., Streiner & Norman, 2008). By developing clinimetric measures in a manner that incorporates information about what patients feel is important to them, areas for desired improvement are inherently embedded in the measure.

Face validity is another aspect of Feinstein's sensibility. He thought that clinimetric measures ought to be judged in terms of the biologic and clinical coherence of its component parts. Face validity has not been considered important in many psychometric circles, perhaps in part because many scales are not intended for routine clinical use.

Finally, sensibility includes feasibility and acceptability, both of which are important for measures used by clinicians. Feinstein believed that the sensibility of an instrument depends, at least in part, on whether it was practicable in clinical settings. In turn, this means that clinimetric instruments should not be lengthy or complicated. As noted by Wright and Feinstein (1992), psychometric measures often include numerous items, many of which are deliberately redundant, but "clinimetric indexes usually contain relatively few items to facilitate ease of usage" (p. 1203).

7.3.b Comparisons of Clinimetric and "Psychometric" Measures

Several researchers have undertaken studies to compare clinimetrically constructed indexes with "psychometric" scales in terms of the measures' content coverage and measurement properties. An early comparative study was conducted by Juniper and colleagues (1997), who developed the Asthma Quality of Life Questionnaire. They began with an item pool of 152 asthma-related impairments and administered the items to a sample of 150 adults with symptomatic asthma. The researchers used both the clinical impact method and factor analysis to select items for a clinimetric and psychometric scale, respectively. The clinical impact method resulted in a 32-item measure, whereas factor analysis resulted in a 36-item scale. Clinicians grouped the clinimetric items into four domains (symptoms, emotional function, physical activity limitations, and problems with environmental stimuli). The factor analysis resulted in a five-factor solution. Of particular interest, seven high-impact items in the clinimetric index were excluded from the psychometric scale (e.g., "Having to avoid dust"), and the psychometric measure included eight items with low-impact rankings (e.g., "Poor concentration"). The researchers concluded that the clinical impact approach yielded a better instrument in terms of "clinical sensibility," although they did not formally compare the measurement properties of the two measures.

Marx and his colleagues (1999a) did, however, undertake such an analysis. They created two 30-item instruments in developing the DASH: a clinimetric version using the clinical impact method and a CTT psychometric version using factor analysis. Like Juniper et al. (1997), they found that the two versions had different items: The versions had only 16 items in common. Despite this fact, total scores on the two measures were similar, and an analysis using a Bland-Altman plot (described in Chapter 10) indicated that patients' scores on the two were comparable. Moreover, both measures performed well in terms of internal consistency (Cronbach's alpha greater than .95 for both).

Similar comparisons have been undertaken by other research teams. For example, Ribera and colleagues (2006) created clinimetric and psychometric versions of the McNew QLMI. They found that both measures performed comparably in terms of internal consistency and responsiveness, but that the clinimetric measure had somewhat better performance on validity tests.

In some respects, these efforts seem anomalous. Formative clinimetric indexes should not be expected to be internally consistent. Clinimetricians may have felt the need to demonstrate that their indexes were not inferior to reflective scales in terms of a criterion held in high esteem in traditional psychometrics, namely internal consistency. However, when comparing clinimetric and psychometric measures, the more relevant measurement properties are reliability (test–retest for patient-reported outcomes [PROs]), criterion (or construct) validity, change score reliability, and responsiveness. Face validity and feasibility also may be relevant in such comparisons.

The fact that internal consistency was found to be high in the clinimetrically developed indexes does not necessarily mean that the items are highly intercorrelated or that the index was homogeneous. Indeed, in most of the examples cited, total scores were derived by adding *all* items together, even though the factor analysis suggested separate domains. The high values for Cronbach's alpha likely reflect the fact that the instruments were long (i.e., had a lot of items). As we will see in Chapter 9, Cronbach's alpha can be increased by adding items, even when item-total correlations are modest.

7.3.c Designing a Clinimetric Study

Researchers interested in constructing a clinimetric index should begin in much the same fashion as in any other instrument project. Early steps include doing a thorough literature review on the construct and undertaking other activities to become an authority, such as consulting with other clinical experts, documenting clinical observations, and conducting open-ended (qualitative) interviews with patients. Constructing a conceptual model or framework that is clinically sound facilitates item development. After an initial pool of items is created, the items should be reviewed for unwanted redundancy, comprehensibility, readability, and so on, as described in Chapter 4.

If the clinical impact method is used to select the final items, a sample of patients from the target population must be recruited to obtain data about the items' impact from their perspective. In many studies, the clinical impact sample has not been particularly large. For example, samples of fewer than 100 patients are not unusual (e.g., Flokstra-deBlok et al., 2009; Jokovic, Locket, & Guyatt, 2006; Marx et al., 1999a; Rutishauser, Sawyer, Bond, Coffey, & Bowes 2001; Visser et al., 2004). However, larger samples are preferred to ensure the stability of the clinical impact ratings. In fact, a rigorous approach would involve a cross-validation. With a sufficiently large sample, the clinical impact scores could be computed for a random half sample and then cross-validated against the rankings of the other half sample. The version of the index resulting from the clinical impact assessment should be carefully reviewed by clinicians (and perhaps a small panel of patients) for content and face validity. This expert panel also could be asked to provide feedback about the instrument's acceptability and the feasibility of implementation in clinical settings.

Clinimetric indexes should not be criticized if they do not have strong internal consistency, or if internal consistency is not even assessed. They are, however, of undetermined quality if reliability is not assessed. To demonstrate the high quality of a clinimetric PRO, a clinimetric study should include an assessment of test–retest reliability. Designs for retest reliability studies, and the issue of identifying an appropriate time interval, are discussed in Chapter 8. Other relevant measurement properties, such as criterion validity and responsiveness, should also be evaluated. As part of a feasibility assessment, researchers should gather data on the amount of time patients need to complete the index.

Not all clinimetric measures are PROs. Clinical measurements that rely on observations and judgments from clinicians (e.g., a measure to diagnose and grade phlebitis) may not involve a clinical impact assessment. For such measures, interrater or intrarater reliability need to be assessed, and the raters require careful training in the use of the instrument.

7.3.d Reporting on Clinimetrically Developed Indexes

In addition to standard descriptions for instrument development papers (e.g., how items were generated, how a sample was selected, characteristics of the sample), the instrument development report should describe in some detail how items were selected because that is fundamentally what makes a clinimetric measure different from other scales. For indexes developed using the clinical impact method, the report should specify the questions and response options used to assess frequency and importance. The method used to score the impact ratings should be explained, for example, whether multiplication or addition was used and whether or not each patient's impact score was computed and then averaged. If a cut point was used to decide the number of items, the cut point should be specified. If clinicians' opinions were used to alter the index, the modifications to the instrument should be explained. Examples of excluded items might be of interest to researchers or clinicians working in the field. Other measurement properties should be described, together with how long, on average, it takes to complete the instrument. The paper should provide readers with an understanding of the population for whom the measure is intended and the applications envisioned for the measure.

References

Apgar, V. (1953). A proposal for a new method of evaluation of the newborn infant. *Current Research in Anesthesia and Analgesia, 32*, 260–267.

Bech, P. (2004). Modern psychometrics in clinimetrics: Impact on clinical trials of antidepressants. *Psychotherapy and Psychosomatics, 73*, 134–138.

Bohn, M. J., Babor, T. F., & Kranzler, H. R. (1995). The Alcohol Use Disorders Identification Test (AUDIT): Validation of a screening instrument for use in medical settings. *Journal of Studies on Alcohol, 56*, 423–432.

Castilhos, R. M., Blank, D., Netto, C., Souza, C., Fernandes, L., Schwartz, I., . . . Jardim, L. (2012). Severity score system for progressive myelopathy: Development and validation of a new clinical scale. *Brazilian Journal of Medical and Biological Research, 45*, 565–572.

Chen, C. L., Wu, K. P., Liu, W., Cheng, H., Shen, I., & Lin, K. (2013). Validity and clinimetric properties of the Spinal Alignment and Range of Motion Measure in children with cerebral palsy. *Developmental Medicine and Child Neurology, 55*, 745–750.

DeVet, H. C. W., Terwee, C. B., & Bouter, L. M. (2003). Clinimetrics and psychometrics: Two sides of the same coin. *Journal of Clinical Epidemiology, 56*, 1146–1147.

Fava, G. A., & Belaise, C. (2005). A discussion on the role of clinimetrics and the misleading effects of psychometric theory. *Journal of Clinical Epidemiology, 58*, 753–756.

Fava, G. A., Giusi, J., Semprini, F., Tomba, E., & Sonino, N. (2010). Clinical assessment of allostatic load and clinimetric criteria. *Psychotherapy and Psychosomatics, 79*, 280–284.

Fava, G. A., Ruini, C., & Radanelli, C. (2004). Psychometric theory is an obstacle to the progress of clinical research. *Psychotherapy and Psychosomatics, 73*, 145–148.

Fava, G. A., Tomba, E., & Sonino, N. (2012). Clinimetrics: The science of clinical measurement. *The International Journal of Clinical Practice, 66*, 11–15.

Fayers, P. M., & Hand, D. J. (2002). Causal variables, indicator variables and measurement scales: An example from quality of life. *Journal of the Royal Statistical Society, 165*, 233–261.

Fayers, P. M., Hand, D. J., Bjordal, K., & Groenvold, M. (1997). Causal indicators in quality of life research. *Quality of Life Research, 6*, 393–406.

Feinstein, A. R. (1982). The Jones criteria and the challenges of clinimetrics. *Circulation, 66*, 1–5.

Feinstein, A. R. (1987). *Clinimetrics.* New Haven, CT: Yale University Press.

Flokstra-deBlok, B. M., van der Meulen, G., DunnGalvin, A., Vlieg-Boerstra, B., Oude Elberink, J., Duiverman, E. J., . . . Dubois, A. (2009). Development and validation of the Food Allergy Quality of Life Questionnaire. *Allergy, 64*, 1209–1217.

Jokovic, A., Locket, D., & Guyatt, G. (2006). Short forms of the Child Perceptions Questionnaire for 11–14-year-old children (CPQ$_{11-14}$): Development and initial evaluation. *Health and Quality of Life Outcomes, 4*, 4.

Jones, T. D. (1944). The diagnosis of rheumatic fever. *Journal of the American Medical Association, 126*, 481.

Juniper, E. F., Guyatt, G. H., Streiner, D. L., & King, D. R. (1997). Clinical impact versus factor analysis for quality of life questionnaire construction. *Journal of Clinical Epidemiology, 50*, 233–238.

Marx, R. G., Bombadier, C., Hogg-Johnson, S., & Wright, J. (1999a). Clinimetric and psychometric strategies for development of a health measurement scale. *Journal of Clinical Epidemiology, 52*, 105–111.

Marx, R. G., Bombadier, C., Hogg-Johnson, S., & Wright, J. (1999b). How should importance and severity ratings be combined for item reduction in the development of health status instruments? *Journal of Clinical Epidemiology, 52*, 193–197.

Raaphorst, J., Beeldman, E., Schmand, B., Berkhout, J., Linssen, W., van den Berg, L.H., . . . de Haan, R. (2012). The ALS-FTD-Q: A new screening tool for behavioral disturbances in ALS. *Neurology, 79*, 1377–1383.

Ribera, A., Permanyer-Miralda, G., Alonso, J., Cascant, P., Soriano, N., & Brotons, C. (2006). Is psychometric scoring of the McNew Quality of Life after Myocardial Infarction questionnaire superior to the clinimetric scoring? A comparison of the two approaches. *Quality of Life Research, 15*, 357–365.

Rutishauser, C., Sawyer, S. M., Bond, L., Coffey, C., & Bowes, G. (2001). Development and validation of the Adolescent Asthma Quality of Life Questionnaire (AAQOL). *European Respiratory Journal, 17*, 52–58.

Streiner, D. L. (2003a). Being inconsistent about consistency: When coefficient alpha does and doesn't matter. *Journal of Personality Assessment, 80*, 217–222.

Streiner, D. L. (2003b). Clinimetrics vs. psychometrics: An unnecessary distinction. *Journal of Clinical Epidemiology, 56*, 1142–1145.

Streiner, D. L., & Norman, G. R. (2008). *Health measurement scales: A practical guide to their development and use* (4th ed.). Oxford: Oxford University Press.

Visser, M., Marinus, J., Stiggelbout, A., & van Hilten, J. (2004). Assessment of autonomic dysfunction in Parkinson's disease: The SCOPA-AUT. *Movement Disorders, 19*, 1306–1311.

Wright, J. G., & Feinstein, A. R. (1992). A comparative contrast of clinimetric and psychometric methods for constructing indexes and rating scales. *Journal of Clinical Epidemiology, 45*, 1201–1218.

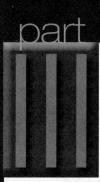

8

Reliability: Test–Retest, Parallel Test, Interrater, and Intrarater Reliability

Chapter Outline

In Parts III to V of this book, we offer a fuller presentation of the measurement properties summarized in Chapter 3. Part III covers the reliability domain (Fig. 3.1), which includes reliability (Chapter 8), internal consistency (Chapter 9), and measurement error (Chapter 10). Although much of our presentation regarding reliability is based on concepts that emerged in the context of classical test theory (CTT), each of the three chapters in Part III has sections that discuss aspects of reliability for scales developed using item response theory (IRT).

Measurement, even when using sophisticated technical equipment to measure physiologic attributes, is seldom perfect. For example, a person's weight may fluctuate somewhat with different measurements *even when his or her weight has not changed* as a result of differences in the calibration or precision of the measuring scale, the person's attire, the time of day, the person who is doing the measurement or recording it, and so on.

Although perfect measurement is essentially impossible, it is an important goal for developers of new measures. The *reliability* of a measure is a key measurement property and needs to be assessed when a new measure is developed and, often, reassessed during its use. This chapter provides guidance on the assessment of a measure's reliability and offers some advice on how to enhance it.

8.1 Basics of Reliability

In Chapter 3, we noted that **reliability** is the extent to which a measurement is free from measurement error. Using the CTT model, any obtained measurement is equal to a hypothetical true score, plus or minus measurement error. The lower the measurement error, the more reliable the measure—that is, the better it is in estimating the true score.

What, exactly, is a **true score**? A common definition is that a person's true score on a measure is the mean of an infinite number of measurements of that person, taken under identical circumstances. Measurement error is what causes obtained scores to fluctuate from one measurement to the next, as in our example of measuring a person's weight. By taking the mean of an infinite number of measurements, errors of measurement are presumed to cancel each other out. Obviously, a true score is a hypothetical construct, but its definition suggests that reliability assessment involves replication.

An extended definition of reliability, adapted from the Consensus-based Standards for the selection of health Measurement Instruments (COSMIN) workgroup (Mokkink et al., 2010b), captures this notion of replication. Reliability is the extent to which scores for people *who have not changed* are the same for repeated measurements, under several situations. One of those situations is the repeating of measurements through the use of multiple items on a composite scale. This aspect of reliability, which concerns *internal consistency*, is discussed in Chapter 9. In this chapter we describe reliability in terms of measurement repetitions at different times or occasions, by different people, or on different versions of a measure. For each approach, there are different potential sources of measurement error that can reduce reliability.

Measurement error will be discussed at greater length in Chapter 10, but because measurement error is what reduces reliability, a few words about it are needed here. Measurement error can be either **systematic** or **random**. Systematic error or bias sometimes affects all measurements equally (e.g., a lenient rater) but sometimes affects some measurements differently than others. For example, if a scale to measure weight is improperly calibrated and makes everyone 2 pounds heavier than they are, this systematic error would be constant across all patients. If the person taking the weight measurement told all women to take off their shoes but did not give such instructions to men, the weights of men would be systematically biased upward relative to the weights of women. Random error might occur if the person recording the weight measurements occasionally entered a value in error (e.g., entering 121 for a person weighing 112 pounds).

Although it is tempting to think of a reliable measure as one that is accurate, such is not necessarily the case. Recalling that a true score is the average of an infinite number of measurements, a weight-measuring scale that is consistently 2 pounds too heavy will, over an infinite number of measurements of a person's weight, yield "true score" weights that are not accurate. As another example, if a person's responses on a scale are biased in the direction of socially acceptable answers due to a social desirability effect, then the bias would presumably persist across an infinite number of measurements. Thus, researchers may have to undertake a separate assessment of bias (see Chapter 4) because bias will not necessarily be revealed in reliability testing.

One of the most important things to keep in mind in computing or interpreting reliability parameters within the CTT framework is that *reliability is not a fixed property of an instrument*. For a given measure, reliability will vary from one population to another or from one situation to another. It is better to think of reliability as a property of a particular set of scores than as a property of a measure itself. Users of an instrument developed using CTT methods need to consider how similar their population is to the population used to compute reliability parameters. If the population is very different, new estimates of reliability should be computed.

8.2   Types of Reliability

In this chapter, we discuss four types of reliability that share some measurement features. In particular, as described later in this chapter, the same reliability parameters can be used to estimate reliability for test–retest, parallel test, interrater, and intrarater reliability. Some special facets of these reliability variants are discussed next.

8.2.a Test–Retest Reliability

In **test–retest reliability**, replication takes the form of administering a measure to the same people on at least two occasions. If a measure yields a good estimate of the true score of an attribute, it should do so comparably on separate administrations. The assumption is that for traits that have not changed, any differences in people's scores on the testings are the result of measurement error. Retest assessments aim to distinguish true score variance from **transient error** that results from time-related fluctuations in people's moods, physiologic states, or information processing mechanisms (Schmidt et al., 2003). When score differences across waves are small, reliability is high. This type of reliability is sometimes called *stability* or **reproducibility**, the extent to which scores can be reproduced on repeated administrations of the measure.

Table 8.1 presents fictitious scores on the 20-item Center for Epidemiologic Studies Depression Scale (CES-D) (Radloff, 1977) for 10 people who were measured 1 week apart. The mean score for Week 1 and Week 2 were 12.20 and 14.20, respectively. A paired t test shows that the change in scores was not significant ($p = .13$). But, do the two sets of scores provide evidence of the scale's reliability? We look at ways to answer this question later in the chapter.

One attractive feature of the retest approach to reliability assessment is that it can be used with most types of measures, including biophysiologic measures, observational measures, single items (e.g., a visual analog scale for pain), reflective scales, and formative indexes. Nevertheless, retest reliability assessment can be problematic. The first problem is that the same measure must be administered to the same people multiple times, which often means that there is attrition on later testings, and attrition could result in biases because attrition is rarely random. Attrition could result in a more homogeneous sample, which would depress reliability coefficients. Moreover, when a scale has to be readministered, it is difficult (although not impossible) to ensure anonymity. For scales that measure traits of a personal

Table 8.1	Fictitious Data for Test–Retest Reliability Example for CES-D Scores		
ID	Week 1	Week 2	Change
1	16	19	3
2	5	8	3
3	8	14	6
4	20	14	−6
5	9	13	4
6	13	19	6
7	17	18	1
8	26	29	3
9	2	5	3
10	6	3	−3

or sensitive nature (e.g., drug use), or that are vulnerable to social desirability bias, anonymity may be essential for encouraging candor.

Estimates of test–retest reliability can be inflated if a measure captures both the focal construct and other personal attributes, such as a social desirability or extreme response bias. A measure of, say, medication compliance could look reliable in a retest situation not because the measure is reliably measuring compliance but rather because it is reliably inducing socially desirable responses.

Another problem for retest reliability stems from the fact that traits do change over time, and sometimes even over a short period of time. In the example in Table 8.1, 8 out of 10 people had higher scores (indicating greater depression) in Week 2 than in Week 1. We must consider the possibility that the mean higher score in Week 2 reflected true change; with only 10 people, the nonsignificance of mean score differences is not totally reassuring.

The possibility of real change in the trait being measured is a major concern. Psychologists have been especially wary of relying on a retest approach to reliability assessment because they feel that it is appropriate only when the attribute being measured is a trait rather than a state (e.g., Nunnally & Bernstein, 1994). A *trait* is an attribute with high temporal stability. Intelligence, for example, is usually considered a trait because it does not fluctuate much over time. A *state* is an attribute with low temporal stability, such as moods. It is usually acknowledged that there is a state–trait continuum rather than a dichotomy, but many attributes of interest to health professionals tend to be more statelike than traitlike. Indeed, a key goal of health care professionals is to improve health states and behaviors through intervention. Thus, many health measures quantify attributes that are expected to change over time.

In general, the longer the time gap between testing waves, the lower the retest reliability, even for traits that are presumed to be stable. Thus, to address the problem of true trait change, it is usually recommended that the time between testings be brief. Yet, new problems can emerge with short time intervals. One issue for patient-reported outcomes (PROs) is that reliability can be inflated by people's memory of how they answered on the first administration and their desire to be consistent—these are so-called **carryover**

effects. For example, there is a risk that someone might answer *rarely or never* to the CES-D item "I felt sad" on a second testing because they gave that response a week earlier and not because their sadness has been constant. Indeed, some people may interpret the entire retest exercise as a test of their ability to be reliable. Another problem is that if people are bored or aggravated with the task when they are measured a second time, they may answer questions haphazardly or perform carelessly, leading to spuriously low estimates of reliability. Another potential factor can depress reliability estimates: For some constructs, the possibility of a *rehearsal effect* or a *learning effect* is relevant (Polit, 2014). For example, on performance tests, people may perform better on the second test than on the first because the first test gave them an opportunity to learn about and reflect on what was expected of them and perhaps motivated them to surpass their initial performance or to refine their response. Yet another potential problem is called **response shift**, which is a change in a person's self-evaluation of the construct, rather than a change on the construct itself, as a result of several forces. The forces can include altered priorities or a reconceptualization of the target construct (Rapkin & Schwartz, 2004; Sprangers & Schwartz, 1999). Finally, regression to the mean can sometimes lower reliability estimates. **Regression to the mean**, it will be recalled, is a statistical phenomenon in which a score that is extreme at an initial measurement tends to be closer to the mean on a second measurement.

These various problems have led some psychometric experts to discourage using the test–retest approach: "We recommend that the retest method generally not be used to estimate reliability" (Nunnally & Bernstein, 1994, p. 255). Health care researchers, however, have disagreed with this viewpoint and have put strong emphasis on retest reliability in CTT measurement, perhaps because of its connection to the definition of a true score and because of its role in interpreting true change in scores. Nevertheless, the many perplexing problems of retest reliability should be kept in mind.

8.2.b Parallel Test Reliability

The development of multi-item *parallel tests* (or *alternative-form tests*) is infrequent in health care, although such tests are common in educational testing. There are, however, a few examples in health care. For instance, the Boston Naming Test is a widely used neuropsychological test that has several parallel short forms (Fastenau, Denburg, & Mauer, 1998). Another example is the latest version of the Mini-Mental State Examination (MMSE-2), which has alternate forms (Folstein, Folstein, White, & Messer, 2010).[1]

Consistent with a domain sampling model, parallel tests can be created by randomly sampling two sets of items from a carefully developed and tested item pool. If the two tests are, indeed, parallel, then they are replicates whose true scores are in theory identical. Having measures that are parallel is useful when researchers expect to make measurements in a fairly short period of time and want to avoid carryover effects such as those described for retest reliability. In practice, however, it is difficult to derive two (or more) totally equivalent measures using the CTT model. Thus, a major source of measurement error in parallel test reliability concerns the sampling of items on the alternate forms.

Similar to test–retest reliability, **parallel test reliability** involves administration of the parallel tests to the same people on two separate occasions and then estimating a reliability parameter. This means that problems such as attrition and lack of anonymity can also be relevant in a parallel test situation. Unlike retest reliability, however, parallel test reliability is appropriate only for reflective multi-item scales. With formative indexes, the specific items are of great importance; they cannot be construed as a random sample of items within a domain sampling model.

---

[1]As another example from cross-cultural research, parallel forms composed of the original language version and a translated version are sometimes administered to a bilingual sample to assess comparability (see Chapter 15).

8.2.c Interrater and Intrarater Reliability

When measurements involve the use of an external clinician or observer who makes scoring judgments, a key source of measurement error can stem from the person making and recording the measurements, as described in Chapter 4. This is a familiar situation for observational instruments (e.g., scales to measure agitation in nursing home residents) and is also true for many performance tests (balance tests) and biophysiologic measures (e.g., skinfold measurement). In such situations, it is important to evaluate how reliably the measurements reflect attributes of the stimulus being rated rather than attributes of the raters. Developers of new observational measures need to know how capable their instruments are of yielding reliable scores with trained observers. Users of such measures—including clinicians and clinical trialists—often want to know whether they or their staff can reliably apply the measure and how much training is needed to achieve adequate reliability. In both reliability assessment situations, replication is necessary.

The most typical approach is to undertake an **interrater** (or *interobserver*) **reliability** assessment, which involves having two or more observers independently applying the instrument with the same people. Reliability involves comparing the observers' scores to see if the scores are consistent.

A less frequently used approach—but one that is appropriate in many clinical situations— is an **intrarater reliability** assessment in which the *same* rater makes the measurements on two or more occasions, blinded to the scores he or she assigned on any previous measurements. Intrarater reliability is an index of self-consistency. It is analogous to retest reliability, except that the focus in retest situations is the consistency of the person *being measured*, and intrarater reliability concerns the consistency of the person *making the measurements*.

Interrater and intrarater reliability can be enhanced in a number of ways. The instrument developer can strive to develop a scoring system that does not require extensive inference and should prepare meticulous instructions with precise scoring guidelines and clear examples. Training sessions are usually necessary, and raters should be given detailed and immediate feedback during training. Training might well involve cognitive interviews (see Chapter 4) in which raters are asked to explain how they arrived at scoring decisions. Such cognitive pretesting, if done during instrument development, might be useful for refining both the instrument and the training materials. If measurements with an instrument are made over an extended time period, recurring reassessments of reliability might be warranted. Finally, in some cases, it might be relevant to screen potential raters for biases that could affect their judgments.

As with all of the reliability assessments discussed in this chapter, timing is a critical factor. For interrater reliability, the ideal situation is to have multiple observers making the measurements simultaneously. This can sometimes be approximated through the use of videotapes or other permanent records such as X-rays. For example, multiple observers could watch segments of videotaped interactions of nursing home residents to score independently for such constructs as confusion, aggression, or agitation. When simultaneous assessment is not possible, the timing between the measurements should usually be short to avoid the possibility of true change in the construct being measured. However, for intrarater assessments, the time interval should not be so short as to risk inflated reliability estimates resulting from memory and carryover effects among the observers. Short time intervals can also risk increasing fatigue and lowering enthusiasm among those being measured, which could lower reliability. Timing from a study design perspective is discussed in Section 8.6.a.

8.2.d Choosing a Type of Reliability to Estimate

As this section hopefully has made clear, those developing a new measure must select the type of reliability to assess. In some cases, the choice will be dictated by the type of instrument that is being developed. For example, the reliability of a formative verbal report index should *only* be assessed through the test–retest method.

In other cases, however, several approaches might be appropriate. For observational measures, interrater or intrarater reliability is essential, but other types of reliability assessment are possible. Our advice is to consider possible sources of measurement error for the specific measure and to then assess as many types of reliability as is meaningful. For example, a multi-item observational scale to assess confusion in the older adults (such as the NEECHAM Confusion Scale; Neelon, Champagne, Carlson, & Funk, 1996) could be evaluated for internal consistency (do the observational items consistently tap the construct of interest?), retest reliability (do elders consistently manifest confusion over a short time interval, as captured by the scale?), interrater reliability (are different raters similar in their evaluation of elders' confusion?), and intrarater reliability (does a rater watching a video of an elder rate confusion consistently in two viewings?). Gathering evidence about *both* intra-rater and interrater reliability is not uncommon. For example, Luby, Bykowski, Schellinger, Merino, and Warach (2006) assessed both interrater and intrarater reliability of ischemic lesion volume measurements for different magnetic resonance imaging sequences.

Because different assessment procedures are designed to deal with different sources of measurement error, researchers should not expect that different reliability parameters will be the same. It might be expected that intrarater reliability would be higher than interrater reliability (Kraemer, 2008), but it is unclear, as Kraemer claimed, that retest reliability would usually be lower than either.[2]

Table 8.2 summarizes key features of different types of reliability, including internal consistency. (Specific parameters relating to IRT are not covered in this table). This table shows that the types of reliability assessments discussed in this chapter are relevant for all types of measurements, including PROs, observations, performance tests, and biophysiologic measures. As this table indicates, the key reliability parameters for the types of reliability being discussed in this chapter are the intraclass correlation coefficient (ICC) and the kappa statistic.

8.3   The Intraclass Correlation Coefficient as a Reliability Parameter

When a measure yields continuous scores, the reliability parameter is the **intraclass correlation coefficient**, or **ICC**. This section provides basic information about this important index, which can be used not only with scales created in a CTT framework but also with performance and biophysiologic measures.

Score variability is at the heart of reliability assessment. Indeed, a reliability coefficient tells us how well people can be differentiated from one another on the target construct, *despite* measurement error. Two or more measurements with a heterogeneous sample are needed to separate true score variance from error variance. It may be recalled from Chapter 3 that the statistical definition of reliability is this: the proportion of total variance in a set of scores that is attributable to "true" differences among the people being measured. This can be summarized in the following equations:

$$R = \frac{\sigma^2_{True}}{\sigma^2_{Observed}} = \frac{\sigma^2_{True}}{\sigma^2_{True} + \sigma^2_{Error}} \tag{8.1}$$

where R = reliability, σ^2_{True} = true score variance, $\sigma^2_{Observed}$ = total observed score variance, and σ^2_{Error} = error variance. The lower the error variance, the closer this proportion will be to 1.0 and the higher the reliability will be.

---

[2]The debate about whether retest reliability or internal consistency yields higher reliability coefficients is discussed briefly in Chapter 9.

Table 8.2 Summary Chart: Reliability and Measurement Error

Measurement Property: Type of Reliability	Measurement Level[a]	Reliability Parameter	Measurement Type				Model		Items		Major Sources of Measurement Error or Confounds	Measurement Error Parameter
			Verbal Report/PRO	Performance Test	Observational	Biophysiologic	Reflective	Formative	Single	Multiple/Composite		
Test–retest (same people, measured 2+ times)	Continuous	Intraclass correlation coefficient (ICC)	X	X	X	X	X	X	X	X	Transient error; carryover (memory) effects; learning/rehearsal; response shift; regression to mean (plus, true change)	Standard error of measurement (*SEM*); Limits of agreement
	Nominal	Kappa	X	X	X	X	X		X			Proportion of agreement[b]
Parallel tests (2+ alternate forms for measuring same attribute, same people)	Continuous	ICC	X	X	X	X	X	X	X	X	Item sampling; transient error	*SEM*; Limits of agreement
Interrater (2+ independent raters using measure) or	Continuous	ICC			X	X	X	X	X	X	Rater biases; non-comparability of stimulus or condition	*SEM*; Limits of agreement
Intrarater (same rater giving ratings 2+ times)	Nominal	Kappa			X	X	X	X	X			Proportion of agreement[b]
Internal consistency (same people, measured with 2+ items)	Continuous (items)	Cronbach's alpha (α)	X	X	X	X	X			X	Item sampling; item heterogeneity	*SEM*
	Nominal (items)	Kuder–Richardson 20 (KR-20)	X	X	X	X	X			X		*SEM*

Note: Does not include item response theory (IRT) parameters.

[a]For ordinal measures, quadratic weighted kappa or ICC can be used for the reliability parameter.

[b]Strictly speaking, there is no parameter of measurement error for categorical variables, but proportion of overall agreement and proportion of positive agreement (PA) and proportion of negative agreement (NA) can be reported.

True score variance is never known, but it can be estimated based on variability between people. Thus, a reliability coefficient can be defined as:

$$R = \frac{\sigma^2_{\text{BetweenPeople}}}{\sigma^2_{\text{BetweenPeople}} + \sigma^2_{\text{Error}}} \tag{8.2}$$

This reliability coefficient is calculated by means of the intraclass correlation coefficient. There are multiple formulas for ICCs. Shrout and Fleiss (1979) described 6 ICCs, and McGraw and Wong (1996) presented 10. Here we discuss the types of greatest relevance to assessing reliability of health measures. Assumptions for the different models vary somewhat, as described in McGraw and Wong. The basic assumption is that the scores for the different people being measured are independent and normally distributed, that the people are randomly selected, and that residual variation (error) is random and independent, with a mean of zero.

8.3.a Intraclass Correlation Coefficient Models for Fully Crossed Designs

For the types of reliability discussed in most of this chapter, score variability can be conceptualized as being of two types: (1) variation from person to person being measured, for N people; and (2) variation from measurement to measurement of each person, for k measurements. In the ICC models discussed in this section, people and measurements are **fully crossed**; that is, each person is rated by k raters (or completes a measure k times), and each rater rates everyone. The value for k is often two: a test and then a retest, two observers' ratings, and so on. However, k can be a larger number, as may be the case for some interrater reliability studies. For simplicity, the examples in this chapter are shown for $k = 2$.

To understand the reliability of a measure, researchers need to partition the total variability in a set of scores into different sources. Beginning with the statistician Ronald Fisher, ICC has been viewed within an analysis of variance (ANOVA) framework. Because the variance being partitioned is for the scores of N people and k measurements in fully crossed designs, a two-way ANOVA for repeated measures is the fundamental model. Because variance in ANOVA is called a *mean square* (MS), and ANOVA software shows values for mean squares, our formulas for the ICCs will include various MS components, following McGraw and Wong (1996).

In selecting an ICC formula for reliability assessment, three things need to be considered. First, the formulas differ for situations in which a single score for each person will be used as the measure versus when an averaged score will be used (e.g., the mean of two blood pressure measurements taken 5 minutes apart).

A second thing to consider—although this affects interpretation rather than calculation of the ICC—is whether the k measurements are viewed as a fixed or random effect. When effects are fixed, all levels of k are included in the analysis, and there is no interest in generalizing the reliability coefficient to other observers or waves of testing. If the k measurements are seen as a random sample of all possible measurements, then a random effects model is appropriate. The developer of a new performance test or observational measure that would be used by others and generalized to other raters would likely conceptualize the ICC as a random effects model.

The third and trickiest issue in selecting an ICC concerns whether the assessment is about consistency of scores, or absolute agreement. **Consistency** in measurement refers to the extent to which the *rankings* of the N people are consistent across the k measurements, regardless of what the actual score values are. **Absolute agreement** is the extent to which scores across the k measurements are identical.[3] Panel A of Table 8.3 shows that

---

[3]Consistency reliability is sometimes referred to as *norm-referenced reliability*, whereas absolute agreement is referred to as *criterion-referenced reliability* (McGraw & Wong, 1996).

Table 8.3	Illustration of ICC Values for Scores Demonstrating High Consistency (Panel A) and Absolute Agreement (Panel B)			
	Panel A Highly Consistent Scores		Panel B Scores in Absolute Agreement	
Person	Observer 1 (k_1)	Observer 2 (k_2)	Observer 1 (k_1)	Observer 2 (k_2)
1	0	2	1	1
2	1	3	2	2
3	2	4	3	3
4	3	5	4	4
5	4	6	5	5
6	5	7	6	6
7	6	8	7	7
8	7	9	8	8
9	8	10	9	9
10	9	11	10	10
	$ICC_{Consistency} = 1.00$		$ICC_{Consistency} = 1.00$	
	$ICC_{Agreement} = .82$		$ICC_{Agreement} = 1.00$	

Note: Using McGraw & Wong (1996) categories, $ICC_{Consistency} = ICC (C,1)$ and $ICC_{Agreement} = ICC (A,1)$.

two observers gave ratings that were not identical, but the rank ordering of the 10 people in the sample was the same for both observers, resulting in scores that were consistent but not in absolute agreement. The ICC for consistency is a perfect 1.00, but the ICC for agreement is .82. In Panel B, both raters gave identical ratings to all 10 people, yielding an ICC of 1.00 for both consistency and agreement. In the widely adopted classification system of McGraw and Wong (1996), the consistency ICCs in Table 8.3 would be called ICC (C,1), with the "C" representing consistency and the "1" indicating that the reliability of a single rather than averaged score was being assessed. The agreement ICCs in Table 8.3 would be classified as ICC (A,1).

The difference between ICCs for agreement versus consistency concerns the value in the denominator of the ICC equation. With agreement estimates, the error term in the denominator is broken into two components: random error and systematic error associated with different raters (interrater or intrarater), waves (test–retest or intrarater), or alternate forms (parallel test). In other words, column variance for the k columns is included in the denominator for $ICC_{Agreement}$. In Panel A of Table 8.3, the scores for Observer 2 are systematically two points higher than those for Observer 1, perhaps indicating that Observer 2 has a leniency bias. When systematic variation across observers or waves is considered relevant, then ICC for agreement should be used. One equation for ICC agreement for a single score, for either random or fixed effects for the k measurements, is:

$$ICC (A,1) = \frac{MS_{Between} - MS_{Residual}}{MS_{Between} + (k-1) MS_{Residual} + (k/n)(MS_{Observers} - MS_{Residual})} \tag{8.3}$$

where $MS_{Between}$ = mean square between people (rows), $MS_{Residual}$ = mean square error or residual, and $MS_{Observers}$ = mean square for columns (raters or waves).[4] Thus, in the denominator for ICC (A,1), total variability is composed of three components: between-people variance, random error variance (residuals), and between-rater (wave) variance, respectively. In the example in Panel A of Table 8.3, we would find[5]:

$$ICC\ (A,1) = \frac{18.33 - 0.00}{18.33 + (1.0)0.00 + (0.20)(20.00 - 0.00)} = \frac{18.33}{22.33} = .821$$

When systematic differences between observers or waves is not considered relevant, then the ICC for consistency can be computed. For consistency estimates, the error term, for both random and fixed effects, comprises random error and column variation:

$$ICC\ (C,1) = \frac{MS_{Between} - MS_{Residual}}{MS_{Between} + (k - 1)\ MS_{Residual}} \tag{8.4}$$

Here, the denominator excludes column variation (i.e., the between-rater or wave variation). In the example in Panel A of Table 8.3:

$$ICC\ (C,1) = \frac{18.33 - 0.00}{18.33 + (1.0)0.00} = \frac{18.33}{18.33} = 1.00$$

Alternative formulas for ICC estimation can be used when variance components are available (e.g., through variance components [VARCOMP] in SPSS). Formula 8.2 can be used directly for ICC (C,1), with the error term being residual variance. For ICC for agreement, the formula is:

$$ICC\ (A,1) = \frac{\sigma^2_{BetweenPeople}}{\sigma^2_{BetweenPeople} + \sigma^2_{Raters/Waves} + \sigma^2_{Error}} \tag{8.5}$$

In our current example for Panel A of Table 8.3, the variance associated with the columns (raters) is 2.00, error variance is 0.0, and between-patient variance is 9.167. Thus, ICC for consistency would be 9.167/9.167 = 1.00 and the ICC for agreement would be:

$$ICC\ (A,1) = \frac{9.167}{9.167 + 2.00 + 0.00} = .821$$

ICC consistency estimates are almost invariably higher than the absolute agreement estimate. Indeed, one way to think of ICC consistency is that it yields values that are *uncorrected* for the lack of agreement between the k raters or k test waves. Some writers have stated that ICC (C,1) is the most widely used formula for assessing reliability (McGraw & Wong, 1996; Suen, 1988). However, it has been argued that in clinical situations, absolute agreement is often more important than consistency (DeVet, Terwee, Mokkink, & Knol, 2011). For example, we are less likely to be concerned with whether a sample of patients is ranked similarly for blood pressure values by two nurses than with whether the nurses have gotten comparable absolute values. Streiner and Norman (2008) suggest that when developing a new scale for which observer reliability must be assessed, it may be more appropriate to use an ICC for absolute agreement and to treat raters as a random factor. They also suggest that the ICC for consistency might be appropriate if the reliability of scores on an *existing* measure were being assessed in connection with a substantive study such as a clinical trial. Weir (2005) recommends examining whether the F test for column differences is significant. When systematic differences between raters or waves are small, as evaluated through a paired t test or repeated measures ANOVA, differences in ICC values for agreement and consistency will be minor.

---

[4]In the Statistical Package for the Social Sciences (SPSS) reliability program in which ICCs are calculated, $MS_{Observers}$ are shown as the mean square between items.
[5]Calculations for the MS components are not shown. They can be obtained using repeated measures ANOVA and are also provided in the reliability analysis in SPSS.

When the score being used for each person is a mean of several scores rather than a single score, different formula than those shown in Equations 8.3 and 8.4 are needed. Without showing the computational formula, we present a consistency formula that illustrates why averaging across measurements reduces measurement error:

$$\text{ICC (averaged)} = \frac{\sigma^2_{\text{BetweenPeople}}}{\sigma^2_{\text{BetweenPeople}} + \left(\dfrac{\sigma^2_{\text{Error}}}{k}\right)} \qquad (8.6)$$

From this equation, it can be seen that the error term in the denominator is divided by the number of measurements being averaged, which increases the value of the reliability coefficient as the value of k increases. The ICC for consistency estimates with score averaging is referred to as ICC (C, k), where k is the number of measurements being averaged. Absolute agreement estimates of averaged scores are designated as ICC (A, k). It might be noted that Cronbach's alpha, the widely used index of internal consistency that we discuss in Chapter 9, is essentially an ICC (C, k) index, where k is the number of items on the scale. The reliability of averaged scores is always higher than that for a single score.

One further note is that none of these ICC formulas provides a mechanism for disentangling interactions between the rows and the columns in the error term. An interaction would be present if, for example, Observer 2 in Table 8.3 gave systematically higher scores for male then for female patients, or if CES-D scores in Table 8.1 systematically improved at retest for a specific subgroup. Variance associated with such interactions are subsumed within the MS error component. When interactions are present within an ICC $(C,1)$ model for fixed effects, reliability tends to be underestimated.

ICCs are considered the appropriate reliability coefficients for the four types of reliability discussed in this chapter, but many researchers compute a Pearson correlation coefficient as the test–retest or interrater reliability parameter. Most measurement experts consider Pearson's r inappropriate for use as a reliability parameter (e.g., DeVet et al., 2011; McGraw & Wong, 1996; Streiner & Norman, 2008). However, values of r when $k = 2$ are essentially the same as those of an ICC $(C,1)$. When k is greater than two, Pearson's r cannot readily be used; r values for all variable pairs would have to be averaged.

Like any other statistic, an ICC is an estimate of a population parameter, and the precision of the estimate should be calculated. As described in a subsequent section, statistical software can compute confidence intervals around ICCs, and the 95% confidence interval (CI) is the usual standard that should be reported. Calculations for the standard error of the reliability coefficient are complex, but readers interested in the formula can consult Streiner and Norman (2008, p. 199).

8.3.b Intraclass Correlation Coefficient Models for Not Fully Crossed Designs

In many assessments of interrater reliability in health research, the measurement designs are not fully crossed, in which case the ICCs described in the previous section are not appropriate. In fully crossed designs, all people in the sample are rated by the same observers. In both panels of Table 8.3, for example, all 10 patients are rated by the same two observers.

There are several other measurement designs, however. For example, suppose we were evaluating interrater reliability for the ratings on a burn scar rating scale, such as the Vancouver Scar Scale (Sullivan, Smith, Kermode, McIver, & Courtemanche, 1990). In a multisite clinical trial in which scar severity was a primary end point, a fully crossed design for evaluating the interrater reliability of scar rating assessments would likely not be feasible. One possible design is a **nested design** in which raters are nested within patients. Table 8.4(A) illustrates such a design, for six raters and six patients. In a nested design, different pairs of raters rate different patients, and there is no overlap (i.e., Raters 1 and 2 always rate the same patients, as do Raters 3 and 4 and Raters 5 and 6). An *unbalanced design*

Table 8.4	Illustrations of a Nested Design (A) and Unbalanced Design (B) for an Interrater Reliability Study												

A. Nested Design: Raters Nested Within Patients							B. Unbalanced Design, Neither Crossed Nor Nested						
	Raters							Raters					
Patients	1	2	3	4	5	6	Patients	1	2	3	4	5	6
1	X	X					1	X			X		
2	X	X					2			X	X		
3			X	X			3			X	X		
4			X	X			4	X				X	
5					X	X	5					X	X
6					X	X	6		X				X

Note: Each "X" corresponds to a rating by the specified rater for the specified patient

is neither crossed nor nested. Such a design involves two raters per patient, but raters are not paired and there is some (but not complete) overlap of patients and raters, as illustrated in Table 8.4(B). Putka, McCloy, and Diaz (2008) called this an *ill-structured* design.

Without elaborating the details, the appropriate reliability coefficient for nested designs such as those shown in Table 8.4(A) is an ICC using a one-way model. In one-way models, variance due to raters and error is collapsed. The same raters do not rate each patient, so it is impossible to segregate rater variance from residual error.[6] Computations of ICCs for one-way models can be performed in many standard statistical software packages such as SPSS, as illustrated in Section 8.3.c.

Unbalanced designs (Table 8.4[B]) are likely to be fairly common in clinical settings, but unfortunately, assessments of interrater reliability for such designs are complex. Putka and colleagues (2008), noted that it is sometimes rationalized that a one-way ICC should be calculated because each patient has a different set of raters. They have demonstrated through simulations, however, that this procedure yields underestimates of reliability, and the degree of underestimation increases as the amount of overlap in raters/rates increases. They proposed a solution that takes the degree of overlap and hence rater variance into account; another solution has been proposed by Narayanan, Greco, and Campbell (2010). Those who wish to use standard software to compute ICCs and who are unable to implement a fully crossed design should consider adopting a nested rather than an unbalanced design.

8.3.c Intraclass Correlation Coefficient Calculation in SPSS

ICCs can be computed in most general-use statistical software packages using a repeated-measures ANOVA analysis or other routines to obtain mean square values. We illustrate here with SPSS using the data from the 1-week retest of the CES-D shown in Table 8.1.

In SPSS, ICCs can be generated in the Reliability Analysis procedure (Analyze → Scale → Reliability Analysis). To begin, the variables corresponding to the *k* measurements

---

[6]A formula for a one-way model is:

$$ICC (1) = \frac{MS_{Between} - MS_{Within}}{MS_{Between} + (k - 1) MS_{Within}}$$

must be inserted in the initial box (labeled "Items"). In our example, the two variables are the Week 1 and Week 2 CES-D scores. Clicking on "Statistics," various options appear, including ones for generating descriptive statistics. To test whether the Week 1 and Week 2 CES-D scores are significantly different (i.e., whether there is significant column variability), an ANOVA F test should be requested. When the box for "Intraclass correlation coefficient" is checked, it is necessary to indicate a Model and a Type. The Model options are "Two-Way Random" (the default), "Two-Way Mixed," and "One-Way Random." The two-way mixed model is "mixed" in that the people in the analysis are assumed to be a random factor, but the measurements (ks) are designated as a fixed factor. In any event, ICC values are identical for fixed and random models, so the default is acceptable. The choices for Type are "Consistency" (the default) and "Absolute Agreement."

Table 8.5 shows what an SPSS table for ICC consistency looks like for the CES-D data in Table 8.1. Table 8.5 indicates that the value for ICC (C,1) is .875; if the CES-D scores for the two waves were averaged, then ICC (C,2) would be higher, .933. SPSS also computes CIs around the ICC estimates, the default being a 95% CI. Because of the small sample size in this example, the 95% CI for the single-score ICC is wide: .577 to .967. Greater precision is achieved for the average scores (95% CI = .732 to .983). Both ICCs are significantly different from .00 ($F = 15.02, p < .001$). We could test whether the value is significantly different from something other than zero as well. McGraw and Wong (1996) suggest that within a reliability context, it is usually safe to assume that the reliability is greater than zero, and so the F test is better used to test whether reliability exceeds some specified nonzero value.

Table 8.6 summarizes additional information relating to the CES-D retest reliability analyses. The ANOVA F test for the mean change of 2.0 from Week 1 to Week 2 was nonsignificant ($F = 2.77, p = .13$). The nonsignificant difference for test waves is consistent with the fact that including column variance in the error term for the ICC did not greatly lower the reliability estimate: ICC (C,1) was .88, compared with .86 for ICC (A,1). Pearson's r was identical to the ICC consistency estimate, .88.

For the sake of illustration, let us suppose that the data in Table 8.1 are not test–retest values for the CES-D but rather are ratings on an observational scale from different pairs of observers in a nested design. In such a situation, a one-way ICC model would be appropriate. Using SPSS to calculate interrater reliability with these data using a one-way random model, we find an ICC of .855, only slightly lower than what was found for the two-way model for agreement (.856) and consistency (.875).

Table 8.5	Information From an SPSS Intraclass Correlation Coefficient Analysis, Two-Way Random Effects Model for Consistency, for 1-Week Test–Retest of CES-D

	Intraclass Correlation[a]	95% Confidence Interval		F Test With True Value 0			
		Lower Bound	Upper Bound	Value	df1	df2	Sig
Single Measures	.875[b]	.577	.967	15.018	9	9	.000
Average Measures	.933	.732	.983	15.018	9	9	.000

Note: Raw data for this analysis are shown in Table 8.1.

[a] Type C ICCs using a consistency definition; between-measure variance is excluded from the denominator variance.

[b] The estimator is the same, whether the interaction effect is present or not.

Table 8.6	Summary of ICC Results for 1-Week Test–Retest of CES-D
Type of Information	**Value**
CES-D Week 1 Mean (*SD*)	12.20 (7.54)
CES-D Week 2 Mean (*SD*)	14.20 (7.67)
Change, Week 2–Week 1: Mean (*SD*)	2.00 (3.80)
F test for change, significance	$F = 2.77, p = .13$
ICC (C,1): Consistency, single score (95% CI)	.88 (.58–.97)
ICC (C,2): Consistency, average of two scores (95% CI)	.93 (.73–.98)
ICC (A,1): Absolute agreement, single score (95% CI)	.86 (.53–.96)
ICC (A,2): Absolute agreement, average of two scores (95% CI)	.92 (.69–.98)
Pearson's *r* between Week 1 to Week 2 scores	.88

Note: Raw data for this table are shown in Table 8.1.
CI, confidence interval; *SD*, standard deviation.

8.3.d Interpretation of Intraclass Correlation Coefficient Values

Several writers have proposed criteria for acceptable ICC values, but many others have taken issue with the criteria, often noting that there is no statistical or conceptual basis for the criteria, only personal opinion. Yet, the criteria are a place for us to begin a discussion of interpreting reliability coefficients.

Although specific recommendations vary from one expert to another, there is neverthe-less agreement that reliability needs to be higher for measures that will be used to make decisions about individual people. Nunnally and Bernstein (1994) suggested that a reliabil-ity of .80 or higher is adequate for group level comparisons (e.g., comparing groups in a clinical trial), but a higher standard is essential for measures used to draw conclusions about individuals. They note that in such situations "A reliability of .90 is the bare minimum, and a reliability of .95 should be considered the desirable standard" (p. 265). Weiner and Stewart (1984) proposed a somewhat lower criterion, .85 or higher, for scores used to make clinical decisions. Recommended minimum reliability values for measures used in group situations are often in the .70 to .75 range (e.g., DeVet et al., 2011; Streiner & Norman, 2008; Terwee et al., 2007).

It could be argued that the standards for reliability might vary according to the situation. For example, Polit (2014) urged developers of *new* measures to aspire to retest reliabilities of .80 or higher. Instrument developers have some control over the testing situation, the defini-tion of the population, and the recruitment of an appropriate sample, and so they should be encouraged to work hard to show how high a reliability coefficient can be under the most favorable conditions. For subsequent assessments with different and perhaps more homo-geneous groups, a lower standard (say .70) might be adequate. When interrater reliability is assessed in clinical studies, a somewhat relaxed standard might also be acceptable because what is being evaluated is not explicitly the measure but rather the raters in their use of the measure (i.e., their ability to give comparable ratings).

In all cases, however, high reliability coefficients are very desirable. An ICC of .70 means that an estimated 70% of the variance in the obtained scores is attributable to true score variance, and 30% is attributable to error. Although there is no consensus on standards for ICCs, no expert has, to our knowledge, suggested that an ICC of .60 (for example) is acceptable, although reliability coefficients this low have been reported as adequate by some scale developers.

When low ICC values are obtained, what might it mean? There are several possible explanations for low ICCs. First and most simply, ICC values can be low even for excellent measures when variability in the N by k data matrix is low. Low variability, in turn, can reflect either a homogeneous sample of people, a "consensual judge set" (Lahey, Downey, & Saal, 1983), or both. When the people in the sample have similar true scores, then ICCs will tend to be low. And, if the k raters (for interrater reliability) are all lenient or all severe in their ratings, variability will also be depressed. Thus, a good place to start when trying to diagnose low ICC values is to look at the score distributions for people and raters. If variability is low, one solution would be to undertake a new reliability assessment with a more heterogeneous sample of people or judges. It might be noted that the converse problem is also true; high ICCs can mask modest consistency when between-people variability is very high. Thus, close inspection of distributional information can be useful for interpretive purposes, regardless of ICC values.

Second, problems with the measurement design could result in low ICCs. For example, if the time interval is faulty in retest studies because the trait itself has changed in the interval, ICC values will be depressed. As another example, if raters are not adequately trained, their ratings may be inconsistent because of poor understanding of the scoring system.

Low ICCs can also be the result of people-by-rater interactions. As previously noted, ANOVA models do not allow estimation of the interaction term independently of the error term. If it is suspected that such interactions exist, however, score distributions for different raters can be plotted, and this might lead to the exclusion of a rater or to a new assessment with different raters.

The fourth explanation of a low ICC is that the measure has low reliability (i.e., that the measure is not capable of yielding consistent scores across raters or waves within the population under study because random error is too high). When this is the case, it must be concluded that the measure is not very good at estimating people's true scores nor at discriminating among people with different levels of an attribute. If low variation, poor design, and people-by-rater interactions can be ruled out as the explanation for low ICC values, then the conclusion is likely to be that the measure is not very reliable.

Interpreting ICCs is further complicated by the fact that different values can be obtained depending on which type of ICC is computed. Consistency estimates can be inflated, relative to agreement estimates, if differences between the k raters or waves are high. Although fixed effects and random effects models yield the same ICC values, generalizability to other raters is most defensible if a random effects model is assumed by using raters who can be construed to be a random sample of raters.

8.3.e Consequences of Low Intraclass Correlation Coefficient Values

High reliability is a desirable measurement property not simply for "aesthetic" or theoretical reasons. Measures that are low on reliability **attenuate** correlations and depress effect size estimates because unreliability inflates error variance. In clinical trials, time and resources can be squandered by using outcome measures with low reliability because such measures may not result in a "fair test" of an intervention's efficacy. Even if an intervention is effective, measures with low reliability may suggest otherwise. Another way to think about this is that a measure's low reliability makes it difficult to detect change: With poor reliability, true change on an attribute is difficult to distinguish from measurement error (see Chapter 17).

The flip side of a potential Type II error is that a larger sample size is needed to detect significant effects with unreliable measures than would be the case with highly reliable ones. This problem, in turn, can affect resources and even the likelihood of getting research funding. The sample size needed to achieve a given power is inversely related to the value of the ICC. For example, if we needed a sample of 100 people per group when ICC was 1.0, 200 per group would be needed if ICC was .50 (Kraemer, 2008). A measure with a reliability of .80 requires a 25% increase in sample size compared to a totally reliable measure.

When clinical decisions are made on the basis of formal measures, low reliability can have harmful consequences. Charter and Feldt (2001) have demonstrated how reliability can result in misclassifications and thus clinical errors. For example, suppose it was decided that 10% of a population in greatest need would be given a special treatment, based on their scores on a measure. If the measure's reliability was .90, 7.8% of the patients would be true positives (i.e., truly in need of treatment). Another 2.2% *not* in need would be false positives and 2.2% in need would be deemed ineligible (false negatives). If the measure's reliability were .70, only 6.0% of patients would be true positives.

Thus, it is well worth the effort to develop highly reliable measures and to select such measures for use in clinical and research settings. But, again, a caution is that a measure shown to have adequate reliability with one population needs to be re-evaluated when used with a different population, with different raters, or in a different type of measurement situation.

8.4   Reliability Parameters for Noncontinuous Variables

Many measurements in health care are not continuous. Indeed, measurements are often dichotomous, such as the presence or absence of a clinical symptom or sign. When there is an interest in assessing the reliability of categorical measurements—that is, assessing the extent to which the categorical "scores" for people who have not changed are the same for repeated measurements—the most frequently used reliability parameter is **Cohen's kappa**. Kappa can be used to assess interrater, intrarater, and retest reliability.[7] For example, multiple raters could examine upper urinary tract computed tomography scans to assess degree of interrater agreement about the presence of tumors or key morphologic features. For intrarater reliability, a radiologist could rate the same scans on more than one occasion. And, for retest reliability, imaging and then reimaging the same people could be undertaken to assess consistency across readings. Various issues relating to kappa and related parameters are discussed in this section. We use interrater reliability in our examples, but the same principles apply to retest and intrarater reliability assessment of categorical measures. It might be noted that there is perhaps more controversy about kappa and its extensions than any other common statistic (e.g., Gwet, 2002; Uebersax, 2011), and yet its use in health research is widely accepted.

8.4.a   Proportion of Agreement

The most basic situation for noncontinuous scores is when two judges provide dichotomous ratings, yielding a two by two contingency table. Table 8.7 shows hypothetical data in which two raters reviewed 100 mammogram images and rated them for presence (malignant) or absence (benign) of a malignancy.

A straightforward index of consistency across raters is the **proportion of agreement**. In the example in Table 8.7, the two raters agreed that the images were benign for 50 patients and that there was a malignancy for 30 patients, so the proportion of agreement is $80/100 = .80$.

The proportion of overall agreement has intuitive appeal as a parameter of agreement, but it does not distinguish between agreement for positive versus negative ratings. Cicchetti

---

[7]In theory, kappa could also be used for parallel test situations, but examples of alternate forms that yield nominal scores are not known to us and seem unlikely.

Table 8.7	Fictitious Ratings by Two Raters for Presence of Malignancy From 100 Mammogram Images			
	Rater 2			
Rater 1	**Benign**		**Malignant**	**Total**
Benign	(a) 50		(c) 5	55
Malignant	(b) 15		(d) 30	45
Total	65		35	100

Proportion in agreement = .80.
Kappa = .588; 95% CI = .427 to .739.
Maximum possible kappa, given marginal distribution = .794.

and Feinstein (1990) pointed out the usefulness of indexes called *proportions of specific agreement*. In our example, agreement regarding malignancy (a positive diagnosis) could be calculated as the *proportion of positive agreement* (PA), in this case $30/100 = .30$. The *proportion of negative agreement* (NA) in this case would refer to agreements about benign ratings, which here would be $50/100 = .50$. During instrument or measurement system development, these indexes of specific agreement provide better information to help understand disagreements and to refine the measurements and rater training than overall agreement or the kappa statistic. This is particularly true if the distribution is severely skewed. For example, if only 1% of a population had a malignancy, PA would be far more important than overall agreement, which would almost certainly be high simply because of the rarity of a positive diagnosis.

Proportion of overall agreement can be calculated even when the ratings are not dichotomous. For example, if we added a middle category so that mammograms could be rated as benign, suspicious, or malignant, the frequencies along the diagonal, divided by the total number of mammograms rated, would yield the proportion of overall agreement. Because it is easily grasped even by those without a statistical background, proportion of agreement should be reported even when other statistics are calculated.

8.4.b Kappa for Dichotomous Ratings by Two Raters

In recognition of the fact that proportion of agreement is almost always high when a distribution is skewed, Cohen (1960) created the kappa statistic (κ). Cohen's intent was to correct for raters' agreement by chance.[8] The reasoning is that, *even without looking at any images*, two raters would agree in their ratings a certain percentage of time, purely by chance. Uebersax (2011) has questioned whether such a correction is necessary in situations in which the two raters are not expected to simply guess, and guessing would rarely be the case for health ratings. Nevertheless, Cohen's kappa remains the most widely used reliability index for situations such as those shown in Table 8.7.

The formula for computing kappa requires the calculation of the proportion of *expected frequencies* in the cells where the raters are in agreement. Expected frequencies are those expected as a result of chance and are based on multiplication of elements in the marginal distributions, as shown in the shaded cells of Table 8.6. For example, the expected frequency for cell (a), based on the marginals for *benign*, is $(55 \times 65)/100 = 35.75$. The

---

[8]Almost all writers describe kappa as chance-corrected agreement, but Uebersax (2011) has written forcefully about why he believes kappa does not correct for chance agreement.

expected frequency in cell (d), based on the marginals for *malignant*, is $(35 \times 45)/100 =$ 15.75. These are the values that are intended to correspond to statistical independence, although strictly speaking, independence is not the case in kappa situations because the raters are rating *the same stimuli*. The expected proportion in agreement (P_e) in this example—the proportion that might be achieved by chance—is .3575 + .1575 = .515. Now kappa can be computed, using the following formula:

$$\kappa = \frac{P_o - P_e}{1 - P_e} \tag{8.7}$$

where P_o = the observed proportion in agreement, and P_e = the expected proportion in agreement. For the data in Table 8.7,

$$\kappa = \frac{.80 - .515}{1 - .515} = .588$$

Use of kappa relies on several assumptions. First, it is assumed that the stimuli (e.g., people) being rated are independent of one another. All ratings should be made by the same k raters. Finally, the rating categories should be independent of one another, which requires careful delineation of the categories. Strictly speaking, kappa also assumes independence of the ratings, which is not totally possible for intrarater reliability. When kappa is used for intrarater reliability, the value is likely to be inflated, but we offer suggestions later in this chapter for designing a study that minimizes memory bias.

Kappa can be easily calculated within SPSS and in myriad free online calculators. Using the data in Table 8.7, we would learn from selecting options within the SPSS Crosstabs procedure that the value of kappa was .588 and that this value was statistically significant at $p < .001$. SPSS calculated the 95% CI around the kappa statistic to be .427 to .739.

When the interest is in refining or understanding rater agreement, Uebersax (2011) recommends also testing for **marginal homogeneity**, which refers to whether the raters distribute their ratings in a comparable fashion. One reason that raters might not have strong agreement is that they might have different propensities to use each category (e.g., a leniency or severity bias). To assess marginal homogeneity, which would be indicated by the lack of significant differences in the distribution of ratings, the simplest test is McNemar's test for a 2×2 table. (The chi-square test would not be appropriate because the ratings are paired rather than independent). In our example, marginal homogeneity was *not* found ($p = .041$). Rater 1 was significantly more likely than Rater 2 to give a malignancy rating (45% vs. 35%, respectively). This difference suggests the need for further investigation and perhaps revisions to the rating protocol or to rater training.

8.4.c Weighted Kappa for Ordinal Ratings

Other methods have been proposed for situations in which the ratings are not categorical, but rather are rank ordered and j (the number of rating categories) is greater than 2. For example, assessment of mammograms using the Breast Imaging Reporting and Data System (BI-RADS) classification involves having radiologists rate lesions using seven categories based on assessed likelihood of malignancy (negative, benign, probably benign, low suspicion of malignancy, intermediate suspicion, moderate suspicion, and highly suggestive of malignancy). In such situations, it is often desirable to give "partial credit" to raters whose ratings are not identical but in close proximity rather than to simply classify all disagreements equally.

With ordinal ratings, one can compute a **weighted kappa**, a statistic that involves multiplying the observed and expected proportions in each cell by a weight prior to calculating kappa. Numerous weighting systems have been used, including ones that rely on expert judgments (Cohen, 1968). *Linear weights* are one option. For example, the weight would be 0 if two raters gave identical ratings, 1 if their ratings were rated in contiguous categories,

2 if the ratings were apart by two categories, and so on. The most widely used weighting scheme is *quadratic weights*, which involves squaring the linear weights. In the example of linear weights of 0, 1, 2, 3, 4, 5, and 6 for the seven-category BI-RAD scheme, quadratic weights would be 0, 1, 4, 9, 16, 25, and 36, respectively.

Crewson (2005) provides a fully worked out example of weighted kappa. Manual computations are laborious, but there are online calculators (e.g., http://vassarstats.net/kappa .html). SPSS does not perform weighted kappa calculations. However, when quadratic weights are used, weighted kappa is mathematically identical to $ICC_{Agreement}$ (Fleiss & Cohen, 1973). Streiner and Norman (2008), in fact, offer this advice: "Our recommendation would be to forget about kappa or weighted kappa for any except the most simple 2 × 2 tables, and use the ICC instead" (p. 188).

8.4.d Multirater Kappa

Thus far we have discussed situations in which the number of raters or measurement replications (k) equals two in designs that are fully crossed. In some cases, however, more than two raters make judgments about the same stimuli. A statistic called **multirater kappa** can be computed with multiple raters for both dichotomous and multicategory ratings (i.e., for $k \times j$ situations).

There are several alternate methods for calculating multirater kappa (e.g., Conger, 1980; Gwet, 2012; Uebersax, 1982), and no consensus about which one is preferable. The two most commonly used multirater kappas were proposed by Light (1971) and Fleiss (1971) in a single issue of the journal *Psychological Bulletin*. Light's approach essentially involves computing kappa for all rater pairs and then taking the mean. A related strategy proposed by Davies and Fleiss (1982) involves using the average expected proportion (P_e) for all rater pairs.

Fleiss's (1971) method, in which a statistic sometimes referred to as *generalized kappa* is computed, uses the average proportion of agreement among pairs of raters. His approach involves arraying information about agreement into a *table of agreement* that summarizes the number of agreements in a patient X classification matrix. For example, suppose there were five raters and three rating categories (e.g., benign, suspicious, malignant for mammograms). If three pairs of raters agreed on a "malignant" rating and two pairs agreed on a "suspicious" category for the first patient, the proportion of all possible pairs (which is $k (k-1) = 20$) in agreement would be .40. One could then compute a mean proportion of agreement across patients and use this value in a kappa formula for P_o. With regard to the expected proportion (P_e), the proportion of classifications in agreement for each of the three diagnostic categories need to be squared and summed. Then, the P_o and P_e values would be used to compute the generalized kappa value using the standard kappa formula.

In SPSS and other general statistical software packages, Light's (1971) method could be used to compute kappa for each pair of raters and the mean then could be calculated. There are also several websites that offer SPSS syntax macros for computing multirater kappa (e.g., Nichols, 1998) as well as a few online calculators. An alternative might be to use ICC in lieu of kappa (Rae, 1988).

8.4.e Kappa in Not Fully Crossed Designs

In the scenarios discussed thus far, every k rater provides ratings for all N patients—that is to say, the design is fully crossed. In some situations, however, multiple raters assess different patients. For example, Rickard and colleagues (2012), in their clinical trial to compare clinically indicated versus routine replacement of peripheral intravenous catheters, used several pairs of nurses in multiple sites to assess the interrater reliability of phlebitis assessments. In such a design, Cohen's kappa is not appropriate. For nested designs (Table 8.4[A]), either Light's (1971) multirater kappa or Fleiss' (1971) generalized kappa could be used. For unbalanced designs (Table 8.4[B]), Fleiss's kappa could be used, but the modification suggested by Uebersax (1982) takes rater overlap into account, whereas Fleiss' method does not.

8.4.f Interpretation of Kappa

Although values for kappa theoretically can range between -1 and $+1$, they are almost always in the 0 to 1 range. A kappa of 1.0 means that all ratings are along the diagonal of the contingency table. Several writers, notably Fleiss (1981) and Landis and Koch (1977), have suggested guidelines for interpreting kappa values. For example, Fleiss describes kappas higher than .75 as "excellent," but Landis and Koch described the same value as "substantial." Landis–Koch guidelines are most often cited: In their scheme, kappas less than .20 are *poor*, .21 to .40 are *fair*, .41 to .60 are *moderate*, .61 to .80 are *substantial*, and .81 and greater are *almost perfect*. Most contemporary writers depict these guidelines as arbitrary, and some have said they are more harmful than helpful (Gwet, 2012) or inappropriate (Uebersax, 2011). Nevertheless, we think that values under .60 might prompt researchers to modify the instrument, the raters, the training protocol, or other aspects of the measurement situation or, at least, to report more detail about the assessment circumstances to facilitate interpretation.

A major reason for being wary about strict criteria for interpreting kappa is that the values are so strongly dependent on the marginal distributions. Kappa is severely reduced if one classification category has a substantially higher prevalence or base rate than others, making it hard to compare kappa values across populations and even across studies with the same population. With skewed distributions, proportion of agreement can be substantial and yet kappa can be low, a phenomenon sometimes referred to as the *kappa paradox* (Cicchetti & Feinstein, 1990). Adjustments to kappa have been proposed by statisticians to take prevalence (Byrt, Bishop, & Carlin, 1993) and rater bias (Siegel & Castellan, 1988) into account, but these adjustments have not been universally endorsed (e.g., DiEugenio & Glass, 2004; Hoehler, 2000). Nevertheless, as suggested by Hallgren (2012), when a distribution is markedly skewed or when a known bias is present, it would be useful to calculate and report both the unadjusted and adjusted values of kappa. Neither adjustment is currently available in SPSS or SAS.

Because of these various issues, when interpreting kappa, it is a good idea to look at values for positive and negative agreement, to consider the case mix and the prevalence of each category, and to examine tests for marginal homogeneity. Also, Dunn (1989) has suggested that the interpretation of kappa can be aided by considering the maximum value for kappa for the set of data in question. This maximum value uses the scores that would be secured for the maximum amount of agreement, given the marginal totals. For example, in Table 8.7, the maximum agreement scores in cells a, b, c, and d would be 55, 10, 0, and 35, respectively. Rater 1 scored 55 images as benign, and so the maximum amount of agreement in cell a would be 55, leaving a value of 0 in cell c. For the data in Table 8.7, the computed value of kappa was .588, and the maximum value, given the marginals, is .794.

8.5 Reliability and Item Response Theory

IRT methods result in statistical indexes relating to precision and reliability that are different from the population-dependent methods discussed in this chapter; although, as we will see in Chapter 9, there are IRT indexes that correspond to CTT-based indexes of internal consistency. In IRT, the concept of *information* is usually used in lieu of reliability. Information, which is population independent, is a conditional expression of measurement precision—that is, it is measurement precision for a single person. The assessment of item and test information in IRT-based measures is discussed in Chapter 10, which focuses on measurement error.

Scales created using IRT techniques can also be assessed for the types of reliability discussed in this chapter, in which case the results are dependent on the group with which the assessments are made. In particular, IRT-derived scales can be evaluated for test–retest and interrater reliability.

Test–retest reliability can be assessed with both static measures developed using IRT methods and with computerized adaptive tests. Such assessments have been used in several initiatives within the Patient Reported Outcomes Measurement Information System (PROMIS®) project. For example, Varni and colleagues (2014) computed 2-week test–retest reliability coefficients for nine pediatric scales created using IRT. In their sample, the retest reliability coefficients for the nine short-form scales (using raw summed scores) ranged from .62 (pain interference) to .77 (mobility). Retest coefficients for the nine scales administered by means of computerized adaptive testing (CAT) were similar, ranging from .65 (pain interference) to .80 (fatigue).

IRT scaling methods have also been used with items that require observational ratings. For example, Yang and colleagues (2013) used IRT to select optimal items to screen for delirium. Several of their dimensions relied on observational judgments (e.g., observational ratings of inattention and disorganized thinking). Application of such IRT-based measures would require interrater reliability assessment to ensure that observers could consistently apply the ratings.

8.6 Designing a Reliability Study

A study to evaluate the reliability of a measure requires careful planning. In this section, we offer some guidance on designing such a study.

8.6.a Study Design

Reliability studies require an overall study design. In many cases, the design is fairly simple—for example, administration of the measure at T1, and then a retest at T2 of everyone in the T1 sample, or, for intrarater reliability, ratings at T1 and then at T2. Few designs with a time component involve more than two measurements per patient.

The design of an interrater reliability study does, however, require careful thought. The most straightforward interrater analyses for ICCs and kappas are with fully crossed designs. When such designs are not feasible, it is probably advantageous, in terms of the analysis of agreement data, to adopt a nested design. Unbalanced designs require more complex statistical work.

Some researchers design their retest studies in such a way that retest reliability is not computed for the full sample; it is calculated based only on a subset of people who report at T2 that their status on the target attribute has not changed or has changed minimally. For example, Yorke and colleagues (2011) evaluated the reliability of a measure of dyspnea, the Dyspnea-12 scale; they calculated retest reliability only for patients who said on a health transition question that their overall health was "about the same" at the time of the 2-week retest as it had been before. Such a procedure has intuitive appeal because it focuses the reproducibility assessment on people who claim to be stable. However, such a study design has certain risks. For example, if a substantial percentage of people report that they *have* changed, this suggests that a flawed decision may have been made about the retest interval. Moreover, it is possible that people who are stable over the interval are more homogeneous than the full initial sample, and greater homogeneity depresses retest reliability. Indeed, in a meta-analysis of factors affecting the retest reliability of back pain scales, Geere, Geere, and Hunter (2013) found that the inclusion of a transition item in the study was associated with significantly lower ICC values. The use of transition scales to create subgroups for retest calculations should be done with caution, especially if the percentage reporting change is substantial.

8.6.b Timing of Measurements

As the foregoing discussion suggests, a critical design decision in a reliability study concerns the timing of the measurements. Ideally, measurements would be simultaneous, because the definition of reliability is the extent to which repeated measurements yield the same score for an attribute that has not changed. Stability can best be ensured if the measurements are made at the same time. Simultaneity is possible in interrater reliability studies when there is a permanent record (e.g., mammogram images) or when it is possible for observers to watch an ongoing event or behavior concurrently, but in such instances, the issue of vantage point might make it questionable to assume that observations were identical. Simultaneous measurements are impossible for test–retest, intrarater, and parallel test reliability. Thus, in most reliability studies, researchers must schedule the measurements at times that enhance the likelihood that extraneous and transient measurement errors will be minimized.

As alluded to earlier in this chapter, timing decisions must balance the risks for different potential sources of error. When the time interval is too brief, carryover effects (the memory of scoring on the previous measurement and the desire to be consistent) can lead to artificially high estimates of reliability. If, on the other hand, people are not paying sufficient attention at the second measurement—due to fatigue, boredom, or irritation—then reliability estimates could be depressed. Other factors, such as the therapeutic effect of the first measurement, learning effects, sensitization, response shift, and regression to the mean, could influence scores on the second measurement. Many experts advise that the time interval between PRO measurements should be in the vicinity of 1 to 2 weeks (e.g., Deyo, Diehr, & Patrick, 1991; Nunnally & Bernstein, 1994; Streiner & Norman, 2008). For physical measurements (e.g., skinfold assessment), even shorter intervals are desirable.

Experimental evidence to support time interval advice for health measurements is rare. Marx, Menezes, Horovitz, Jones, and Warren (2003) conducted a randomized controlled trial (RCT) in which patients who completed a battery of health status measurements were randomly assigned to a retest interval of 2 days or 2 weeks. The researchers found no significant differences for the two time intervals on ICCs and measurement error statistics. Their conclusions of no differences have, however, been challenged (Stratford, 2004) because of their small sample size. Additional evidence from RCTs regarding the interval for widely used health constructs could be useful.

It appears that researchers sometimes opt for "intervals of convenience" (Watson, 2004) in retest research or base their decision on generic advice about appropriate intervals. Finding the right time interval to balance the myriad concerns of retest research will probably require some effort. For example, the researchers' conceptualization of the construct could include a vision of how the construct would evolve over time and what factors would affect the timing and amount of change. Experts who are knowledgeable about the theoretical or clinical aspects of the construct could be asked to recommend an appropriate interval—for example, in the context of a content validity study. Another strategy is to undertake a small substudy in which a health transition question regarding change is asked several times over a period of time (e.g., weekly for 1 month) as a way of estimating the trajectory of change for the attribute. Polit (2014) has offered several suggestions for strategies to improve decision making about the retest interval and for basing decisions on evidence or theory about an attribute's stability rather than on assumptions. Whatever timing decision is made, the time interval between measurements should always be reported, together with a rationale for the decision.

8.6.c Other Design Issues in Reliability Studies

Meticulous attention to other aspects of a reliability study can help to minimize risks of improper estimation of reliability parameters. Among the many issues to consider, the following are especially important:

■ *Blinding.* For interrater reliability, raters should make their ratings independently and be blinded to the scoring of other raters. In test–retest, intrarater, and parallel test reliability, respondents or observers should be blinded to their original responses or ratings and overall scores.

■ *Comparable measurement circumstances.* To the extent possible, everything about the measurement replications should be identical. For example, in a retest situation, if the original instrument was completed in a hospital, the retest instrument should ideally be administered in the same location and at the same time of day using the same measurement procedures and personnel.

■ *Training.* Everyone involved in the collection of reliability data should be carefully trained in the use of the measure. If interrater reliability is being assessed, all raters or observers should have the same level of experience and training.

■ *Attrition.* Because most reliability studies unfold over time, there is a risk of study participants' attrition from the study. Loss of participants can lower the precision of reliability estimates and make it necessary to discard the first measurement instance, and, of course, attrition can result in a biased and likely more homogeneous sample. Numerous strategies can be used to encourage ongoing participation in a study, but the evidence suggests that a particularly important strategy is to offer incentives (especially monetary incentives) for study retention in multiwave research (e.g., Collins, Ellickson, Hays, & McCaffrey, 2000; Gates et al., 2009; Henderson, Wight, Nixon, & Hart, 2010).

■ *Ordering.* For intrarater reliability studies, it might be advantageous to randomly order the study participants on each rating occasion to enhance the independence of the k ratings. In retest studies of PRO scales, the ordering of items could be ordered differently on the two testings, unless there is a theoretically relevant ordering. And in parallel test assessment, respondents should be randomly assigned to different orderings of the alternate forms.

■ *A priori standard.* A minimum standard for ICC or kappa values should be specified prior to data collection to resist the temptation of calling any reliability estimate "adequate" after the analysis.

8.6.d Sampling in Reliability Studies

Sampling is a key issue in the design of a reliability study. To the extent possible, the people being measured should be representative of the population for whom the measure is designed, and, if relevant, the raters should also be representative of a population of potential raters.

With regard to those being measured, it is important to use a heterogeneous sample from the population of interest, because with a homogeneous sample, the reliability estimates will be depressed. It is not, however, appropriate to artificially inflate variability by including members of a different population. For example, if a patient-reported scale is designed to assess fatigue in patients with cancer, then a retest reliability study should not include patients without cancer. Reliability estimates would almost certainly be higher because of the increased heterogeneity, but the estimate would tell us nothing about how reliably the scale could discriminate among patients with cancer.

A lot has been written about sample size for reliability studies, but there is no consensus about the strategy to use for estimating sample size requirements. Some have proposed methods to estimate sample sizes needed to achieve statistical significance (e.g., Donner & Eliasziw, 1987). However, the purpose of a reliability study is to draw conclusions about how reliable a measure is (i.e., how close the value is to 1.0), not to draw conclusions about whether it is statistically different from zero. Thus, this approach is not recommended.

Others have suggested a fixed number for reliability studies, but the problem is that the recommended numbers vary widely, ranging from 50 to several hundred. Cicchetti (1976) argued that increasing the sample size much above 50 was not worth the added cost. Streiner and Norman (2008) also noted that "going above 50 subjects . . . in many situations is probably overkill" (p. 201). DeVet and colleagues (2011) recommend using 50 people as "the starting point for negotiations" (p. 127).

A method that has particular appeal is to base sample size estimates on the confidence interval around an estimated reliability coefficient (e.g., Giraudeau & Mary, 2001). To arrive at N, researchers need to estimate the value of the reliability coefficient, specify the desired precision of the estimate, and know how many measurement replications (k) there will be. Using the formula from Giraudeau and Mary, we have created a table displaying sample size requirements for some likely scenarios for ICCs (Table 8.8).

As an illustration, Table 8.8 shows that if the expected ICC were .75 and we were willing to tolerate a 95% CI of ± .10 (i.e., from .65 to .85), a sample of 74 participants would be needed for a simple test–retest situation or a two-rater interrater reliability assessment. Only 50 people would be needed if the estimated ICC were .80 for a two-measurement situation with the same level of precision, and this is perhaps what DeVet and colleagues were considering as a "starting point." However, some have urged researchers to use much larger samples to improve the level of precision of reliability estimates; for example, 95% CIs of ± .05 (Polit, 2014; Watson, 2004).

Table 8.8 makes clear that sample size requirements decrease when (1) the anticipated ICC is larger, (2) lower precision is required, and (3) there are more measurements. In test–retest, intrarater, and parallel test situations, k is typically 2. For interrater reliability, smaller Ns are needed to achieve a given level of precision when there are more than two raters.

Table 8.8	Sample Size Requirements (N) for Specified Estimated Values of the Intraclass Correlation Coefficient, 95% CIs, and Number of Measurements (k)			
		Number of Measurements (k)		
Estimated ICC	95% CI: ±	2	3	4
.70	.05	400	266	222
	.10	100	67	56
	.15	45	30	25
.75	.05	295	200	170
	.10	74	50	42
	.15	33	22	19
.80	.05	200	139	119
	.10	50	35	30
	.15	22	15	13
.85	.05	119	84	73
	.10	50	35	30
	.15	13	9	8

Note: Estimates of N are based on the formula in Giraudeau and Mary (2001).

For those whose scenarios differ from those in Table 8.8, we offer this formula, which we have simplified from Giraudeau and Mary (2001) to facilitate computation for a 95% CI:

$$N = \frac{30.73 \, (1.0 - \text{ICC})^2 \, [1 + (k - 1) \, \text{ICC}]^2}{k \, (k - 1.0) \, w^2}$$

where N = estimated needed sample size, ICC = estimated intraclass correlation coefficient, k = number of measurement replicates, and w = the *total* width of the 95% CI (i.e., $w = .10$ for CI $\pm$ .05). Thus, for 95% CIs at $\pm$ .05, $\pm$ .10, and $\pm$ .15, (as in Table 8.8), the value of w^2 would be .01, .04, and .09, respectively.

We think it is advantageous to use large samples when this is possible. Researchers may be tempted to estimate the ICC as the value they hope to achieve, not as the value they can reasonably expect. Also, although it may be appealing to allow a $\pm$ .10 or greater 95% CI around an ICC estimate, this margin leaves open a very wide and possibly unacceptable range of possible values for the reliability estimate. Clearly, smaller confidence intervals inspire greater trust that reliability is adequate.

Sample sizes for kappa are difficult to estimate because information is needed not only about the expected value of kappa but also about the expected proportion of positive ratings. In general, the more skewed the distribution of positive versus negative ratings, the larger the sample must be. A table with some examples for kappa at different estimated values, for different proportions of positive ratings, and for different lower bounds to a confidence interval has been prepared by Sims and Wright (2005). To illustrate, their table indicates that to detect a kappa estimated to be .70 with a lower bound of .50 and power = .80, a sample size of 380 is needed when the expected proportion of positive ratings is .90 (or .10), but a sample size of 148 would suffice for 50–50 proportions. Higher estimated values of kappa correspond with smaller sample size needs. Thus, if kappa is estimated to be .90 with a lower bound of .70, the sample size needed would be 273 and 101, respectively, for the proportions in the previous example (i.e., 90–10 and 50–50). Other advice on sample size for kappas is offered by Flack, Afifi, Lachenbruch, and Schouten (1988) and Cantor (1996).

8.7   Achieving Adequate Reliability

For PROs and observational scales, the inclusion of carefully developed and tested items is essential to achieving good reliability. Advice on how to develop robust scales was offered in Chapter 4, and different strategies for selecting strong items were described in Chapters 5 to 7. A useful scale construction strategy to inform item selection for a PRO, from the point of view of test–retest reliability, is to evaluate the degree to which item responses are stable over the designated interval. This implies that a retest assessment would be scheduled even before the scale is finalized (Chapter 4).

A useful way to think about reliability as captured by the ICC is that it is analogous to an ANOVA situation in which the goal is to maximize between-patient variability while minimizing error variability. Between-patient variability can be increased by selecting a heterogeneous sample from the target population, as noted earlier. It can also be made larger by adding more items to a multi-item scale or by combining the scores of multiple raters. In Chapter 9 we explain the *Spearman–Brown prophecy formula*, which can be used to estimate how many more items (or how many more raters) would need to be added to achieve a desired reliability.

With regard to error variance, a general overall strategy is to consider in advance what the possible sources of measurement error might be. What factors might affect the measurements and add "noise" to the scores? If sources of measurement error can be envisioned, then steps should be taken to minimize those threats. For example, if it is suspected that scores on a performance test might decline over the course of the day, then everyone should be given the test at the same time of day. Our advice for designing a reliability study (Section 8.6) offers some suggestions for how to enhance reliability values. For example, care in training personnel and in standardizing the measurement protocols can help to reduce extraneous measurement error. During training for an interrater reliability study, if some raters are found to be consistently more extreme than others, it might be advisable to remove them from the study or replace them with other raters.

Sophisticated methods have been developed to tease out sources of measurement error and thus focus on ways to reduce error variance. These methods derive from **generalizability theory** (or *G theory*), an approach developed by psychometrician Lee Cronbach and colleagues (Cronbach, Gleser, Nanda, & Rajaratnam, 1972). Generalizability theory is the framework for a *G study*, the goal of which is to more precisely analyze sources of variation in measurements. In a G study, sources of variation—referred to as *facets*—may include patients, raters, items, time, settings, and so on. The purpose of a G study is to quantify the amount of error variance associated with each facet and with interactions among facets. Results from a G study can be used in an inquiry aimed at making measurement decisions—a so-called *D study*. As an example, we have seen that using averaged scores rather than single scores results in higher ICC values. In a D study, a researcher could explore whether having more measurements or more raters results in a greater improvement to reliability. Full explication of generalizability theory is beyond the scope of this book, but interested readers are encouraged to consult Streiner and Norman (2008) for a brief introduction or lengthier treatments by Brennan (2010) or Cardinet, Johnson, and Pini (2010).

8.8 Reporting a Reliability Study

When preparing a paper to describe a reliability study, researchers must share many of the details of their work, including design and sampling decisions, the population studied, statistical analyses undertaken, and reliability estimates. Here are some of the questions that researchers should consider addressing in their papers, some of which are relevant for only certain types of reliability assessment:

- *Type of reliability.* What type of reliability was assessed (e.g., interrater, test–retest, etc.)? Why was this type selected? What types of measurement error were of special concern? Why were other types *not* addressed?

- *Nature of the measure.* What type of instrument or measure is being assessed? If the measure is a multi-item instrument, is it a formative index or a reflective scale? What type of scores does it yield in terms of level of measurement? What types of application of the measure are envisioned?

- *Population.* For whom was the measure developed? What are the key demographic and clinical characteristics of the target population?

- *Sample.* How was the sample recruited? What efforts were made to recruit a heterogeneous and representative sample? What percentage of people invited to participate actually participated? What are the key demographic and clinical characteristics of the sample? If there are any known biases in the sample, relative to the population, what are they?

- *Sample size.* How large was the sample? How was the sample size decision made? What parameter estimates were used in estimating sample size requirements?

- *Attrition.* What percentage of people who started the study failed to complete it? What efforts were made to minimize attrition? How do the characteristics of those who withdrew from the study differ from the characteristics of those who remained?

■ *Timing.* When were measurements made? What was the time interval between measurements, and what was the rationale for this schedule? If measurements were simultaneous, what was done to ensure similar vantage points?

■ *Raters.* How many raters were there and what were their characteristics? How were they trained, and what prior experience was required of them? In the measurement design, were raters and people being rated fully crossed, and, if not, what design was used and why?

■ *Procedures.* How were the measurements made, and under what circumstances? What efforts were made to maintain constancy across measurements? Who was blinded, and to what were they blinded? Was the ordering of the measurements controlled, and, if so, how and why?

■ *Data preparation.* How extensive were missing values? What strategies were used to address missing data problems?

■ *Statistical decisions.* Which reliability parameter was estimated? If an ICC was used, was ICC for consistency or agreement computed, and why? Was a fixed or random effects model specified? If the design was not fully crossed, was the appropriate ICC model used? Were single or averaged measurements used to compute the ICC? If kappa was computed, was it Cohen's kappa, Fleiss's kappa, or another version of kappa? Was marginal homogeneity examined? For ordinal data, were the scores weighted prior to calculating kappa? If yes, what weighting scheme was used, and what was the rationale? In a multirater kappa situation, was reliability estimated through a multirater kappa statistic or through an ICC?

■ *Statistical results.* For ICCs and kappas, what were the reliability values, and what were the confidence intervals around the estimates? For kappa, what was the proportion of agreement, and (for $k = 2$) what proportion was positive and negative agreement? Was there marginal homogeneity? Were adjusted kappas computed, and, if so, what were the values? What statistic was used if there were more than two raters?

■ *Interpretation.* What might the reliability estimates mean? How might they be improved? What effect might any known biases have had on the estimates? What steps would be needed to replicate the results in other studies?

Answers to many of these questions help readers to draw conclusions about an important aspect of a measure's quality—namely, its reliability. For those evaluating reliability reports, one level of assessment involves determining whether the researchers addressed the appropriate questions from this list (e.g., did they state the time interval between measurements?). Another level of assessment involves evaluating the researchers' decisions (e.g., was the time interval justifiable, and to what extent might that interval have depressed or inflated the reliability estimate?). And the third level involves an evaluation of the results: Do the ICC or kappa values support an inference of good reliability?

Many important evaluative questions with regard to reporting and study design have been incorporated into the COSMIN checklists (DeVet et al., 2011; Mokkink et al., 2010a; Terwee et al., 2012). For evaluating reliability evidence, Box B, which lists 15 assessment questions, should be considered. Although the checklists were designed primarily for those evaluating measurement studies, they can be usefully applied to a self-evaluation of a manuscript for a measurement study prior to submission.

References

Brennan, R. L. (2010). *Generalizability theory*. New York, NY: Springer–Verlag.

Byrt, T., Bishop, J., & Carlin, J. B. (1993). Bias, prevalence, and kappa. *Journal of Clinical Epidemiology, 46*, 423–429.

Cantor, A. B. (1996). Sample-size calculations for Cohen's kappa. *Psychological Methods, 1*, 150–153.

Cardinet, J., Johnson, S., & Pini, G. (2010). *Applying generalizability theory using EduG*. New York, NY: Routledge.

Charter, R. A., & Feldt, L. (2001). Meaning of reliability in terms of correct and incorrect clinical decisions: The art of decision-making is still alive. *Journal of Clinical and Experimental Neuropsychology, 23*, 530–577.

Cicchetti, D. V. (1976). Assessing interrater reliability for rating scales: Resolving some basic issues. *British Journal of Psychiatry, 129*, 452–456.

Cicchetti, D. V., & Feinstein, A. R. (1990) High agreement but low kappa: II. Resolving the paradoxes. *Journal of Clinical Epidemiology, 43*, 551–558.

Cohen, J. (1960). A coefficient of agreement for nominal scales. *Educational and Psychological Measurement, 20*, 37–46.

Cohen, J. (1968). Weighted kappa: Nominal scale agreement with provision for scaled disagreement or partial credit. *Psychological Bulletin, 70*, 213–220.

Collins, R. L., Ellickson, P., Hays, R., & McCaffrey, D. (2000). Effects of incentive size and timing on response rates to a follow-up wave of a longitudinal mailed survey. *Evaluation Review, 24*, 347–363.

Conger, A. J. (1980). Integration and generalization of kappas for multiple raters. *Psychological Bulletin, 88*, 322–328.

Crewson, P. E. (2005). Reader agreement studies. *American Journal of Roentgenology, 184*, 1391–1396.

Cronbach, L. J., Gleser, G. C., Nanda, H., & Rajaratnam, N. (1972). *The dependability of behavioral measurements: Theory of generalizability for scores and profiles.* New York, NY: John Wiley & Sons.

Davies, M., & Fleiss, J. L. (1982). Measurement agreement for multinomial data. *Biometrics, 38*, 1047–1051.

DeVet, H. C. W., Terwee, C., Mokkink, L. B., & Knol, D. L. (2011). *Measurement in medicine: A practical guide.* Cambridge, MA: Cambridge University Press.

Deyo, R. A., Diehr, P., & Patrick, D. L. (1991). Reproducibility and responsiveness of health status measures: Statistics and strategies for evaluation. *Controlled Clinical Trials, 12*(4 Suppl), 142S–158S.

DiEugenio, B., & Glass, M. (2004). The kappa statistic: A second look. *Computational Linguistics, 30*, 95–101.

Donner, A., & Eliasziw, M. (1987). Sample size requirements for reliability studies. *Statistics in Medicine, 6*, 441–448.

Dunn, G. (1989). *Design and analysis of reliability studies.* London, United Kingdom: Edward Arnold.

Fastenau, P. S., Denburg, N., & Mauer, B. (1998). Parallel short forms for the Boston Naming Test: Psychometric properties and norms for older adults. *Journal of Clinical & Experimental Neuropsychology, 20*, 828–834.

Flack, V. F., Afifi, A., Lachenbruch, P., & Schouten, H. (1988). Sample size determinations for the two-rater kappa statistic. *Psychometrika, 53*, 321–325.

Fleiss, J. L. (1971). Measuring nominal scale agreement among many raters. *Psychological Bulletin, 76*, 378–382.

Fleiss, J. L. (1981). *Statistical methods for rates and proportions.* (2nd ed.). New York, NY: John Wiley & Sons.

Fleiss, J. L., & Cohen, J. (1973). The equivalence of weighted kappa and the intraclass correlation coefficient as measures of reliability. *Educational and Psychological Measurement, 33*, 613–619.

Folstein, M., Folstein, S., White, T., & Messer, M. (2010). *MMSE-2: User's manual.* Lutz, FL: PAR.

Gates, S., Williams, M., Withers, E., Williamson, E., Mt-Isa, S., & Lamb, S. (2009). Does a monetary incentive improve the response to a postal questionnaire in a randomised controlled trial? The MINT incentive study. *Trials, 10*, 44.

Geere, J. H., Geere, J. L., & Hunter, P. R. (2013). Meta-analysis identifies Back Pain Questionnaire reliability influenced more by instrument than study design or population. *Journal of Clinical Epidemiology, 66*, 261–267.

Giraudeau, B., & Mary, J. Y. (2001). Planning a reproducibility study: How many subjects and how many replicates per subject for an expected width of 95 percent confidence interval for the intraclass correlation coefficient? *Statistics in Medicine, 20*, 3205–3214.

Gwet, K. (2002). Kappa statistic is not satisfactory for assessing the extent of agreement between raters. *Statistical Methods for Interrater Reliability Assessment Series, 1*, 1–6.

Gwet, K. (2012). *Handbook of interrater reliability* (3rd ed.). Gaithersburg MD: Advanced Analytics.

Hallgren, K. A. (2012). Computing interrater reliability for observational data. *Tutorials in Quantitative Methods for Psychologists, 8*, 23–34.

Henderson, M., Wight, D., Nixon, C., & Hart, G. (2010). Retaining young people in a longitudinal sexual health survey: A trial of strategies to maintain participation. *BMC Medical Research Methodology, 10*, 9.

Hoehler, F. K. (2000). Bias and prevalence effects on kappa viewed in terms of sensitivity and specificity. *Journal of Clinical Epidemiology, 53*, 499–503.

Kraemer, H. C. (2008). Interrater reliability. In *Wiley encyclopedia of clinical trials.* Hoboken, NJ: John Wiley.

Lahey, M. A., Downey, R. G., & Saal, F. (1983). Intraclass correlations: There's more there than meets the eye. *Psychological Bulletin, 93*, 586–595.

Landis, J. R., & Koch, G. G. (1977). The measurement of observer agreement for categorical data. *Biometrics, 33*, 159–174.

Light, R. J. (1971). Measures of response agreement for qualitative data. Some generalizations and alternatives. *Psychological Bulletin, 76*, 365–377.

Luby, M., Bykowski, J., Schellinger, P., Merino, J., & Warach, S. (2006). Intrarater and interrater reliability of ischemic lesion volume measurements on diffusion-weighted, mean transit time and fluid attenuated inversion recovery MRI. *Stroke, 37*, 2951–2956.

Marx, R., Menezes, A., Horovitz, L., Jones, E., & Warren, R. (2003). A comparison of two time intervals for test–retest reliability of health status instruments. *Journal of Clinical Epidemiology, 56*, 730–735.

McGraw, K. O., & Wong, S. P. (1996). Forming inferences about some intraclass correlation coefficients. *Psychological Methods, 1*, 30–46.

Mokkink, L. B., Terwee, C., Patrick, D., Alonso, J., Stratford, P., Knol, D. L., … de Vet, H. C. W. (2010a). The COSMIN checklist for assessing the methodological quality of studies on measurement properties of health status instruments: An international Delphi study. *Quality of Life Research, 19*, 539–549.

Mokkink, L. B., Terwee, C., Patrick, D., Alonso, J., Stratford, P., Knol, D. L., . . . de Vet, H. C. W. (2010b). The COSMIN study reached international consensus on taxonomy, terminology, and definitions of measurement properties for health-related patient-reported outcomes. *Journal of Clinical Epidemiology, 63*, 737–745.

Narayanan, A., Greco, M., & Campbell, J. (2010). Generalisability in unbalanced, uncrossed and fully nested studies. *Medical Education, 44*, 367–378.

Neelon, V. J., Champagne, M. T., Carlson, J., & Funk, S. (1996). The NEECHAM Confusion Scale: Construction, validation, and clinical testing. *Nursing Research, 45*, 324–330.

Nichols, D. P. (1998). SPSS: Choosing an intraclass correlation coefficient. *SPSS Keyworks*, 67.

Nunnally, J., & Bernstein, I. H. (1994). *Psychometric theory* (3rd ed.). New York, NY: McGraw-Hill.

Polit, D. F. (2014). Getting serious about test–retest reliability: A critique of retest research and some recommendations. *Quality of Life Research, 23*(6), 1713–1720.

Putka, D. J., Le, H., McCloy, R. A., & Diaz, T. (2008). Ill-structured measurement designs in organizational research: Implications of estimating interrater reliability. *Journal of Applied Psychology, 93*, 959–981.

Radloff, L. S. (1977). The CES-D scale: A self-report depression scale for research in the general population. *Applied Psychological Measurement, 1*, 385–401.

Rae, G. (1988). The equivalence of multiple rater kappa statistics and intraclass correlation coefficients. *Educational and Psychological Measurements, 48*, 367–374.

Rapkin, B. D., & Schwartz, C. E. (2004). Towards a theoretical model of quality-of-life appraisal: Implications of findings from studies of response shift. *Health & Quality of Life Outcomes, 2*, 14.

Rickard, C. M., Webster, J., Wallis, M. C., Marsh, N., McGrail, M., French, V., . . . Whitby, M. (2012). Routine versus clinically indicated replacement of peripheral intravenous catheters: A randomized controlled equivalency trial. *Lancet, 380*, 1066–1074.

Schmidt, F. L., Le, H., & Ilies, R. (2003). Beyond alpha: An empirical examination of the effects of different sources of measurement error on reliability estimates for measures of individual differences constructs. *Psychological Methods, 8*, 206–224.

Shrout, P. E., & Fleiss, J. L. (1979). Intraclass correlations: Uses in assessing rater reliability. *Psychological Bulletin, 36*, 420–428.

Siegel, S., & Castellan, N. J. (1988). *Nonparametric statistics for the behavioral sciences*. Boston, MA: McGraw-Hill.

Sims, J., & Wright, C. C. (2005). The kappa statistic in reliability studies: Use, interpretation, and sample size requirements. *Physical Therapy, 85*, 257–268.

Sprangers, M. A., & Schwartz, C. E. (1999). Integrating response shift into health-related quality-of-life research: A theoretical model. *Social Science & Medicine, 48*, 1507–1515.

Stratford, P. W. (2004). Comment on the comparison of test–retest reliability for 2-day and 2-week intervals. *Journal of Clinical Epidemiology, 57*, 993–994.

Streiner, D. L., & Norman, G. R. (2008). *Health measurement scales: A practical guide to their development and use* (4th ed.). Oxford: Oxford University Press.

Suen, H. K. (1988). Agreement, reliability, accuracy, and validity. *Behavioral Assessment, 10*, 343–366.

Sullivan, T., Smith, J., Kermode, J., McIver, E., & Courtemanche, D. (1990). Rating the burn scar. *The Journal of Burn Care & Rehabilitation, 11*, 256–260.

Terwee, C. B., Bot, D. S., de Boer, M., van der Windt, D., Knol, D. L., Dekker, J., de Vet, J. C. (2007). Quality criteria were proposed for measurement properties of health status questionnaires. *Journal of Clinical Epidemiology, 60*, 34–42.

Terwee, C. B., Mokkink, L. B., Knol, D. L., Ostelo, R., Bouter, L. M., & DeVet, H. C. W. (2012). Rating the methodological quality in systematic reviews of studies on measurement properties: A scoring system for the COSMIN checklist. *Quality of Life Research, 21*, 651–657.

Uebersax, J. (1982). A generalized kappa coefficient. *Educational and Psychological Measurement, 42*, 181–183.

Uebersax, J. (2011). *Statistical methods for rater and diagnostic agreement*. Retrieved from http://john-uebersax .com/stat/agree.htm

Varni, J. W., Magnus, B., Stucky, B., Lin, Y., Quinn, H., Thissen, D., . . . DeWalt, D. (2014). Psychometric properties of the PROMIS pediatric scales: Precision, stability, and comparison of different scoring and administration options. *Quality of Life Research, 23*(4), 1233–1243.

Watson, D. (2004). Stability versus change, dependability versus error: Issues in the assessment of personality over time. *Journal of Research on Personality, 38*, 319–350.

Weiner, E. A., & Stewart, B. (1984). *Assessing individuals: Psychological and educational tests and measurements*. Boston, MA: Little, Brown.

Weir, J. P. (2005). Quantifying test-retest reliability using the intraclass correlation coefficient and the SEM. *Journal of Strength and Conditioning Research, 19*, 231–240.

Yang, F. M., Jones, R., Inouye, S., Tommet, D., Crane, P., Rudolph, J., . . . Marcantonio, E. R. (2013). Selecting optimal screening items for delirium: An application of item response theory. *BMC Medical Research Methodology, 13*, 8.

Yorke, J., Swigris, J., Russell, A., Moosavi, S. H., Kwong, G. N. M., Longshaw, M., & Jones, P. W. (2011). Dyspnea-12 is a valid and reliable measure of breathlessness in patients with interstitial lung disease. *Chest, 139*, 159–164.

9

Internal Consistency

Chapter Outline

The extended definition of reliability presented in Chapter 3 supports the inclusion of internal consistency as a measurement property within the reliability domain of the measurement taxonomy shown in Figure 3.1:

■ Reliability is the extent to which scores for patients who have not changed are the same for repeated measurements (Mokkink et al., 2010)

For the four types of reliability discussed in Chapter 8, repeated measurements involve multiple measurement *instances*—for example, a test and then a retest, or a measurement by different observers. For internal consistency, replication takes the form of completing multiple items in a composite scale during a single administration. Whereas reliability estimates described in the previous chapter assess a measure's degree of consistency across time, across forms, or across raters, internal consistency captures consistency across items.

Internal consistency concerns the degree to which the items on a scale or subscale are all measuring the same underlying latent trait, and for this reason, it is sometimes referred to as *homogeneity*. As shown in the reliability summary table in the previous chapter (Table 8.2), internal consistency is a relevant measurement property only for multi-item reflective scales and not for formative indexes. Such scales are typically self-reports (patient-reported outcomes [PRO]) but could also be multi-item observational scales. Typically, internal consistency is evaluated for every subscale of a multidimensional scale.

As discussed in Chapter 5, a good reflective multi-item scale created using classical test theory (CTT) methods is one in which the items are highly intercorrelated. Almost all scale developers who use "traditional" methods of scale construction assess their scales for internal consistency and employ it as a tool for final item selection. The term "internal consistency" is seldom used by those who use item response theory (IRT) techniques but, as we shall see, there are analogous concepts within IRT.

9.1 Internal Consistency and Measurement Error

In CTT, an observed score on a multi-item scale is conceptualized as a person's true score, plus or minus error. In reliability estimates, the sources of measurement error vary across types (see Table 8.2). For example, in retest reliability, error could stem from memory and other carryover effects, rehearsal, and so on. In estimating internal consistency, a major source of measurement error stems from the sampling of items.

A single item is often inadequate for measuring a construct; indeed, that is the reason for constructing multi-item scales. In responding to an item, people are influenced not only by the underlying latent trait but also by their interpretation of the item wording and the personal meanings attributed to the words. Measurement error on items results from the influence of forces that are irrelevant to the latent trait. By sampling multiple items with various wordings, item irrelevancies are expected to cancel each other out.

Like other types of reliability, estimates of internal consistency conceptually involve distinguishing variability in a set of scores due to true variation on the construct across patients and error variability. This will become clearer later in the chapter when we demonstrate the relationship between the intraclass correlation coefficient (ICC) and the central parameter of internal consistency, coefficient alpha.

9.2 Parameters of Internal Consistency

Assessments of internal consistency in multi-item tests and scales date back over 100 years. We begin with a brief discussion of an early parameter of internal consistency because early formulas and concepts led to some important insights.

9.2.a Split-Half Reliability

Early in the 20th century, interest in reliability arose in the context of concerns about consistency in measuring intelligence. Psychometricians initially conceptualized reliability as the correlation between two parallel tests (Brennan, 2001). Two independent and comparable tests of the same construct were not always available, so an approximation was achieved by splitting the items on a scale in two, scoring each half-test, and then computing a correlation coefficient between the two. The underlying assumption is that if the half-tests are measuring the same construct (as in two parallel tests), then scores on the two halves should correlate highly. This **split-half reliability** thus yields an estimate of the internal consistency of a multi-item scale.

In 1910, two psychometricians, Charles Spearman and William Brown, independently published a formula for an index of split-half reliability in the *British Journal of Psychology*. The formula represented a formal recognition of the fact that the correlation between two half-tests underestimates the reliability of a full test because longer tests are more reliable than shorter ones. The formula has come to be known as the **Spearman–Brown prophecy formula** because it "predicts" what the reliability would be for a full scale based on the correlation between two half-scales.

Although internal consistency is no longer estimated in this manner, the Spearman–Brown formula is nevertheless useful for other purposes. The formula is:

$$R_{SB} = \frac{k'R}{1 + (k' - 1)R} \tag{9.1}$$

Where R_{SB} = the Spearman–Brown reliability estimate, k' = the factor by which a scale will be increased (or decreased),[1] and R is the original reliability estimate. In the context of a split-half assessment, k' equals 2, and R is the correlation between the two half-tests. So, for example, if the correlation between scores on two halves of a 10-item scale were .60, then the estimated full-test internal consistency would be:

$$R_{SB} = \frac{2\,(.60)}{1 + (2 - 1)\,.60} = \frac{1.20}{1.60} = .75$$

Thus, the formula "prophecies" that the internal consistency for the full 10-item scale would be .75, given that the correlation between the two five-item half-scales is .60.

Traditionally, split-half reliability was estimated using a division of odd versus even items. In our example, R would be calculated by correlating the summed scores for Items 1, 3, 5, 7, and 9 with those for Items 2, 4, 6, 8, and 10. One problem with the split-half approach to estimating an internal consistency parameter, however, is that a multi-item scale can be split in half in many ways. For example, our 10-item scale could be divided 126 different ways.[2] The value of R for different splits can vary markedly. Another limitation of the split-half method is that the procedure provides no diagnostic information about which item or items may be reducing the consistency estimate.

The term "index of reliability" was first used in the 1920s to refer to the coefficient generated in a split-half analysis (Traub, 1997). However, new approaches to estimating internal consistency were developed in recognition of problems with the split-half approach. The widespread availability of computers and statistical software has made these approaches more appealing than using split-half methods.

9.2.b Kuder–Richardson KR-20

In 1937, psychometricians G. Frederic Kuder and Marion Richardson published an article in the journal *Psychometrika* that had a large impact on the assessment of internal consistency. Kuder and Richardson offered formulas for estimating the internal consistency of a single test, without any need to split the items into half-tests. Their most widely known formula is the **KR-20** (Kuder–Richardson, equation 20). The KR-20 formula is appropriate only for scales or tests with items that can be scored dichotomously, such as correct/incorrect, yes/no, present/absent, and so on.

The formula for the KR-20 coefficient is:

$$\text{KR-20} = \frac{k}{k-1}\left(1 - \frac{\Sigma p_i q_i}{\sigma^2_t}\right) \tag{9.2}$$

where k is the number of items on the scale or test, p_i is the proportion of people answering positively (or correctly) to item i, q_i is the proportion of people answering negatively (or incorrectly) to item i, and σ^2_t = the variance of the total scale or test score. Values for KR-20 range from 0.0 for no consistency among items to 1.0 for a totally consistent scale.

Table 9.1 presents fictitious data that we can use to illustrate the calculation of KR-20. Suppose (purely for the sake of illustration) that we devised a simple four-item scale designed to assess children for attention deficit hyperactivity disorder (ADHD). The items represent four parent-reported symptoms and behavior problems associated with ADHD, and 10 parents have completed the scale. Items are coded 1 if the symptom is present and 0 if it is absent. Table 9.1 shows item responses, values for p and q for each item, products for

---

[1] k' is computed as the new test length (number of items), divided by the old test length (original number of items).
[2] The number of splits possible for a k-item test (for ks that are an even number) is $k! \div 2[(k/2)!]^2$.

Table 9.1	Data for KR-20 Example				
Child	**Item A**	**Item B**	**Item C**	**Item D**	**Total Score**
1	1	1	1	0	3
2	1	0	0	0	2
3	0	1	0	1	2
4	0	1	1	1	3
5	1	1	1	1	4
6	1	0	1	1	3
7	0	0	0	0	1
8	0	0	0	0	0
9	1	1	1	0	3
10	1	1	0	1	3
p	.60	.60	.50	.50	$M = 2.20$
q	.40	.40	.50	.50	$\sigma^2 = 1.76$
p^*q	.24	.24	.25	.25	

Note: These fictitious data are shown for parental reports of four children's symptoms and behaviors relating to ADHD, for $N = 10$ children. Data are coded 1 = symptom present, 0 = symptom absent. KR-20 = .591.

$p \times q$, and the variance for the total scale scores. Calculating KR-20 to assess the internal consistency of this scale, we find:

$$\text{KR-20} = \frac{4}{3}\left(1 - \frac{.24 + .24 + .25 + .25}{1.76}\right) = .591$$

Much like the reliability index described in Chapter 8 (the ICC), values close to 1.0 are desirable. The KR-20 value of .591 is thus disappointing. We can, however, use the Spearman–Brown prophecy formula, to guide us during scale development. Suppose that we wanted our ADHD scale to have an internal consistency coefficient of .80. By using the Spearman–Brown formula, we could estimate how many items we would need to add to achieve this level of internal consistency. The formula can be rearranged to arrive at an estimate of desired scale length:

$$k' = \frac{R_{SB}\,(1 - R)}{R\,(1 - R_{SB})} \tag{9.3}$$

In our example, then, we would estimate test length to achieve a KR-20 of .80 as:

$$k' = \frac{.80\,(1 - .591)}{.591\,(1 - .80)} = 2.77$$

Here, k′ is the factor by which the number of items must be increased, so to achieve a KR-20 of .80, the prediction formula suggests that we would need a scale with about 11 items tapping the same construct (2.77 × 4 = 11.08). After adding 7 more items, the internal consistency of the scale would then be re-evaluated.

9.2.c Coefficient Alpha

In 1951, Lee Cronbach published an influential paper in which he presented a formula for testing the internal consistency of a scale comprised of items that are not necessarily dichotomous. This index of internal consistency, usually referred to as **coefficient alpha** (or *Cronbach's alpha*), is essentially an extension of KR-20 to scales with items of any type. Most typically, alpha is computed with Likert-type items that are on an ordinal scale.

One formula for alpha illustrates how it is an extension of the KR-20 formula:

$$\alpha = \frac{k}{k-1}\left(1 - \frac{\Sigma\sigma^2_i}{\sigma^2_t}\right) \qquad (9.4)$$

where k is the number of items, σ^2_i = the variance of individual i items, and σ^2_t = the variance of the total scale or test score. It can be seen that the only difference between equations 9.2 and 9.4 is that the formula for α includes item variances in lieu of $p \times q$ values. Indeed, an item variance for a dichotomous variable *is $p \times q$*, and so the formulas are totally equivalent. Coefficient alpha can be used with dichotomous and ordinal items, and so it is never really necessary to compute KR-20. When we used statistical software to compute coefficient alpha with the data in Table 9.1, the result was an α equal to .591.

Coefficient alpha relies on several assumptions. One of these is an assumption of what is called *tau equivalency*. In psychometrics, scales can be classified in a hierarchy that concerns the degree of similarity among the scale's items or subparts. At the pinnacle of this hierarchy are scales that are *classically parallel*, followed by ones that are *tau-equivalent*, *essentially tau equivalent*, and then *congeneric*.[3] Without elaborating the details of this hierarchy, we note that tau equivalency assumes equal item variances, an assumption that is frequently violated. Streiner and Norman (2008) have pointed out that few scales can demonstrate tau equivalence but rather are congeneric. With congeneric scales, coefficient alpha can be considered a lower bound of internal consistency (Brennan, 2001; Graham, 2006; Miller, 1995).

Another assumption for coefficient alpha is that measurement error for the items are uncorrelated. This assumption implies that errors for items are random, which is not always the case. For example, sometimes early scale items affect responses to subsequent items. Subconsciously, respondents to a scale may strive for consistency and thus may not respond to later items in a totally independent manner. As another example, transient factors (e.g., fatigue) may affect item responses in a consistent manner, thus resulting in correlated errors. The assumption of uncorrelated error is generally ignored when computing coefficient alpha. This has led to criticisms of coefficient alpha, and the advocacy by some of pursuing other strategies, such as structural equation modeling, to estimate internal consistency (e.g., see Green & Yang, 2009; Gu, Little, & Kingston, 2013; Raykov, 1997a, 1997b).

Nevertheless, coefficient alpha is at the moment perhaps the most widely used index relating to scale reliability for multi-item reflective scales in the health and social sciences. It is an index that can readily be calculated in most general-purpose statistical software packages.

To illustrate, we use the Statistical Package for the Social Sciences (SPSS) reliability procedure (within the Scale program) to compute coefficient alpha. We use data from a sample of 1,000 low-income women who completed various health scales, including the Center for Epidemiologic Studies Depression Scale or CES-D (Radloff, 1977). In Chapter 5, we used these data in describing scale construction procedures using a CTT model and illustrated inter-item correlations, item-total correlations, and exploratory factor analysis (EFA) with a subset of 9 of the 20 CES-D items (see Tables 5.2 and 5.6). During scale construction using CTT, internal consistency analysis is almost always undertaken to further guide the selection of items for a scale.

---

[3]For greater elaboration on the hierarchy of scale similarity, readers can consult Brennan (2001), Feldt and Brennan (1989), or Lord and Novick (1968).

A. Reliability statistics for 9 CES-D Items (N = 961)

Cronbach's Alpha	Cronbach's Alpha based on standardized items
.826	.829

B. Item-Total statistics

Item	Scale mean if item deleted	Scale variance if item deleted	Corrected item-total correlation	Squared multiple correlation	Cronbach's Alpha if item deleted
1. More bothered by things than usual	8.23	30.030	.560	.351	.805
3. Couldn't shake off blues	8.34	28.751	.650	.452	.794
5. Trouble keeping mind on things	8.38	30.016	.577	.394	.803
6. Felt depressed	8.20	27.720	.756	.608	.781
7. Felt everything required effort	7.79	32.585	.255	.120	.842
11. Sleep was restless	8.17	29.277	.574	.359	.803
12. Was happy (reversed)	8.26	31.158	.434	.377	.819
16. Enjoyed life (reversed)	8.45	31.764	.364	.349	.827
18. Felt sad	8.34	29.143	.652	.461	.795

C. Scale statistics

Mean	Variance	Std. deviation	N of items
9.27	37.222	6.101	9

D. Intraclass correlation coefficient

	Intraclass correlation[b]	95% Confidence interval		F Test with True Value 0			
		Lower bound	Upper bound	Value	df1	df2	Sig
Single measures	.345[a]	.320	.372	5.748	926	7408	.000
Average measures	.826	.809	.842	5.748	926	7408	.000

Two-way random effects model where both people effects and measures effects are random.

[a]The estimator is the same, whether the interaction effect is present or not.

[b]Type C intraclass correlation coefficients using a consistency definition-the between-measure variance is excluded from the denominator variance.

Figure 9.1

Internal consistency analysis (SPSS) for nine CES-D items in sample of low-income women (nine items subjected to exploratory factor analysis, Chapter 5).

Panel A of Figure 9.1 shows that coefficient alpha for the nine-item CES-D short scale is .826. Panel B shows a wealth of information regarding each scale item. Of particular note, the far-right column of this panel shows what the value of coefficient alpha would be if an item were deleted entirely. Deleting Item 6 (*I felt depressed*), which was a marker variable in the EFA, would lower the scale's internal consistency from .826 to .781. By contrast, deleting Item 7 (*I felt that everything I did was an effort*), which we identified as a problematic item in the EFA, would increase internal consistency ($\alpha = .842$). Based on all the evidence from the analyses in Chapter 5 and these internal consistency analyses, if we were developing this depression scale from scratch for use with a population of low-income women, we would recommend dropping Item 7. It might also be noted that when we ran the reliability analysis for the two-half samples with nearly 500 women in each, the value of alpha was .826 and .827 for samples 1 and 2, respectively, and in both cases, the value of alpha increased when Item 7 was deleted.

Panel C of Figure 9.1 shows some scale statistics for the nine-item CES-D scale (mean, *SD*, and variance). The final panel (D) demonstrates the relationship between coefficient alpha and the ICC. For a single item on this nine-item scale, the ICC (C, 1) is only .345.

However, for the measure averaged across nine items, ICC $(C, 9) = .826$, exactly the same as coefficient alpha. This can be illustrated by offering another formula for alpha:

$$\alpha = \frac{\sigma^2_{BetweenPeople}}{\sigma^2_{BetweenPeople} + \left(\dfrac{\sigma^2_{Error}}{k}\right)} \qquad (9.5)$$

Thus, the formula for alpha is identical to that for ICC consistency, with the error term in the denominator averaged across k items, the same formula that applies to measurements averaged across raters or time periods. From this equation, it is easy to see that increasing k—that is, adding items—will increase the value of α. In our example, instructing the computer to show the ICC $(C, 9)$ provided us with information about the 95% confidence interval (CI) around the coefficient. In the full sample, the 95% CI around the coefficient of internal consistency was .809 to .842.

It may be recalled that in Chapter 5, the factor analysis suggested two subscales—a seven-item subscale that we labeled "Depressed affect" and a two-item subscale (Items 12 and 16) that we called (lack of) "Positive affect." The reliability analysis for the two subscales resulted in alphas of .833 and .719, respectively (not shown in tables). If we wanted to "beef up" internal consistency on the Positive affect subscale, we could use the Spearman–Brown formula to estimate how many items we would need in the subscale. For example, if we wanted an alpha of .80 for the positive affect scale, we would compute the following:

$$k' = \frac{.80 (1 - .719)}{.719 (1 - .80)} = 1.56$$

In other words, the number of items on this subscale of positive affects should be increased by at least 50% to three or four items rather than two ($1.56 \times 2 = 3.13$) to achieve a high level of internal consistency.

9.3   Internal Consistency (Alpha) and Retest Reliability (ICC)

For scales developed within CTT, psychometricians who discuss reliability are usually referring to internal consistency. Psychometricians have tended to be wary of retest assessments due to the many potential hazards of this approach (see Section 8.2.a), although devotion to internal consistency within the field of psychology is far from universal (e.g., McCrae, Kurtz, Yamagata, & Terracciano, 2011). Medical researchers, on the other hand, have valued retest reliability to a greater degree, perhaps in part because of its importance in the measurement of change (see Chapter 17). In this section, we describe some of the similarities and differences between internal consistency (as assessed using coefficient alpha) and retest reliability (as assessed using the ICC).

In terms of similarity, we have already seen that alpha and ICC$_{Consistency}$ (averaged) are mathematically equivalent. Both indexes are estimated by contrasting variability between people against total variability, which includes random measurement error. Coefficient alpha, like the ICC, communicates the degree to which people can be differentiated from one another on the target attribute, *despite* measurement error. Values for both indexes range from 0.0 to 1.0, representing (in CTT) an estimate of the proportion of true score variance that is present in a set of obtained scores. In both cases, similar criteria for excellence have been proposed, although, as discussed in Chapter 8, many commentators argue against having fixed standards because the value of the index is dependent on factors other than the instrument itself, such as sample heterogeneity. Nevertheless, a value of .70 to .75 or higher is often considered acceptable for both alpha and the ICC for group-level comparisons (DeVet, Terwee, Mokkink, & Knol, 2011), but several psychometric experts have advocated a minimum value of .80 or higher (e.g., Carmines & Zeller, 1979; Nunnally & Bernstein, 1994).

Another similarity is that the reliability and internal consistency of an instrument are not properties of the instrument itself but rather of the instrument used with a particular population of patients under certain conditions. When a measure is used with a population different from that used in the instrument development sample, new reliability values should be estimated. One final similarity is that estimates of both retest reliability and internal consistency can be inflated if a measure captures both the focal construct and other personal attributes, such as a social desirability bias. A measure of, say, drug compliance might look internally consistent not because the items on the scale are consistently measuring compliance but rather because they are consistently inducing socially desirable responses. The same bias would likely be in play for retest reliability estimates.

There are also many differences, a major one being that the sources of measurement error differ for internal consistency and retest reliability, as previously discussed and as shown in Table 8.2. Other important ways in which the two measurement properties differ include the following:

■ *Types of measures.* Retest reliability can be assessed for all types of measures, not just multi-item PROs. By contrast, internal consistency is only appropriate for estimating the homogeneity of a set of items in multi-item reflective scales. Internal consistency is not relevant in formative indexes because each item typically captures different constructs.

■ *Number of administrations.* Coefficient alpha can be computed based on responses to items in a single administration, which makes internal consistency easier to estimate than retest reliability. In calculating the coefficient alpha based on responses at one point in time, researchers do not worry about real change in the construct, nor about carry-over effects, response shift, attrition bias, or other potential sources of error. However, this means that internal consistency does not provide information about transient error.

■ *Role in instrument development.* For multi-item reflective scales constructed within a CTT framework, coefficient alpha plays a key role in instrument development. Diagnostic information about items, such as that presented in Figure 9.1 (Panel B), augments the item analyses and factor analyses that guide final selection of items. By contrast, retest reliability is seldom used as a diagnostic tool for item selection, although we would argue that examining retest item performance can be very valuable for enhancing retest reliability (see Section 4.3.b, Chapter 4).

■ *Reassessments.* Retest reliability is assessed infrequently in the life of a multi-item scale. Researchers who develop a new scale should ideally assess retest reliability, but some do not, especially if their training has been in traditional psychometrics. Other researchers seeking confirmation that an existing scale applies to a different population, or researchers who adapt or translate a scale, should also reassess retest reliability. Typically, however, users of an existing scale do not evaluate retest reliability; they administer the scale only once, or only before and after a real change on the construct is expected to occur. By contrast, virtually everyone who creates a multi-item reflective CTT scale assesses its internal consistency, and most researchers who use an existing scale in a new study re-compute coefficient alpha with their own data. Indeed, reassessment of coefficient alpha with each use of an instrument is advisable. Thus, retest reliability is typically assessed only within the context of methodologic work, whereas internal consistency is assessed in both methodologic and substantive research. This, in turn, means that there typically is far more evidence about a scale's internal consistency than there is about its reproducibility.

■ *Upper criterion.* As noted, values exceeding .70 for both the ICC and alpha are often recommended. However, no *maximum* retest reliability value has been advocated; an ICC of 1.0 would be ideal, albeit virtually unattainable. By contrast, some have advised against alpha values exceeding .90 (e.g., DeVet et al., 2011; Streiner & Norman, 2008). This is because alphas in excess of .90 may be the result of overredundancy of items and may create excessive respondent burden. When alpha exceeds .90, it might be prudent to remove an item or two using the Spearman–Brown formula to estimate how many items would be needed to achieve an alpha of, say, .85 or .90.

One final issue concerns the long debate in psychometric circles about upper bounds of reliability. As mentioned earlier, because underlying assumptions are typically violated, coefficient alpha has been shown to be a lower bound for estimates of internal consistency. Some, however, have asserted that coefficient alpha yields an upper limit for reliability estimation in comparison with other types of reliability. That is, it has been claimed that values of internal consistency indexes generally can be expected to be higher than for retest reliability coefficients (e.g., Brennan, 2001). There are inherent problems with such a proposition, however. If, for example, we had a five-item scale to measure self-efficacy and then added five items that were really measures of, say, fatigue, internal consistency would surely be lowered, but the addition of five irrelevant items to a self-efficacy scale might do little to alter retest reliability. Many examples of studies in which retest reliability is higher than internal consistency can readily be found. For example, Chin and Huang (2013) developed and assessed the Diabetes Foot Self-Care Behavior Scale (DFSBS) in a sample of nearly 300 patients with diabetes and peripheral neuropathy. The internal consistency of their seven-item scale was alpha = .73, and the 2-week retest assessment yielded an ICC consistency of .92.

In the final analysis, the decision on whether to assess both internal consistency and retest reliability for a CTT scale will rest on the nature of the construct and the uses to which the instrument are likely to be put and the type of generalizations one wishes to make. Internal consistency supports generalization over items, whereas retest reliability supports generalizations over time. For multi-item reflective scales, assessments of internal consistency are usually pro forma. Retest reliability should be evaluated when a CTT scale will be used in assessments of change because it will be important to distinguish random and transient error from true change in the construct. It is likely to be prudent to assess both retest reliability and internal consistency for most reflective scales used in health care research and in clinical settings.[4]

9.4   Correction for Attenuation

For over 100 years, psychometricians have known that imperfect reliability (measurement error) attenuates or dampens correlation coefficients between variables. In 1904, Charles Spearman wrote a paper in which he presented a formula to "correct for" measurement error when examining the relationship between two imperfectly measured variables. His argument was that scientists are interested in understanding the relationships among constructs in their pure or true form—but that, in practice, we must study relationships of interest using actual measures. Because actual measures contain errors of measurement, estimates of the true correlation between constructs are biased downward.

Spearman's **disattenuation correction** can be either single (correcting for unreliability in the measurement of one of the variables) or double (correcting for the unreliability of both measures). For the double correction, the formula is:

$$\rho_{xy} = \frac{r_{xy}}{\sqrt{R_x}\,\sqrt{R_y}} \tag{9.6}$$

where ρ_{xy} is the corrected correlation, estimating the true correlation, between variables X and Y; r_{xy} is the observed correlation between the two variables; R_x is the reliability of the measure of X; and R_y is the reliability of the measure of Y. For example, if the correlation

---

[4]Some efforts have been made to develop a reliability estimate that takes both internal consistency and stability into account (e.g., Green, 2003), but this work has received little attention among scale developers.

between a measure of self-efficacy (X) and perceived quality of life (Y) in patients with heart failure was .50 and the reliability of the measures of both variables was .80, then the "corrected" correlation between the two constructs would be:

$$\rho_{xy} = \frac{.50}{\sqrt{.80}\ \sqrt{.80}} = .62$$

Such disattenuated correlations are best interpreted as *estimates*, rather than corrections, of how highly two constructs might be correlated if it were possible to measure them with perfect reliability. Double corrections are sometimes used to help understand the upper limits of a measure's validity in assessments of construct validity (Muchinsky, 1996).

A single correction is most often used when a scale is used to predict a criterion, and it is the criterion whose measurement error is typically corrected. The argument for a one-sided correction is that it is a perfectly reliable criterion that one wants to predict on the basis of an imperfect measure (Guilford, 1954). The formula for the single correction puts only one reliability coefficient in the denominator:

$$\rho_{xy} = \frac{r_{xy}}{\sqrt{R_x}} \tag{9.7}$$

where R_x is the reliability of the one measure for which measurement error is being corrected. So, for example, if we used the values from our previous example but corrected only one measure, the original correlation of .50 would be .56 after disattenuation.

The correction for attenuation has been the topic of many debates. One debate that raged for decades in the early part of the 1900s was which reliability estimate to use in the formula—internal consistency or retest reliability. Johnson (1950), for example, argued for using retest reliability, whereas Nunnally and Bernstein (1994) advocated using internal consistency. We have included a discussion of disattenuation is this chapter, rather than in Chapter 8, in part because we think there is some merit to Cureton's (1958) position that the correction applied to coefficient alpha can be used as a diagnostic tool in making decisions about adding, subtracting, or improving items. (Nunnally and Bernstein suggested using the formula to estimate the increased correlation between two variables if the reliability were increased to a particular amount.) However, if the correction is used, it should be applied to the type of reliability estimate that deals with the most relevant type of measurement error for the construct under consideration (Schmidt & Hunter, 1996).

Debates about the disattenuation correction have been reinvigorated by its use in meta-analytic estimates of correlations among variables. For example, Rhodes and Smith (2006) examined personality constructs as correlates of physical activity, and they corrected for attenuation stemming from scale unreliability in the measures used in the primary studies. Muchinsky (1996) has noted several difficulties with such applications of the correction. In particular, issues arise when reliability estimates of the measures used in a primary study are not reported or when reliability estimates are a mixture of retest reliability and internal consistency.

Problems with the correction, such as the possibility that a correction could result in correlations greater than 1.0, have led to debates about whether the correction should be used at all. Muchinsky (1996), in his summary of issues relating to disattenuation, urged "caution" in both the use of the correction and, especially, interpretation of the results, echoing Nunnally's concerns about the risk of "fooling oneself" about the value of correlations.[5] Interest in correcting for measurement error underscores an important precept: Always strive to make measures as reliable as possible.

---

[5]Despite problems, interest in correcting for attenuation has persisted. For example, Behseta, Berdyyeva, Olson, and Kass (2009) proposed a Bayesian correction, which they illustrated with correlations of neuronal spike count data. They concluded that their approach was "far superior" to Spearman's method in terms of accuracy of the correction.

9.5   Item Response Theory and Person Separation

IRT provides another framework for constructing multi-item reflective scales of unidimensional constructs. As noted in earlier chapters, IRT scale developers are typically interested in estimating measurement precision for particular items and for particular respondents, generating parameter estimates that are presumed to be population independent. They have been less focused on sample-dependent indexes such as coefficient alpha. Nevertheless, scale developers who have applied IRT methods sometimes report values for alpha for their development sample, perhaps because it is an index that is widely understood. For example, Wilcox and colleagues (2013) developed the Shortness of Breath with Daily Activities (SOBDA) questionnaire using Rasch model analysis and estimated coefficient alpha for their 24-item measure ($\alpha = .87$).

A few IRT experts have advocated for the estimation of group-level reliability (internal consistency) as a useful supplement to usual IRT estimates of precision. Raju and Oshima (2005), for example, expressed their belief that "an overall measure of the degree of accuracy of ability estimates . . . may be needed to summarize the data for a group of examinees" (p. 362). Kim (2012) noted that when the interest is on measuring interindividual differences, then group-dependent consistency is more relevant than test information. Nicewander and Thomasson (1999), who proposed methods to estimate reliability for computerized adaptive tests, pointed out that IRT reliability estimates can be used to compare tests and item banks and for quantifying the strength of the relationship between an observed score and the latent trait (theta).

Reliability in IRT is conceptualized as the squared correlation between theta (θ, the latent trait) and the estimate of theta ($\hat{\theta}$), which in turn corresponds to the ratio of variance for the "true" theta value to the variance of the estimate. This is essentially the same as the basic reliability equation shown in Chapter 8, in which true variance is contrasted with observed variance, which in turn represents true variance plus error variance (formula 8.1).

Formulas for estimating the reliability of IRT-based trait estimates were proposed many years ago (e.g., Lord, 1983; Samajima, 1994). One formula for the estimating the reliability of theta for a sample of respondents is as follows:

$$R_\theta = \frac{\sigma^2_\theta}{\sigma^2_\theta + E\,(SEM^2)} \tag{9.8}$$

where σ^2_θ is the variance of the theta estimate, E is the expectation operator, and *SEM* is the standard error of measurement for the group (*SEM*s are discussed in Chapter 10). The variance is the variance of the theta estimates for a given group. The expectation of the squared *SEM*s is estimated by first computing the *SEM* for each person in the sample and then computing the mean of all the squared *SEM*s (Raju & Oshima, 2005).

Sample-dependent reliability in IRT has gotten most attention in the Rasch modeling literature. Software for Rasch model analysis often provides estimates of two indicators of reliability for the analysis sample. The first is called *person reliability* (or sometimes *person separation reliability*). The second is an index called the *person separation index*.

Person reliability is an index that indicates how effectively a set of items can discriminate among a group of people who are measured. Like alpha, a person reliability index can range from 0.0 to 1.0. The link between person reliability and internal consistency reliability has been explained in detail by Wright and Stone (1999). The formula for Rasch person reliability is strongly similar to formula 9.4 for coefficient alpha:

$$\text{Rasch } R_{Person} = \frac{k}{k-1}\left(1 - \frac{MSE_p}{SD_p^{\,2}}\right) \tag{9.9}$$

where k is the number of items, MSE_p is the average error of measurement variance for the sample of people (p) in logits, and $SD_p^{\,2}$ is the sample variance of the linear logit measures.

Unlike alpha, the person reliability index uses *individual* standard errors of measurement, which are squared and summed to produce a more accurate average error variance for the sample. As this formula indicates, person reliability, like alpha, increases with more items[6] and with more heterogeneous samples. When the items and the person are well aligned on the theta continuum, and when there are no extremes (items or persons), then coefficient alpha and person reliability are typically close in value.

The second index that is frequently reported in the Rasch literature is the **person separation index (PSI)**,[7] which can be directly calculated from the person reliability estimate:

$$PSI = \sqrt{\left(\frac{R_{Person}}{1 - R_{Person}}\right)} \tag{9.10}$$

The PSI, which typically ranges from 1.0 to 3.0, is essentially an index that provides an estimate of the signal-to-noise ratio, the ratio of "true" variance to error variance. For example, a PSI of 3.0 means that the sample is three times more variable than the test is "noisy." The PSI can be described as the number of different performance levels that the set of items measures in a particular sample (i.e., how much *separation* is possible). The PSI must equal 2.0 to attain a person reliability of .80 and must equal 3 to attain a person reliability of .90. A PSI of 1 corresponds to a reliability coefficient of only .50. PSIs of 2.0 or greater are considered desirable.

One advantage of the PSI is that it is possible to estimate separations for new samples. Wright and Stone (1999) provide the following formula

$$PSI_{Estimated} = SD \div SEM \tag{9.11}$$

where *SD* is the estimated standard deviation of the target sample and *SEM* is the estimated standard error of measurement for the target sample. The *SEM* can "almost always be well approximated" by multiplying the square root of the number of items by 2.5 (Wright & Stone, 1999, p. 162).

As an example of how researchers have used separation indexes to draw conclusions about scales and reduced item sets, Mallinson, Stelmack, and Velozo (2004) compared different versions of the VF-14, a measure of visual functioning widely used in assessments relating to cataract surgery. The researchers applied Rasch model analysis to the original VF-14 and to six other 7-item short form versions (two of which involved explicitly adding items to cover important gaps in item locations). The PSI was highest for one of the new VF item sets (2.67), compared to 2.15 for a published short-form version and 2.60 for the original 14-item set. Alphas were also computed, and the internal consistency estimates largely led to the same conclusions.

Raju and Oshima (2005) predicted that as experience with IRT expands, so, too, will interest in group-dependent measures of reliability (i.e., internal consistency).

9.6   Other Issues Relating to Internal Consistency

In this concluding section, we talk briefly about factors to consider in achieving adequate internal consistency as well as design and reporting issues in connection with internal consistency. Most of this discussion is appropriate primarily for the internal consistency of scales constructed within the traditional CTT model.

---

[6]Linacre (1995) offers a nomogram that graphically shows predicted person reliability (and person separation) for tests of different length. Raju and Oshima (2005) offer prophecy formulas, analogous to the Spearman–Brown formula, for estimating the impact of adding or subtracting items in IRT models.

[7]Wright and Stone (1999) refer to the PSI index as *G*. Mallinson et al. (2004) use the term *separation ratio* (SR) in lieu of PSI. Some writers (e.g., Streiner & Norman, 2008) use the term *person separation index* to refer to the index we have called *person reliability*. One can draw conclusions about which index is being referenced by its value. Person reliability as we define it ranges from zero to one, and the PSI ranges from one to three.

9.6.a Achieving Adequate Internal Consistency

As with retest reliability, it is important to strive for high internal consistency in measures that will be used both in research and clinical practice. Low internal consistency coefficients can increase the risk of a Type II error, for example, and put an upper limit on the value of validity coefficients for both criterion validity and construct validity.

Three factors play an especially important role in the value of coefficient alpha estimates. The first is the number of items. For example, assuming an average inter-item correlation of .40, a four-item scale will yield a coefficient alpha of .73, whereas an eight-item scale with the same average inter-item correlation will increase alpha to .84. Thus, all else equal, longer scales are more internally consistent than shorter ones, but there are diminishing returns as more and more items are added.

A second factor is the value of the inter-item correlations. If the average inter-item correlation of our eight-item scale were increased from .40 to .60, coefficient alpha would go up from .84 to .92. Thus, the degree to which the items are capturing the same construct plays a strong role in internal consistency estimates.

The third factor has to do with total score variance. As with the ICC, estimates of coefficient alpha are depressed when variability is constrained.

9.6.b Study Design and Internal Consistency

When a multi-item reflective scale is being developed using CTT methods, an assessment of the scale's internal consistency should always be undertaken. Such an assessment typically occurs as part of the process of finalizing scale items, which includes those methods described in Chapter 5. As we advised in that chapter, the development sample should be rather large to support factor analytic work—ideally, a sample of at least 300 people would be used to avoid risks of spurious inter-correlations. Moreover, because instrument development samples are almost always samples of convenience, larger samples may increase the likelihood that the sample will be heterogeneous (Ponterotto & Ruckdeschel, 2007), and heterogeneous samples are desirable.

For most multi-item health scales that will be used to evaluate changes in an attribute—for example, changes resulting from an intervention—both internal consistency and retest reliability should be assessed. Such dual assessments sometimes occur within the development sample. For example, a large, heterogeneous sample could be used to assess internal consistency, and then a sizeable subsample (or the entire sample) could be asked to complete the scale again for retest assessment. However, to increase the potential for a scale to have both high internal consistency and retest reliability, we encourage using the development sample to examine item quality for both measurement properties. If item analysis suggests that many items need to be revised or replaced, then reassessment of the scale's internal consistency and retest reliability might be needed.

9.6.c Reporting Internal Consistency

In describing the internal consistency of a new measure, coefficient alpha (or KR-20) should be computed and reported for each subscale (and sometimes for the entire scale, if it is defensible to add subscale scores together). Although it is not standard to do so, researchers should consider reporting the confidence interval around estimates of internal consistency. If a retest reliability assessment has been undertaken with the development sample, alphas should be reported for both the initial test and the retest, for the sample that completed the scale twice.

When multi-item scales are used for research purposes, it is common to calculate coefficient alpha. Assuming that the value of alpha is similar to that reported in the development sample, reporting a scale's internal consistency will provide readers with some evidence that the scale has maintained its utility for a new sample of people.

9.6.d Evaluating Internal Consistency

The Consensus-based Standards for the selection of health Measurement Instruments (COSMIN) group has offered guidelines and a scoring system for evaluating evidence regarding a scale's internal consistency (Terwee et al., 2012). The COSMIN website (www.cosmin.nl) lists 11 questions in Box A that concern internal consistency, focusing primarily on the quality of reporting and the rigor of the study itself rather than on the quality of the scale. For example, there are items about the adequacy of the sample size and whether evidence supporting unidimensionality (e.g., from a factor analysis) was reported.

The COSMIN questions do not guide an evaluation of the actual internal consistency results nor of the evidence regarding the unidimensionality of the scale or subscale. Those evaluating a scale for possible use in research or clinical settings will need to draw conclusions about whether the scale was adequate in terms of its internal consistency and unidimensionality, based on the results presented in the report. They will also have to evaluate the extent to which the researchers' description of the sample and the target population are sufficiently detailed to draw conclusions about the appropriateness of using the measure in another study.

References

Behseta, S., Berdyyeva, T., Olson, C., & Kass, R. (2009). Bayesian correction for attenuation of correlation in multi-trial spike count data. *Journal of Neurophysiology, 101*, 2186–2193.

Brennan, R. L. (2001). An essay on the history and future of reliability from the perspective of replications. *Journal of Educational Measurement, 38*, 295–317.

Brown, W. (1910). Some experimental results in the correlation of mental abilities. *British Journal of Psychology, 3*, 296–322.

Carmines, G., & Zeller, A. (1979). *Reliability and validity assessments.* Thousand Oaks, CA: Sage.

Chin, Y. F., & Huang, T. T. (2013). Development and validation of a Diabetes Foot Self-Care Behavior Scale. *Journal of Nursing Research, 21*, 19–25.

Cronbach, L. J. (1951). Coefficient alpha and the internal structure of tests. *Psychometrika, 16*, 297–334.

Cureton, E. E. (1958). The definition and estimation of test reliability. *Educational and Psychological Measurement, 18*, 715–738.

DeVet, H. C. W., Terwee, C., Mokkink, L. B., & Knol, D. L. (2011). *Measurement in medicine: A practical guide.* Cambridge, MA: Cambridge University Press.

Feldt, L. S., & Brennan, R. L. (1989). Reliability. In R.L. Linn (Ed.), *Educational measurement* (3rd ed., pp. 105–146). New York, NY: Macmillan.

Graham, J. M. (2006). Congeneric and (essentially) tau-equivalent estimates of score reliability: What they are and how to use them. *Educational and Psychological Measurement, 66*, 930–944.

Green, S. B. (2003). A coefficient alpha for test-retest data. *Psychological Methods, 8*, 88–101.

Green, S., & Yang, Y. (2009). Commentary on coefficient alpha: A cautionary tale. *Psychometrika, 74*, 121–135.

Gu, F., Little, T. D., & Kingston, N. M. (2013). Misestimation of reliability using coefficient alpha and structural equation modeling when assumptions of tau-equivalence and uncorrelated errors are violated. *Methodology: European Journal of Research Methods for the Behavioral and Social Sciences, 9*, 30–40.

Guilford, J. P. (1954). *Psychometric methods* (2nd ed.). New York, NY: McGraw Hill.

Johnson, H. G. (1950). Test reliability and correction for attenuation. *Psychometrika, 15*, 115–119.

Kim, S. (2012). A note on the reliability coefficients for item response model-based ability estimates. *Psychometrika, 77*, 153–162.

Kuder, G. F., & Richardson, M. W. (1937). The theory of estimation of test reliability. *Psychometrika, 2*, 151–160.

Linacre, J. M. (1995). Reliability and separation nomograms. *Rasch Measurement Transactions, 9*, 420–421.

Lord, F. M. (1983) Unbiased estimators of ability parameters, of their variance, and of their parallel forms reliability. *Psychometrika, 48*, 233–245.

Lord, F. M., & Novick, M. R. (1968). *Statistical theories of mental test scores.* Reading, MA: Addison-Wesley.

Mallinson, T., Stelmack, J., & Velozo, C. (2004). A comparison of the separation ratio and coefficient alpha in the creation of minimum item sets. *Medical Care, 42*(Suppl.), I17–I24.

McCrae, R. R., Kurtz, J. J., Yamagata, S., & Terracciano, A. (2011). Internal consistency, retest reliability, and their implications for personality scale validity. *Personality and Social Psychology Review, 15*, 28–50.

Miller, M. B. (1995). Coefficient alpha: A basic introduction from the perspectives of classical test theory and structural equation modeling. *Structural Equation Modeling, 2*, 255–273.

Mokkink, L. B., Terwee, C., Patrick, D., Alonso, J., Stratford, P., Knol, D.L., . . . de Vet, H. C. W. (2010). The COSMIN study reached international consensus on taxonomy, terminology, and definitions of measurement properties for health-related patient-reported outcomes. *Journal of Clinical Epidemiology, 63*, 737–745.

Muchinsky, P. M. (1996). The correction for attenuation. *Educational and Psychological Measurement, 56*, 63–75.

Nicewander, W. A., & Thomasson, G. L. (1999). Some reliability estimates for computerized adaptive tests. *Applied Psychological Measurement, 23*, 239–247.

Nunnally, J., & Bernstein, I.H. (1994). *Psychometric theory* (3rd ed.). New York, NY: McGraw-Hill.

Ponterotto, J. G., & Ruskdeschel, D. (2007). An overview of coefficient alpha and a reliability matrix for estimating adequacy of internal consistency coefficients with psychological research measures. *Perceptual and Motor Skills, 105*, 997–1014.

Radloff, L. S. (1977). The CES-D scale: A self-report depression scale for research in the general population. *Applied Psychological Measurement, 1*, 385–401.

Raju, N. S., & Oshima, T. C. (2005). Two prophecy formulas for assessing the reliability of item response theory-based ability estimates. *Educational and Psychological Measurement, 65*, 361–375.

Raykov, T. (1997a). Estimation of composite reliability for congeneric measures. *Applied Psychological Measurement, 21*, 173–184.

Raykov, T. (1997b). Scale reliability, Cronbach's coefficient alpha, and violations of essential tau-equivalence with fixed congeneric components. *Multivariate Behavioral Research, 32*, 329–353.

Rhodes, R. E., & Smith, N. E. (2006). Personality correlates of physical activity: A review and meta-analysis. *British Journal of Sports Medicine, 40*, 958–965.

Samajima, F. (1994). Estimation of reliability coefficients using the test information function and its modifications. *Applied Psychological Measurement, 18*, 229–244.

Schmidt, F. L., & Hunter, J. E. (1996). Measurement error in psychological research: Lessons from 26 research scenarios. *Psychological Methods, 1*, 199–223.

Spearman, C. (1904). The proof and measurement of association between two things. *American Journal of Psychology, 15*, 72–101.

Spearman, C. (1910). Correlation calculated from faulty data. *British Journal of Psychology, 3*, 271–295.

Streiner, D. L., & Norman, G. E. (2008). *Health measurement scales: A practical guide to their development and use* (4th ed.). Oxford: Oxford University Press.

Terwee, C. B., Mokkink, L. B., Knol, D. L., Ostelo, R., Bouter, L. M., & DeVet, H. C. W. (2012). Rating the methodological quality in systematic reviews of studies on measurement properties: A scoring system for the COSMIN checklist. *Quality of Life Research, 21*, 651–657.

Traub, R. E. (1997). Classical test theory in historical perspective. *Educational Measurement: Issues and Practices, 16*, 8–14.

Wilcox, T. K., Chen, W., Howard, K., Wiklund, I., Brooks, J., Watkins, M., . . . Crim, C. (2013). Item selection, reliability and validity of the Shortness of Breath with Daily Activities (SOBDA) questionnaire: A new outcome measure for evaluating dyspnea in chronic obstructive pulmonary disease. *Health & Quality of Life Outcomes, 11*, 196.

Wright, B., & Stone, M. (1999). *Measurement essentials* (2nd ed.). Wilmington, DE: Wide Range.

Measurement Error

Chapter Outline

Measurement error is the systematic and random error that occurs when a score obtained through a measuring process differs from a hypothetical "true" score of a latent trait. As shown in the measurement taxonomy in Figure 3.1, measurement error is a component within the reliability domain. The concepts of measurement error and reliability are inextricably connected, and yet measurement error parameters yield information that reliability coefficients alone cannot provide.

As noted in our measurement parameter summary table (Table 8.2), there are no measurement error parameters when variables are categorical. Thus, this chapter focuses on major methods of summarizing measurement error for continuous variables, mostly within the classical test theory (CTT) framework. This includes the standard error of measurement and Bland–Altman limits of agreement,[1] which are relevant for measures of any type—reflective and formative patient-reported outcomes (PROs), observations, performance measures, and biophysiologic measures. A separate section discusses measurement error for multi-item scales developed with item response theory (IRT) models.

10.1 Basic Concepts of Measurement Error

Differences between observed scores and true scores reflect measurement error. As discussed in Chapter 8, an intraclass correlation coefficient (ICC) reliability coefficient communicates the degree to which people can be differentiated from one another using a

---

[1]A third parameter of measurement error, the *coefficient of variation* (CV) is not often encountered in connection with reliability assessments in most health fields, except in laboratory assays, and is not described in detail here. The CV, which requires ratio-level measurements, yields a percentage error. The CV is the standard deviation divided by the mean, multiplied by 100 to result in a percentage.

measure, *despite* the presence of measurement error. Unless a reliability coefficient is 1.0 (which is virtually never the case), measurement error is present.

Measurement errors lower reliability, yet reliability can be reasonably high even when measurement error is not negligible. Conversely, low measurement error cannot guarantee an acceptable reliability parameter. The explanation for this seeming paradox concerns the heterogeneity of the sample. As we discussed in Chapter 8, reliability parameters (except IRT-based measures) are depressed with homogeneous samples because reliably differentiating people is more challenging when people are similar on the attribute being measured.

To illustrate, we have plotted the Center for Epidemiologic Studies Depression Scale (CES-D) depression scores from our example of test–retest reliability described in Chapter 8. The raw data for 10 patients were presented in Table 8.1 and are reproduced in Table 10.1. Graph A of Figure 10.1 shows a scatterplot for the original data. $ICC_{Consistency}$ for this sample is .88 (.875), and the standard error of measurement (to be discussed subsequently) is 2.69. The standard error of measurement (*SEM*) is an index that tells us about the **precision** of a given measurement; the lower the *SEM* value, the greater the degree of precision. When scores for each person across two waves in a retest study are close in value, the dots cluster close to the diagonal line and the *SEM* tends to be low. In Graph A, the score values across the test and retest are not strongly similar, and yet the reliability is very respectable, .86. The reason for the high ICC in Graph A is that variability in the sample is high. In Week 1, patients' scores range from a low of 2 (virtually no risk of depression) to 26 (high risk of depression), and the *SD* is 7.54.

In Figure 10.1, Graph B, precision has increased, as illustrated by tight clustering around the diagonal. The *SEM* is now only 1.69, substantially lower than the *SEM* in Graph A. Yet, the ICC value remains the essentially same (.86). The reason that the ICC has not improved despite lower measurement error is that sample heterogeneity declined. The range

Table 10.1	Fictitious Data for Test–Retest Reliability Example for CES-D Scores		
ID	Week 1	Week 2	Change
1	16	19	3
2	5	8	3
3	8	14	6
4	20	14	−6
5	9	13	4
6	13	19	6
7	17	18	1
8	26	29	3
9	2	5	3
10	6	3	−3
Mean	12.20	14.20	2.00
SD	7.54	7.67	3.80

SD, standard deviation.

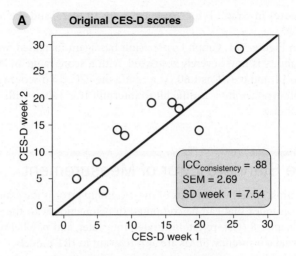

A   **Original CES-D scores**

$ICC_{consistency}$ = .88
SEM = 2.69
SD week 1 = 7.54

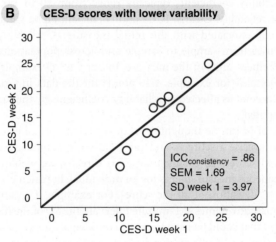

B   **CES-D scores with lower variability**

$ICC_{consistency}$ = .86
SEM = 1.69
SD week 1 = 3.97

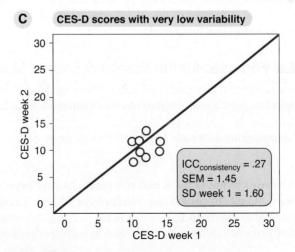

C   **CES-D scores with very low variability**

$ICC_{consistency}$ = .27
SEM = 1.45
SD week 1 = 1.60

Figure 10.1

Fictitious CES-D Scores for 1-week test–retest reliability with different ICCs and standard errors of measurement (*SEM*s).

of scores in Graph B for Week 1 is only 10 to 23, and the *SD* for all scores has dropped to 3.97.

In Figure 10.1, Graph C, precision has again increased, with an *SEM* of 1.45. However, variability is now severely restricted, with a score range in Week 1 of only 5 points, from 10 to 14, and the *SD* is 1.60. As a result, the ICC is a discouraging .27. Hopefully this example illustrates why it is difficult to interpret ICC values without information about sample variability.

10.2 The Standard Error of Measurement

The most widely used index of measurement error is the **standard error of measurement**. It is an index that can be computed in connection with the reliability estimates discussed in Chapter 8 (test–retest, intrarater, interrater, and parallel test reliability), as well as with internal consistency. *SEM*s are also relevant in IRT models.

Reliability coefficients typically range from 0.0 to 1.0, with higher values indicating greater reliability. Clearly, ICCs and coefficient alpha values are not in the units of measurement associated with the actual measure. A reliability coefficient is a *relative* index that varies from sample to sample and across populations. *SEM*s, by contrast, are in the measurement units of the measure. In our CES-D example, the *SEM* was in points on the CES-D scale—for example, 1.45 points for the data in Graph C of Figure 10.1. The *SEM* values are not as affected as reliability coefficients by the sample within which the estimate is computed.

The *SEM* can be thought of as quantifying "typical error" on a measure. It is an index of how precise a score is, and can be used to compute confidence intervals (CI) around obtained scores. To calculate an *SEM* directly, we would need a large number of near-simultaneous measurements for an individual, in which case the *SEM* would simply be the standard deviation of all the scores. For example, if a patient's heart rate were measured 500 consecutive times at 1-minute intervals, the *SD* of the heart rate values would constitute the *SEM* that could be used to create confidence intervals around the mean heart rate value. In practice, consecutive measurements such as this do not happen, and so the *SEM* must be estimated. The remainder of this section discusses the *SEM* for measures other than those created within an IRT framework.

10.2.a Formulas for the Standard Error of Measurement

*SEM*s are estimated using the same data as those used to compute reliability coefficients. For example, data from a test–retest or interrater situation, or data used for internal consistency estimates, can be used in equations for estimating the *SEM*.

The most general formula for the *SEM* estimate is:

$$SEM = \sqrt{\sigma^2_{error}} \tag{10.1}$$

Alternative formulas for actual computations have been developed, which we will illustrate using the 10-person test–retest of the CES-D (i.e., the data shown in Table 10.1 and graphed in Figure 10.1A). First, when $k = 2$ (e.g., two raters, or a test then a retest), the standard error of a difference can be used to estimate the *SEM*:

$$SEM = SD_{Difference} \div \sqrt{2} \tag{10.2}$$

With our CES-D data, the mean score for Week 1 was 12.20, and the mean for Week 2 was 14.20. The mean difference, then, was 2.00, and the $SD_{Difference}$ was 3.801, as shown in Figure 10.2. Thus, for this example,

$$SEM = 3.801 \div \sqrt{2} = 3.801 \div 1.414 = 2.69$$

Paired samples T-test

| | Paired differences | | | | | | | |
| | Mean | Standard deviation | Standard error mean | 95% Confidence interval of the difference | | t | df | Sig. (2-tailed) |
				Lower limit	Upper limit			
CES-D wk 2 – CES-D wk 1	2.000	3.801	1.202	-.719	4.719	1.664	9	.130

Figure 10.2

Paired t-test analysis of test–retest CES-D data (SPSS).

The second *SEM* formula is the one that is most widely provided in textbooks, and it can be used in many situations[2]:

$$SEM = SD \sqrt{(1 - R)} \tag{10.3}$$

where R is the reliability estimate (the ICC or coefficient alpha) and *SD* is the standard deviation for the sample in which the reliability was calculated. The use of the standard deviation in this formula essentially "cancels out" the between-patient variability that was used in calculating the reliability coefficient, which helps to explain why *SEMs* are more stable from sample to sample than ICCs. When using formula 10.3 to estimate the *SEM*, care should be taken in deciding which standard deviation to use. When ICCs are used as the reliability coefficient, there are multiple *SDs*—one for each k measurement—and these should be pooled. When $k = 2$, as in our CES-D example, the pooled *SD* can be computed using the following formula:

$$SD_{\text{Pooled}} = \frac{(SD_1 + SD_2)}{2} \tag{10.4}$$

In the CES-D example, the *SD* for Week 1 was 7.54 and the SD for Week 2 was 7.67, and so in this example:

$$SD_{\text{Pooled}} = \frac{(7.54 + 7.67)}{2} = 7.605$$

Using this pooled *SD* value in our *SEM* formula, given that the ICC estimate was .875, we find that:

$$SEM = 7.605 \sqrt{(1 - .875)} = 7.605 \sqrt{(.125)} = 2.69$$

This *SEM* is the same value as obtained earlier, using the formula with the standard deviation of difference scores. Equation 10.3, however, is one that can be used when R is estimated using coefficient alpha. In this situation, the *SD* is simply the *SD* for the total scores for the sample. Using the example of the coefficient alpha estimate for CES-D scores of 1,000 low-income women (alpha = .826), as described in Chapter 9, we would compute the *SEM* to be:

$$SEM = 6.101 \sqrt{(1 - .826)} = 2.56$$

The third approach to estimating the *SEM* comes directly from the computation of ICCs. In Chapter 8, we explained that reliability is estimated based on the ratio of variability between people to the ratio of total variability, which includes error:

$$R = \frac{\sigma^2_{\text{BetweenPeople}}}{\sigma^2_{\text{BetweenPeople}} + \sigma^2_{\text{Error}}} \tag{8.2}$$

---

[2]DeVet, Terwee, Mokkink, and Knol (2011) caution against using this formula when it is applied using *SDs* from a sample other than the one used for estimating reliability.

As indicated in Equation 10.1, the *SEM* is estimated by taking the square root of the second term in the denominator, the error term. Within an analysis of variance (ANOVA) context, the error term is the mean square error (mean square residual in SPSS printouts), multiplied by $k - 1$. In the SPSS printout for our CES-D data (not shown), the mean square residual was 7.222, and $k - 1 = 1$. So, we would find that

$$SEM = \sqrt{\sigma^2_{error}} = \sqrt{(MS_{Residual})(k - 1)} = \sqrt{(7.222)(1)} = 2.69$$

Thus, all three approaches yield the same *SEM* value for the CES-D retest data shown in Table 10.1 (i.e., 2.69).

Readers may recall that there are multiple formulas for the ICC and, in particular, that the ICC for agreement and the ICC for consistency have different error terms. The three calculations shown here all yielded estimates of *SEM* for consistency. For agreement estimates, we would need to add in the column variation associated with different raters or different waves, as shown in the formula for $ICC_{Agreement}$, Equation 8.3 (p. 117). Just as error variance attributable to column variance reduces the value of the ICC, that additional error variance increases the value of the *SEM*. A simple method of estimating $SEM_{Agreement}$ is to use formula 10.3, with $R = ICC_{Agreement}$. In our CES-D example, $ICC_{Agreement}$ was .856 and the pooled *SD* was 7.605, and therefore:

$$SEM_{Agreement} = 7.605 \sqrt{(1 - .856)} = 7.605 \sqrt{(.144)} = 2.89$$

As expected, the ICC for agreement is lower than that for consistency, and the *SEM* value is greater. When *SEM*s are reported, they are typically for $SEM_{Consistency}$, although this information is seldom made explicit.

10.2.b Confidence Intervals Around Observed Scores

The *SEM* is often easy for users of a measure to understand because it is in units that may be clinically relevant. For example, for people who routinely use the CES-D and are aware that a score of 16 is the cutoff score designating *at risk for depression*, an *SEM* of 2.69 helps to put a patient's score of, say, 14 in perspective. As other examples, the *SEM* for scores on the 6-minute walk test would be in meters, the *SEM* for waist circumference measurements would be in centimeters, and the *SEM* for low-density lipoprotein (LDL) cholesterol values would be in milligrams per deciliter. Clinicians familiar with a measure may thus find it easy to interpret its *SEM*.

*SEM*s are often used to construct confidence intervals around individual scores. The "traditional" approach (Charter & Feldt, 2002) is to use the obtained score as the estimate of a true score, and then apply the following formula, here for a 95% CI:

$$95\% \text{ CI around } X = X \pm 1.96 \, (SEM) \tag{10.5}$$

where X is an individual score and 1.96 is the *z* value associated with the 95% CI. In our CES-D example, Patient 1 had a score of 16 at Week 1, so we would estimate that the 95% CI around that score would be:

$$95\% \text{ CI} = 16 \pm 1.96 \, (2.69) = 16 \pm 5.3 = 10.7 \text{ to } 21.3$$

Charter and Feldt (2002) explained how to interpret such CIs. As an example using CES-D scores, if we administered the depression scale to 100 patients, for 95 of them, the 95% CI could be expected to include the respective patient's true score. For an individual score (such as Patient 1's CES-D score of 16), we can say that we are 95% confident that the true score is somewhere between 10.7 and 21.3.

By building confidence intervals around individual scores using the *SEM*, it is clear why it is risky to use instruments with moderate reliabilities when making individual decisions (e.g., eligibility for an intervention). Suppose in our CES-D example that we were to use a cutoff score of 25 to initiate a certain intervention. (Of course, this example is contrived to illustrate a point: Health care decisions would not be made on the basis of CES-D scores). At Time 1, two patients in our sample obtained a score whose 95% CI included 25. For example, Patient 4 had a T1 score of 20, so the 95% CI is 14.7 to 25.3. If reliability had been stronger (e.g., .95), the precision of the confidence interval would be improved; in this example, the *SEM* would be reduced to 1.70. With this level of precision, the upper limit of the 95% CI for Patient 4 would be 23.3, and we would be more confident that this patient was not in need of treatment. Conversely, consider the possibility that ICC was .70, a criterion that is sometimes suggested as an acceptable reliability value. With an ICC of .70, the 95% CI around patients' scores would be the observed score ± 8.16; now three patients might be considered in need of treatment. For example, Patient 7 had a T1 score of 17. With ICC = .70, we would be 95% confident that this patient's true score was between 8.84 (relatively low depression) and 25.16 (substantial risk for depression).

Two issues about these confidence interval calculations should be noted. The first is that these computations assume that the *SEM* is the same for everyone, when in fact this is almost never the case. Typically, the data are *heteroscedastic*, which means that the measurement error is not uniform across scale values. When an individual score is near the mean for the measure, the true *SEM* tends to be smaller, whereas more extreme scores have larger *SEMs* (Feldt, Steffan, & Gupta, 1985). This limitation is eliminated in multi-item measures from an IRT analysis.

A second issue is that the CIs are built around observed scores. In many cases, this approach is sufficient, and this confidence interval is easy to compute once the *SEM* is known. Sometimes, however, confidence intervals are built around estimated true scores.

10.2.c Confidence Intervals Around True Scores

Unless the reliability of a measure is perfect, obtained scores are biased approximations of true scores. In particular, extreme scores tend to be biased outward from the mean. True scores are never known, but an estimated true score can be calculated. The formula is:

$$X_{ET} = R(X - M) + M \tag{10.6}$$

where X_{ET} is an estimated true score, R is the reliability coefficient, X is an observed score, and M is the mean for the distribution of scores. In our example for Patient 1, whose initial obtained score was 16, we would find:

$$X_{ET} = .875(16 - 12.20) + 12.20 = 15.53$$

In every case, unless $R = 1.0$, the estimated true score will be closer than the observed score to the mean of the overall distribution. Because this reflects regression to the mean, centering confidence intervals on the estimated true score is often referred to as a *regression-based approach*.

In this true-score method, the confidence intervals are not based on the *SEM* but rather on another index called the **standard error of estimate (SEE)**. The formula for estimating the SEE is as follows:

$$SEE = SD \sqrt{R(1 - R)} \tag{10.7}$$

Again using the CES-D scores from Table 10.1 and the pooled *SD* as the example, we would obtain:

$$SEE = 7.605 \sqrt{.875(1 - .875)} = 7.605 \sqrt{.109} = 2.52$$

Thus, in our example, an observed score of 16 using this true-score method would have a 95% CI of 15.53 ± (1.96 × 2.52), or 95% CI = 15.53 ± 4.93. Unless R = 1.0, the 95% CI will be narrower using the regression-based approach using estimated true scores than those using the traditional approach using obtained scores.

Although both the traditional and regression-based methods are acceptable, the interpretation is different. For the method just described, we would say that for all the people in the tested population whose score on the CES-D was 16, 95% of them would have true scores falling between 10.60 and 20.46. Thus, the two approaches to computing CIs around scores can be used for different purposes. The traditional approach can be used to interpret an individual person's obtained score, and the regression-based approach can be used to interpret the scores of all people with a given score. Manuals for standardized tests created within a CTT model typically use the latter approach.

10.2.d Debates about the Standard Error of Measurement

There are differences of opinion about whether the *SEM* is appropriate when Cronbach's alpha (internal consistency) rather than ICC (test–retest or interrater reliability) is used as the reliability coefficient. The Consensus-based Standards for the selection of health Measurement Instruments (COSMIN) group asserts that the *SEM* should not be calculated based on a single measure: " . . . the calculation of the *SEM* based on Cronbach's alpha is considered not appropriate, because it does not take the variance between time points into account" (Mokkink et al., 2012, p. 29). However, psychometricians have been calculating *SEM* with Equation 10.3 using alpha as the reliability coefficient for decades (e.g., Nunnally & Bernstein, 1994). In fact, some have claimed that it is inappropriate to build confidence intervals around an observed score using the *SEM* if the reliability coefficient is based on a test–retest or interrater reliability assessment (Charter & Feldt, 2002).

If a measurement is not made with a multi-item reflective scale (e.g., biophysiologic measurements, performance tests, formative indexes), then the only possibility is to base the *SEM* on test–retest reliability information. When a measurement is made with a multi-item scale, it may be advantageous to estimate both internal consistency and test–retest reliability and to compare the resulting *SEM*s. When the reliability of change scores is of interest (Chapter 17), then it is likely to be important to distinguish short-term fluctuations from true change, and so test–retest reliability should be estimated.

10.3 Limits of Agreement

Scatterplots such as those shown in Figure 10.1 provide some insight into the degree to which two sets of scores are comparable—in this case, scores on a test and then a retest of the CES-D. When there is no measurement error, all the points align on the diagonal. Bland and Altman (1986) devised another way to plot two sets of scores, and the plot and its associated parameter (limits of agreement) are used in health care research to understand and display measurement error.

10.3.a Bland–Altman Plots and Limits of Agreement

The **Bland–Altman plot** was created originally to show agreement and comparability in a criterion validity situation, in which one of two measurements was the "gold standard" and the other was an alternate measure designed to approximate gold standard scores in a more efficient manner. However, the Bland–Altman plots are widely used in connection with reliability assessments and, as we will see in a later chapter, in connection with the measurement of change. The basic requirement is that there be two measures of the same attribute, with scores on the same measurement scale. This situation thus applies to most of the situations discussed in Chapter 8 (i.e., test–retest, intrarater reliability, etc.) when $k = 2$ and measurements are on a continuous scale.

Bland–Altman plots are designed to show systematic error (e.g., differences in scores resulting from biased raters) distinct from random error. To illustrate, we turn again to our 10-person example of CES-D test and retest at a 1-week interval. Values from a paired *t* test are used in the construction of a Bland–Altman plot. For our CES-D data (Table 10.1), paired *t* test information is shown in Figure 10.2. As this figure indicates, the mean difference between scores on Week 1 and Week 2 was 2.00 (i.e., slightly greater depression in Week 2), and the *SD* of the difference was 3.801.

Figure 10.3 presents a Bland–Altman plot for these CES-D data. In a Bland–Altman plot, the X-axis is used to graph the mean of the two scores for each person. To illustrate, Patient 10 had a score of 6 on Week 1 and a score of 3 on Week 2. The mean score is thus 4.5, which is where the point for Patient 10 is plotted on the X-axis. The Y-axis is used to plot

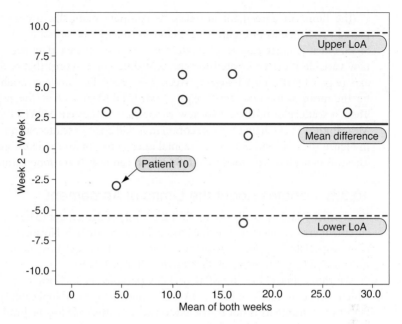

Figure 10.3
Bland–Altman plot for fictitious CES-D scores, 1-week test–retest situation.

the score difference for each person. Patient 10's difference score is −3 (3 − 6), and so the point for this patient is at the intersection of 4.5 (X-axis) and −3.0 (Y-axis). Values for all 10 patients are plotted similarly.

Information from the paired t test is then superimposed on these plotted scores. The solid horizontal line, labeled *Mean difference*, is the value of the mean difference in the two sets of scores. In our example shown in Figure 10.2, the line (sometimes represented as $\bar{d}$) is drawn at 2.0 on the Y-axis. Note that this difference is not statistically significant ($p = .13$), and the 95% CI around the mean of two includes zero (−4.72 to 0.72). Nevertheless, the value of two is our estimate of systematic error. Thus, the difference between zero on the Y-axis (no difference in scores) and the mean difference of 2.0 graphically represents estimated systematic error between the two sets of CES-D scores.

Random error is shown in the area between $\bar{d}$ and the two sets of dashed lines, which are the **limits of agreement (LOA)**. The LOA designate the confidence interval around the mean difference and can be computed by multiplying the relevant z (1.96 for the 95% CI) by the $SD_{\text{Difference}}$,[3] which in this case is 3.801. Thus, the LOAs in this example are:

$$\text{Upper LOA} = 2.00 + (1.96 \times 3.801) = 2.00 + 7.45 = 9.45$$
$$\text{Lower LOA} = 2.00 - (1.96 \times 3.801) = 2.00 - 7.45 = -5.45$$

If the distribution of scores is normal, then 95% of all points will fall within these two limits.[4]

Ideally, what one hopes to find in a Bland–Altman plot is (1) a mean difference line close to 0.0; (2) limits of agreement that are close to $\bar{d}$, indicating greater precision (less measurement error); (3) no major outliers; (4) similar differences above and below $\bar{d}$—that is, randomly distributed; and (5) score differences on the Y-axis that do not change with increasing mean values on the X-axis—that is, the data are not markedly heteroscedastic. Patterns are more discernible when there are more data points, but the plot in Figure 10.3 does not seem problematic except for the wide range of the LOA, which is consistent with the fairly high *SEM*.

---

[3]An alternative formula for computing the LOA, based on the *SEM*, is presented in Chapter 17.
[4]When the mean difference is not statistically different, the mean is often set to zero, and the LOA estimate is then $SD_{\text{Difference}}$ times ±1.96.

The limits of agreement are easy to compute manually, using information from a paired *t* test such as in Figure 10.2. Bland–Altman plots cannot be created directly within SPSS, but it is fairly easy to generate them with some easy data transformations. First, a new variable must be created to represent differences scores that will be used on the Y axis (e.g., COMPUTE Change = Week 2 − Week 1). Another variable must be created for the mean of the two scores (e.g., COMPUTE MeanBoth = Mean [Week 1, Week 2]). Then, a scatterplot of these two new variables is requested (SCATTERPLOT [BIVAR] = MeanBoth WITH Change). These commands will create a scatterplot such as the one shown in Figure 10.3, but without the horizontal lines drawn in for the LOAs and mean difference. These lines need to be added manually, which can readily be done within SPSS.

10.3.b Debates About the Limits of Agreement

Psychometricians typically do not find the limits of agreement to be a useful index of measurement error, preferring the *SEM* instead (e.g., Streiner & Norman, 2008). Even in medicine—especially in sports medicine—there have been debates about which parameter is most useful (e.g., Atkinson, 2000; Hopkins, 2000a, 2000b).

We think that either the *SEM* or LOA parameters, or both, can be useful. The *SEM*, which can be used to compute LOA, has somewhat greater applicability because the number of measurements is not restricted to two, as is the case for the limits of agreement. For example, the *SEM* can be calculated in interrater studies with three or more raters. Also, *SEM*s can be calculated with coefficient alpha, but LOA cannot. Bland–Altman plots are useful for graphically distinguishing systematic and random error. These plots can also help to identify problems of heteroscedasticity. Thus, the use to which the information is put can help determine which measurement error parameter to calculate.

10.4   Item Response Theory and Measurement Error

Measurement error as discussed in the previous sections is relevant for most types of measures, including non-PROs and multi-item scales constructed using CTT. Measurement error for items and scales using IRT models requires a separate discussion.

As noted in Chapter 6, a major difference between CTT and IRT is the manner in which measurement error is conceptualized. CTT-based analyses yield reliability estimates and a standard error that is the same for everyone in a sample, and reliability values are sample dependent. In IRT, however, measurement error can be assessed for each item, each scale (or set of items), and each person and is not sample dependent. Proponents of IRT methods have pointed out that it is more realistic to admit that a measure provides different amounts of precision for people who are at different points along a latent trait continuum. As mentioned earlier in this chapter, the *SEM* in a CTT framework is based on an assumption of homoscedasticity, but this rarely holds true; measurement error is typically higher for people at the extremes of a scale than for those near the middle. Thus, measurement error in IRT models is seen as more realistic and also more precise because it can be estimated for each person.

In IRT, the concept of **information** usually replaces the concept of reliability. Item information indicates how well an item can discriminate among people who are at different levels of the latent trait theta (θ). As noted in Chapter 6, an item response function can be transformed into an **item information function (IIF)**. In one-parameter logistic (1-PL) and two-parameter logistic (2-PL) models, an item's information is at its maximum at its difficulty level, and the *amount* of information an item yields is a function of discrimination. Highly discriminating items provide more information.

These features are illustrated in Figure 10.4, which shows item information curves for three items with different difficulty and discrimination values. Items A and B have high and

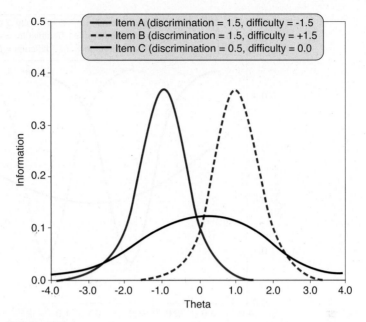

Figure 10.4

Item information functions for three items differing in item difficulty/location and item discrimination.

comparable information (as shown on the Y axis), but item information for the two items is maximized at different locations. Item A provides the most information for theta level −1.5, whereas Item B provides the most information at theta level +1.5. Item C, by contrast, has low discrimination ($a = 0.5$) and consequently has low information. Less discriminating items have wider and flatter information curves than items with good information, which are narrow and peaked.

For illustrative purposes, we present the following equation for an IIF for dichotomous item i in a 2-PL model:

$$I_i(\theta) = a_i^2\, p_i(\theta)\, q_i(\theta) \tag{10.8}$$

where item information for item i is a function of the probability of a positive response p_i times the probability of a negative response q_i times the square of a_i, the discrimination parameter. This equation clearly shows that discrimination (a) plays a pivotal role in item information, which is a key factor in measurement error in IRT.

The standard error (SE) for an item is, in fact, the reciprocal of the amount of item information. When the SE for an item is plotted against theta, the SE curve for a high information item is sharply U-shaped, as illustrated in Figure 10.5, which plots the standard error for the same three items as in Figure 10.4. The high-information Items A and B achieve a low standard error at the items' location on the theta continuum. By contrast, Item C has a higher SE at most difficulty levels.

We illustrate IIFs further with an actual example, using the data set of nearly 1,000 low-income women who completed the 20-item CES-D (Polit, London, & Martinez, 2001). In our IRT analysis described in Chapter 6, we used seven CES-D items to create a short "Depressed Affect" subscale. Figure 10.6 presents the item information for two of these items, Item 6 ("I felt depressed") and Item 7 ("I felt everything I did was an effort"). It may be recalled from Chapter 6 (Table 6.3) that Item 6 had the highest discrimination value ($a = 3.67$) and Item 7 had the lowest ($a = 0.73$). Figure 10.6 shows that the location of both items was near 0.0 on the latent trait, but Item 6 had a high level of information, peaking at about 1.7, whereas Item 7 had relatively little information.

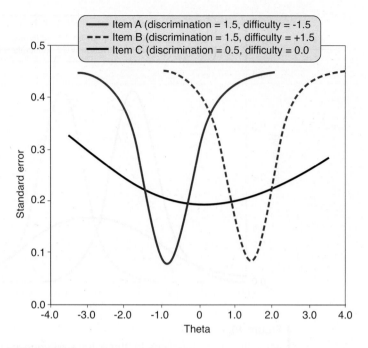

Figure 10.5

Standard error curves for three items differing in item difficulty/location and item discrimination.

Item information is additive across items, and so the IIFs can be added together to yield a **test** (or scale) **information function (TIF)**. Thus, the more information contributed by individual items, the greater the overall information of the set of items will be. The TIF indicates how the items, taken together, function in terms of measurement precision. This allows researchers to evaluate information for different sets of items, and for smaller or larger numbers of items, which is useful when developing a short form from an existing scale. Figure 10.7 displays the test information function for the seven-item CES-D Depressed Affect subscale from our data set of 1,000 women.

With an IRT-derived scale, people who complete the set of items have different *SEMs* depending on their location on the theta continuum because scales, like items, can provide different amounts of information (and lower measurement error) at different levels of the latent trait. The *SEM* at any trait level is the inverse of the square root of the overall information function, summed across items. As an illustration, the equation for a 2-PL model with dichotomous items is:

$$SEM\ (\theta) = \frac{1}{\sqrt{I\ (\theta)}} = \frac{1}{\sqrt{\sum a_i^2\ p_i\ (\theta)\ q_i\ (\theta)}} \qquad (10.9)$$

SEM functions for scales are also U-shaped, with lowest levels of error at the point on the theta continuum where the collection of items has maximal information. This means that a scale developer can select information-rich items to establish the point along the continuum where highest levels of precision are most desired. Typically, that point is near zero, with error increasing at the extremes. However, for some clinical and screening applications, a scale that discriminates best at high (or low) levels of the trait might be desirable, especially if there is a critical cutpoint for decision making.

An IRT analysis of different measures of depression illustrates this principle (Olino et al., 2012). The TIF for the CES-D, which is a measure of depression frequently used in epidemiologic studies with general populations, was highest near zero on the latent depression

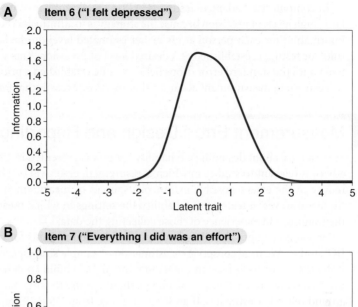

Figure 10.6
Item information function for two CES-D items.

continuum, and the *SEM* was consequently lowest at that point. (This is similar to what we found in our IRT analysis, as shown in Figure 10.7). By contrast, the Beck Depression Inventory, which is more often used with clinical samples and in treatment studies, was found in the Olino study to provide more information at higher levels of depression severity, peaking near 2.0 on the latent trait continuum.

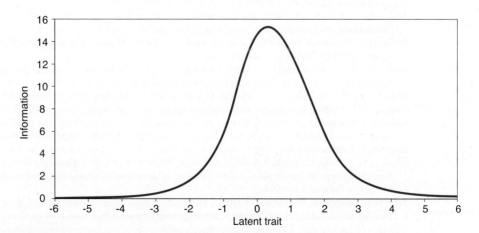

Figure 10.7
Test information curve for seven CES-D items.

In computerized adaptive testing (CAT), a small number of items can yield scores with fairly high levels of precision because the strategy is to administer those items with maximum information for each person at his or her estimated level on the latent trait. The "stopping rule" for testing is established at a desired level of precision. That is, the items are administered until the standard error drops below a value established a priori. As a result, small item sets can attain measurement accuracy that meets or exceeds that for longer static tests.

10.5 Measurement Error: Design and Reporting

Some advice about designing a reliability study was presented in Chapters 8 and 9, and that advice is relevant to studies in which measurement error will be estimated. A key goal is to reduce to the extent possible extraneous sources of measurement error, be that from the timing of waves in test–retest reliability, the settings in which measurements take place, or the training and experience of those collecting the data.

Previous chapters also discussed sample size requirements for reliability studies and for IRT studies. We urge conservative estimation of sample size, especially with regard to ICCs, if the ICC estimate is used in calculating the *SEM* to build confidence intervals around individual scores. In particular, researchers should aspire to fairly narrow confidence intervals around reliability estimates. If an ICC can range from .65 to .95 around an estimated value of .80, then it is difficult to put a lot of faith in confidence intervals around individual scores.

Many researchers who undertake a reliability study do not report on measurement error. Because information about measurement error can help clinicians to understand and interpret scores, we urge those who describe a new instrument to report a parameter of measurement error, as does the COSMIN group (DeVet et al., 2011). The influential *Standards for Educational and Psychological Testing* (American Educational Research Association, American Psychological Association, & National Council on Measurement in Education, 2014) also recommends that the *SEM* be reported in instrument development papers, although those who have adhered to traditional psychometric methods often do not do so.

References

American Educational Research Association, American Psychological Association, & National Council on Measurement in Education. (2014). *Standards for educational and psychological testing*. Washington, DC: American Psychological Association.

Atkinson, G. (2000). Typical error versus limits of agreement. *Sports Medicine, 30*, 375–381.

Bland, J. M., & Altman, D. G. (1986). Statistical methods for assessing agreement between two methods of clinical measurement. *Lancet, 327*, 307–310.

Charter, R. A., & Feldt, L. S. (2002). The importance of reliability as it relates to true score confidence intervals. *Measurement and Evaluation in Counseling and Development, 35*, 104–112.

DeVet, H. C. W., Terwee, C., Mokkink, L. B., & Knol, D. L. (2011). *Measurement in medicine: A practical guide*. Cambridge, MA: Cambridge University Press.

Feldt, L. S., Steffan, M., & Gupta, N. (1985). A comparison of five methods for estimating the standard error of measurement at specific score levels. *Applied Psychological Measurement, 9*, 351–361.

Hopkins, W. G. (2000a). Measures of reliability in sports medicine and science. *Sports Medicine, 30*, 1–15.

Hopkins, W. G. (2000b). Typical error versus limits of agreement: Reply. *Sports Medicine, 30*, 375–378.

Mokkink, L. B., Terwee, C., Patrick, D., Alonso, J., Stratford, P., Knol, D., . . . DeVet, H. (2012). *COSMIN checklist handbook*. Retrieved from http://www.cosmin.nl/images/upload/files/COSMIN%20checklist%20manual%20v9.pdf

Nunnally, J., & Bernstein, I. H. (1994). *Psychometric theory* (3rd ed.). New York, NY: McGraw-Hill.

Olino, T., Yu, L., Klein, D., Rohde, P., Seeley, J., Pikonis, P., & Lewinson, P. (2012). Measuring depression using item response theory: An examination of three measures of depressive symptomatology. *International Journal of Methods in Psychiatric Research, 21*, 76–85.

Polit, D. F., London, A., & Martinez, J. (2001). *The health of poor urban women: Findings from the Project on Devolution and Urban Change*. New York, NY: Manpower Demonstration Research Corporation.

Streiner, D. L., & Norman, G. R. (2008). *Health measurement scales: A practical guide to their development and use* (4th ed.). Oxford: Oxford University Press.

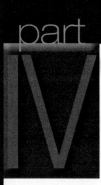

part IV

THE VALIDITY DOMAIN

chapters

11

Content Validity and Face Validity

Chapter Outline

Part IV of this book is devoted to the **validity** domain of measurement. Part IV includes this chapter on content and face validity as well as chapters on criterion validity (Chapter 12), hypothesis-testing construct validity (Chapter 13), structural validity (Chapter 14), and cross-cultural validity (Chapter 15).

As noted in Chapter 3, validity is one of four broad domains for assessing the quality of a measure. Consensus-based Standards for the selection of health Measurement Instruments (COSMIN) defined validity as "the degree to which an instrument measures the construct(s) it purports to measure" (Mokkink et al., 2010, p. 743). The key validity question is: To what extent does evidence support the inference that this measure is indeed measuring the target construct? The validity question can be addressed in various ways, bringing to bear several different kinds of evidence. In all cases, however, the central issue is whether an instrument is truly measuring the attribute that users of the instrument believe is being measured. For relatively concrete attributes, this may not be a problem; for the attribute *height*, for example, few doubt that a measuring rod is really measuring height rather than, say, weight. For many health constructs, however, especially abstract constructs measured as health-related patient-reported outcomes (HR-PROs), the validity question is not easy to answer. How do we know, for example, that a scale to measure patients' resilience, such as the Resilience Scale (Wagnild & Young, 1993), is really measuring *resilience* (a trait associated with a person's ability to adapt to challenging life circumstances)? How do we know the scale is not really measuring a similar construct with a different label, such as coping, hardiness, or flexibility?

This chapter discusses how to gather and evaluate evidence relating to two types of validity, face and content validity. COSMIN defined **content validity** as "the degree to which the content of an HR-PRO instrument is an adequate reflection of the construct to be measured"

(Mokkink et al., 2010, p. 743). We think that content validity is relevant for measures other than PROs, and so we would define content validity more broadly as the extent to which an instrument's content adequately represents the focal construct. This definition implies that content validity is relevant primarily for measures that involve multiple components. This is because the term "adequate reflection" implies that the key issues are content relevance (Are the components of the measure relevant to the construct?) and content comprehensiveness (Are all aspects of the construct represented in the measure?).

Thus, content validity is an especially important aspect of validity for multi-item scales and indexes, including PROs, composite observational scales, and complex classification or staging rules. Content validity is a special concern for formative indexes because, as discussed in Chapter 2, the components of an index *define* the attribute.

Unlike other types of validity assessment, content validity is usually explored during instrument development, as part of item selection and refinement processes, rather than after a measure has been finalized. However, in its guiding document regarding the use and evaluation of PROs in clinical trials to assess a medical product, the U.S. Food and Drug Administration (U.S. FDA, 2009) recommended that a separate content validation be undertaken if researchers choose an existing PRO that was finalized without any content validation. And, as we shall see, efforts to create item banks using item response theory (IRT) methods have led to some content validity assessments after items have been psychometrically tested.

Face validity is defined by COSMIN as the degree to which an HR-PRO (measurement instrument), indeed, looks as though it is "an adequate reflection of the construct to be measured" (Mokkink et al., 2010, p. 743). This chapter offers advice on ways to enhance content and face validity and how to assess and report them.

11.1   Content Validity

In the FDA's guiding document (2009) on measuring PROs, more attention was paid to content validity than to any other type of validity. Yet, content validity has not always been held in high esteem as a means of assessing an instrument's validity, perhaps because content validity involves subjective judgments. It is increasingly recognized, however, that evaluating and enhancing a measure's content validity is a critical early step in enhancing the construct validity of an instrument (Haynes, Richard, and Jubany, 1995; Strauss & Smith, 2009; Vogt, King, and King, 2004). If the content of an instrument is a good reflection of a construct, then the instrument has a greater likelihood of achieving its measurement objectives.

A measure can, however, be found to have good construct validity without necessarily being adequate in terms of its content validity. For example, Park, Reilly-Spong, and Gross (2013) recently observed that scales to measure *mindfulness* (a construct that has emerged as an important health concept because of evidence that mindfulness interventions can improve health-related quality of life) have considerable evidence of hypothesis-testing construct validity despite the absence of evidence that the scales are comprehensive in their coverage of the construct. A strong effort at conceptualizing the construct at the outset is essential.

Content validity, like other forms of validity, involves a process of evidence building, and so the more evidence that can be assembled, the more confident users of a measure will be. Like other forms of validity, content validity is not a fixed property of an instrument. In particular, content validity may vary from one population or context to another. Users of a measure should consider the degree of similarity between their population and context and those used in the developmental efforts to validate it. If similarity is weak, a new measurement study might be needed.

Content validity efforts have been described as a two-part process. One part involves developing an adequate conceptualization of the construct, and a second involves gathering evidence from external sources to support the inference that the instrument reflects that conceptualization. It is important to recognize, however, that the two steps typically are iterative rather than linear: A good conceptual model improves the measure's content validity, but efforts to gather evidence of content validity often lead to modifications and refinements of the conceptualization (Strauss & Smith, 2009). This iterative process is illustrated by work with the Patient Reported Outcomes Measurement Information System (PROMIS®) item banks (Riley et al., 2010), as discussed in a later section.

11.1.a Understanding the Construct: Conceptual Models

For all validity efforts, it is essential to have a thorough and comprehensive understanding of the construct being measured, including its complexity, factors that are likely to impinge on its presence and intensity, factors that affect its stability, and other constructs from which it needs to be distinguished. Chapter 4, which described challenges in scale development, emphasized the value of a careful conceptualization of the construct as an initial step in creating items.

An explicit conceptual framework is important for guiding content validity efforts as well. For complex constructs, the framework typically includes a visual diagram (a conceptual model) of the construct as well as conceptual definitions of key concepts. Two types of conceptual model are relevant to measurement assessments. The first type, which is consistent with the one recommended in the FDA guidelines (their Figure 4), focuses squarely on the construct and its dimensionality—that is, the domains subsumed under a broad construct. Models of this kind are valuable in content validation and in assessments of the structural validity of multidimensional instruments, as discussed in Chapter 14. A second and more comprehensive type of model depicts presumed interrelationships among the target construct and its subparts on the one hand and clinical and other factors influencing it on the other hand. Because this second type inherently suggests hypothesized relationships, such models are excellent tools for assessing construct validity (Chapter 13).

Figure 11.1 presents an example of a conceptual model portraying the domains (dimensions) encompassed in a complex construct, *postpartum depression*. In this model,

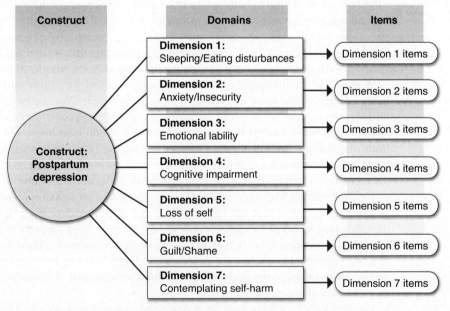

Figure 11.1
Conceptual model for postpartum depression.

Beck and Gable (2000, 2001) conceptualized postpartum depression as having seven domains, and items for the Postpartum Depression Screening Scale (PDSS) were developed to map onto these domains. Each dimension was conceptually defined. For example, the domain "Cognitive impairment" was defined as follows: "A mother's loss of control over her thought processes leaves her frightened that she may be losing her mind" (Beck & Gable, 2001, p. 206). In the 35-item final scale, 5 items tapped each dimension. Examples of items to measure the cognitive impairment dimension include: "I had a difficult time making even a simple decision" and "I thought I was going crazy."

Methods for developing conceptual models for instrumentation purposes are diverse and may depend in part on the maturity of the construct. For constructs that have been subjected to considerable empirical inquiry, instrument developers may depend on a thorough review of the literature, perhaps reinforced by discussions with or review by experts. For example, Rasmussen, Dunning, Hendrieck, Botti, and Speight (2013) developed the Pregnancy and Postnatal Well-being in T1DM Transition scale to measure the social and psychological well-being of women with Type 1 diabetes. Their conceptual framework was based on a detailed literature review, and the framework and resulting items were reviewed by an expert panel of professionals with backgrounds in endocrinology, psychology, and nursing, as well as members of consumer advocacy groups. As noted in Chapter 4, it is often productive to have an external review of the framework and domain specifications, even prior to item generation.

Sometimes, a formal **concept analysis** is the basis for creating a framework. Concept analysis is a methodology that has been used to analyze many health concepts and has been especially prominent in several health specialties, including public health and nursing. Numerous approaches to concept analysis have been established (e.g., Rodgers & Knafl, 2000; Wilson, 1963), but they typically involve a systematic and staged process of identification and analysis aimed at definitional and dimensional clarity and boundary-setting for a construct. Lang, Goulet, and Amsel (2003), for example, developed the Lang and Goulet Hardiness Scale to measure hardiness in parents following the death of their fetus or infant. The scale dimensions were based on a concept analysis that identified three domains of parental hardiness.

In-depth qualitative inquiry can be extremely helpful in understanding the dimensionality of a construct. In such studies, researchers probe deeply into people's experiences relating to the construct and use the themes and patterns that emerge to develop a conceptual model. This was the approach used in the construction of Beck and Gable's (2000) Postpartum Depression Screening Scale, which relied heavily on three qualitative inquiries (two phenomenologic studies and one grounded theory study) that Beck had undertaken with women who were experiencing postpartum depression.

The conceptual model or framework forms the basis for initial item generation. A carefully constructed framework can thus contribute to content validity right from the start. As described in Chapter 4, items should be subjected to close scrutiny and pretesting using strategies that overlap with content validation. Before describing some specific strategies, we discuss the focus of content validation and the issue of who the "experts" for a content validity study should be.

11.1.b The Focus of Content Validation

Content validation concerns the extent to which a measure is an "adequate reflection" of the attribute being measured and involves obtaining input from external reviewers. Three issues are pertinent in a content validation: relevance, comprehensiveness, and balance.

■ *Relevance.* An assessment for relevance involves feedback from experts on the relevance of both individual items and the overall set of items. For each item, one needs to know: Is this item relevant to the construct, or to a specific domain (dimension) of the construct? Another important consideration, at both the item and aggregate level, is whether the items have relevance for the target population, and for the type of situation envisioned for the use of the measure. For example, in a measure of dietary intake that involves asking about food consumption, food items should be relevant to diverse ethnic groups if the target population is multicultural.

■ *Comprehensiveness.* The flip side of asking experts about whether items are relevant to a construct is to ask them if there are notable omissions. To be content valid, a measure should encompass the full dimensionality of the construct.

■ *Balance.* An instrument that is content valid represents the domains of the construct in a balanced manner. For example, in Beck's Postpartum Depression Screening Scale, the scale might not be considered content valid if, for example, only one item measured the cognitive impairment domain, but 10 items measured the emotional lability domain. In a multi-item scale, a sufficient number of items is needed for each dimension to ensure high internal consistency (or, in IRT, a high test information function) of the subscales. Balance across domains is especially important when subscale scores are summed to yield a total score.

11.1.c Content Validity Experts

Many of the strategies for assessing a new instrument's content validity involve a review of the relevance and comprehensiveness of scale items with an appropriate group. Often, the "appropriate group" is patients themselves, especially when the construct concerns attributes about which patients are themselves the "experts." For example, for a construct involving preferences, symptoms, and burdens, patients (or their family caregivers) are likely to have a good understanding of the construct and its dimensions. The FDA guidelines (2009) emphasize the importance of client input in content validity efforts for PROs used to support labeling claims in conjunction with medical product development.[1] If product developers claim that their product "lessens pain" or "increases quality of life," for example, then patients are usually in the best position to evaluate the content validity of a scale to measure these attributes.

For some constructs, however, clinicians or substantive specialists might have a broader or more objective view of a construct's manifestations and dimensions than patients. For example, if a construct is abstract or theoretical (e.g., *resilience*), then it is likely that the judgments of professionals who have pertinent clinical or academic expertise would be appropriate in a content validity study. When such experts are involved, instrument developers typically share with them not only a draft of the new instrument but also a fairly detailed description of the conceptual model, the target population, and uses to which the instrument would be put. Of course, there are many measures for which it would be advantageous to obtain content validity feedback from both lay people and professionals.

11.1.d Content Validity: Qualitative Strategies

Content validation often involves obtaining opinions from experts using qualitative methods. Qualitative researchers have devised several strategies for collecting rich in-depth information from people. These strategies typically involve the use of semistructured or unstructured interviews in which the interviewers make little attempt to constrain the flow of communication. Questions are *open ended* (i.e., there are no response options from which to choose), and the interviews tend to be conversational. In-depth interviews are typically tape-recorded and then transcribed for subsequent analysis. Such a procedure allows

---

[1]The 2009 FDA document gives the following warning: "Without adequate documentation of patient input, a PRO instrument's content validity is likely to be questioned" (p. 12). The document further notes that "evidence of other types of validity (e.g., construct validity) or reliability (e.g., consistent scores) will not overcome problems with content validity because we evaluate instrument adequacy to measure the concept represented in the labeling claim" (p. 12).

interviewers to listen more attentively than would be the case if they were recording notes, and to devise suitable probes and follow-up questions to obtain richer and more complete data. Advice on how to conduct and analyze qualitative data is available in many research method textbooks (e.g., Merriam, 2009; Patton, 2002; Tracy, 2013), and specific advice about the application of qualitative methods to content validity efforts was offered by Brod, Tesler, and Christensen (2009).

Conducting focus group interviews is a widely used approach to exploring content validity issues with patients (Vogt et al., 2004). As described in Chapter 4, focus group interviews involve in-depth questioning, usually with a group of 5 to 10 people from the target population, to dialogue about the construct and its dimensions or to review drafts of individual scale items and the overall instrument. For example, Vakil and colleagues (2012) conducted four focus group interviews with 32 patients diagnosed with gastroesophageal reflux disorder (GERD) during an exploratory content validity phase for constructing the Reflux Symptom Questionnaire (RESQ). Patient statements were coded to identify symptom concepts, and two expert gastroenterologists reviewed and confirmed symptom selection.

One-on-one interviewing is also a common strategy and is often referred to as *cognitive interviewing* even though the goal is somewhat different from what we described in Chapter 4 in connection with efforts to understand how patients interpret questions and select an answer. The FDA guidance on content validity explicitly mentions cognitive interviews and *cognitive debriefing* as a content validity strategy. Indeed, the FDA recommends that "repeating cognitive interviews" (presumably as the instrument is revised) "can help confirm content validity" (p. 16). As an example of cognitive interviewing for content validity purposes, Crawford, Stanford, Wong, Dalal, and Bayliss (2011) developed the Experience with Allergic Rhinitis Nasal Spray Questionnaire (EARNS-Q) to assess experience and preference of intranasal corticosteroids in patients with allergic rhinitis. Patient focus groups helped to inform the conceptual framework and initial selection of items. Cognitive interviews (lasting an average of 2 hours) were then conducted. In the first part, patients were allowed to suggest attributes to be included in the questionnaire, and then in the second part, they were asked to comment on the content and relevance of items on the draft instrument.

When professional experts rather than patients are invited to participate in content validity investigations, they may be asked for formal ratings, as described in the next section, or they may be asked simply to provide feedback regarding how relevant the items are, whether additional items are needed to reflect the construct thoroughly, and whether there is an appropriate balance of items for measuring different domains.

11.1.e Content Validity: Quantitative Strategies

Some quantitative information about content validity can be gleaned from pretesting a draft instrument with a small sample from the target population (Chapter 4). For example, if there are large amounts of missing data for a scale item on a pretest, this might suggest that the item was confusing or that patients found the item irrelevant for them (U.S. FDA, 2009, Table 1). Follow-up interviews with the pretest sample could help to diagnose the reason for missing data.

Quantitative assessments of content validity most often take the form of ratings of item relevance from a panel of experts—most often professionals but sometimes members of the target population. Various approaches have been devised, notably in the field of personnel psychology, all of which are based on assessments of the degree to which experts agree on the items' relevance (Lindell & Brandt, 1999). For example, as early as 1975, Lawshe proposed an index of interrater agreement called the *content validity ratio*, or CVR. In health fields, quantitative assessments of expert agreement are typically performed using the **content validity index (CVI)**, whose development has been attributed to an educational psychometrician (Martuza, 1977). Polit, Beck, and Owen (2007) noted that the CVI is preferable to other available CVIs because (1) it provides expert assessment data at both the item and scale level, (2) it is easy to compute, and (3) it is the only index that captures agreement *in one direction*. With respect to the last attribute, the various CVIs in the field of personnel psychology can yield values of 1.00 (perfect agreement) if there is universal agreement that an item is *not* relevant, which does not seem desirable for summarizing the extent of content validity for a set of items. The CVI, which will be described subsequently, only takes agreement about the relevancy of items into account.

In a typical study using the CVI, a panel of experts is invited to complete a content validity questionnaire that elicits both qualitative and quantitative feedback about the items. Qualitative feedback can be solicited about the adequacy of the conceptual framework and conceptual definitions, the need for additional items to thoroughly represent the construct, and the appropriateness of item balance in the item set. The experts are also asked to rate each draft item for its relevance to the construct, typically on a 4-point scale. Points on the scale are often labeled as follows: 1 = not relevant, 2 = somewhat relevant, 3 = quite relevant, and 4 = highly relevant (Polit et al., 2007). Table 11.1 presents an example of a portion of a content validity questionnaire for the measurement of one dimension (assertiveness) of the construct *safe sexual behaviors among adolescents*. In an actual content validity study, the construct and its domains would need to be fully explicated, and additional information about the scale (e.g., the intended target population, intended use of the measure, how items were developed, readability statistics) would be provided to the review panel.

In terms of scoring, **item-level CVIs (I-CVIs)** are computed as the proportion of experts who agree that the item is either "quite" or "highly" relevant. This is analogous to what Cicchetti and Feinstein (1990) called *proportions of specific agreement* (Chapter 8). So, if there were eight raters and seven of them gave a rating of either 3 or 4 for an item, the I-CVI for that item would be .875. Information from the I-CVIs can be used to compute a **scale-level content validity index (S-CVI)**. There are two methods of calculating an S-CVI (Polit & Beck, 2006), and the methods almost always yield different values. The preferred method is to compute the S-CVI as the average of all the I-CVIs.

One criticism of the CVI is that it throws away information. The four-point rating essentially boils down to a dichotomous judgment of relevance versus irrelevance. However, the more finely graded ratings, together with open-ended comments and suggestions, can be used to inform decisions about item revision and rewording. For example, the content validity questionnaire can ask experts to explain why they rated any item as less than "highly relevant."

Critics of the CVI have been especially concerned with the fact that the I-CVI is essentially an index of proportion in agreement and is not corrected for chance agreement in a manner analogous to Cohen's kappa (Chapter 8). Indeed, some have proposed replacing the I-CVI with multirater kappa, which does take chance agreement into account (e.g., Wynd, Schmidt, and Schaefer, 2003). However, kappa traditionally is calculated based on agreement of any kind, which in this situation would mean agreement about irrelevance as well as relevance. Polit et al. (2007) proposed a modified kappa for one-sided agreement and then constructed a table to show how I-CVI values map onto the modified kappa values. Using criteria suggested by Fleiss (1981), in which kappa values in excess of .75 are deemed "excellent," Polit and colleagues (2007) demonstrated that any I-CVI value in excess of .78 would translate to a modified kappa greater than .75 and so could be considered evidence of adequate item relevance. They also proposed that S-CVI values of .90 or higher provide evidence of strong content validity of the overall scale.

Typically, a first round of expert judgments leads to modifications to the scale, including the revision of some items, the deletion of others, and the development of new items. Thus, unless the initial panel has few criticisms, the content validity exercise as described ideally should be undertaken twice, wherein experts evaluate a draft version of the instrument, and then assess a near-final version once revisions have been made. Occasionally, a Delphi-type approach is used in which judgments from the first round are shared with the full panel so that consensus can be achieved. For example, Remijn and coresearchers (2013) involved 15 expert speech therapists in a three-round Delphi content validation in developing an

Table 11.1	Example of a Portion of a Content Validity Questionnaire

The scale items that follow have been developed to measure one of five dimensions of the construct of **Safe sexual behaviors among adolescents**, namely **Assertiveness**, as described in our conceptual model. Please read each item and score it for its relevance in representing the Assertiveness domain.

Assertiveness is defined as the use of verbal and interpersonal skills to negotiate protection during sexual activities.

Item	Item Relevance Rating			
	Not Relevant	Somewhat Relevant	Quite Relevant	Highly Relevant
A1. I ask my partner about his/her sexual history before having intercourse.	1	2	3	4
A2. I don't have sex without asking the person if he/she has been tested for HIV/AIDS.	1	2	3	4
A3. When I am having sex with someone for the first time, I insist that we use a condom.	1	2	3	4
A4. I don't let my partner talk me into having sex without knowing something about how risky it would be.	1	2	3	4
A5. I have the will power to resist my partner if I feel uncomfortable about having sex.	1	2	3	4
A6. I am strict about knowing the background of anyone I have sex with.	1	2	3	4

Please comment on any of these items, including possible revisions or substitutions, or your views about why an item is not relevant to the concept of assertiveness within the construct of safe sexual behaviors in adolescents.

Comments/Suggestions

A1
A2
A3
A4
A5
A6

Please suggest any additional items you feel would improve the measurement of assertiveness, or make any further comments to help us improve this subscale.

observational measure of the children's chewing ability, the Mastication Observation and Evaluation Instrument.

The CVI has been used to evaluate content validity in many health-related instrument development studies. For example, Takasaki, Johnston, Treleaven, and Jull (2012) developed the Neck Pain Driving Index (NPDI) to assess perceived driving difficulty for patients with whiplash-associated disorders. Preliminary items, which included driving tasks and symptoms, were assessed for content validity by a 15-member expert panel that included researchers and clinicians in medicine, physiotherapy, and chiropractic. Items with an I-CVI less than .80 were discarded. The experts suggested adding several items, and so a second content validity assessment was undertaken for the new items. The authors did not report the scale-level CVI, but I-CVI information in the article permitted us to calculate the S-CVI value to be .89 for the driving task item subscale and .95 for the symptom item subscale.

11.1.f Content Validity and IRT-Derived Measures

When IRT methods are used to select items for measuring a construct efficiently, many preliminary items are typically discarded during IRT testing, and this is particularly true when the goal is to prune items for an item bank such as PROMIS®. For example, in creating the PROMIS® item banks for measuring three domains of emotional distress, the initial item pool of 1,404 items was reduced to 168 based on content validity work such as described in this chapter (as well as efforts to improve readability and eliminate redundancies). The final item banks of 28, 29, and 29 items (total = 86) to measure depression, anxiety, and anger, respectively, were calibrated using IRT methods (Pilkonis et al., 2011).

Item reduction in IRT usually reflects a variety of concerns that are not content related. For example, items may be eliminated because of differential item functioning (DIF), insufficient unidimensionality, local dependence, disordered response thresholds, and poor IRT model fit. Such item pruning may cause a potential threat to the content validity of the final item bank because the set of items is no longer reflective of the conclusions drawn during initial content validation with respect to comprehensiveness and balance. For example, in the emotional distress item banks, a total of 82 items of the 168 tested items were eliminated, all of which had had previous evidence of content validity.

The strategy recommended by the PRO task force of the International Society for Pharmacoeconomics and Outcomes Research (ISPOR) is that patient interviews or focus groups be used after item selection to evaluate the content importance of items that were eliminated versus those that were retained (Rothman et al., 2009). In such situations, the researchers would not be able to simply reinsert omitted items deemed to be content-important into the item bank because of their psychometric deficiencies. Rather, new items covering the same content would have to be devised and reevaluated.

Because such an endeavor would be time consuming and resource-intensive, Riley and colleagues (2010) proposed an alternative—or at least an interim—strategy. In their work with PROMIS®, their approach to improving the content validity of the item banks was to reevaluate the domain names and definitions so that the items and domains would be better aligned. They relied on reviews from content experts to revise conceptual definitions of all domains. For example, the revised definition for the domain of "Anxiety" stipulates what the item bank covers (e.g., fear, anxious misery, hyperarousal, and somatic symptoms) as well as what it does not (behavioral fear avoidance).

Although the effects of item pruning on content validity is especially worrisome for IRT-derived measures, concerns may also be relevant to scales developed within CTT. Whenever a large number of items are eliminated based on psychometric requirements, the content validity of the remaining items may need to be reevaluated. If short forms are developed from previously validated instruments, such an assessment is advisable.

11.2 Face Validity

Face validity, which refers to whether a measure "looks like" it is measuring the right attribute, is not always considered an important attribute. Indeed, there are some measures—such as the projective Rorschach inkblot test—that are designed *not* to have face validity. Nevertheless, it is usually desirable to use measures that can be viewed as appropriate for the target population, just on the face of it.

The important parties to consider in assessing face validity are the people who are being measured and, in clinical settings, the people who decide to make the measurements. Face validity has special relevance when there is concern that about potential hesitation to administer the measure (e.g., clinicians) or reluctance to be measured (e.g., patients). Thus, an instrument being developed for routine adoption by clinicians should be assessed for face validity and for other feasibility issues (e.g., ease of administration, usefulness) by asking for clinicians' input.

Face validity is also a concern for many public health researchers who rely on the cooperation of a general population of people. Response rates to general public health surveys are typically low in any event, so it is important to ensure that potential responders are not "turned off" by a seemingly inappropriate set of questions. For cxample, Sarmugam, Worsley, and Flood (2013) developed a Salt Knowledge Questionnaire designed to assess knowledge about dietary salt consumption in a general population. Their 25-item measure was assessed for face validity.

Assessments of face validity often overlap with evaluations of content validity, and many of the same qualitative strategies are used for both. It might, however, be noted that face validity is relevant for a broader range of measures, including ones that are not multicomponent, such as one-item PROs and simple performance measures.

As we saw in Chapter 7, face validity is considered especially important in clinimetrics. Efforts to assess face validity with patients and clinicians are usually undertaken during the development of clinimetric instruments. For example, Howell and Concato (2004) used clinimetric methods to develop patient satisfaction items for obstetric patients and sought to identify items with high face validity.

Typically, face validity assessments are based on qualitative feedback from a small number of people (patients, clinicians, or other experts) about whether the measure seems to be measuring the right attribute. Such assessments often focus on the suitability of the overall measure, but item-level face validity can also be scrutinized. Item face validity is sometimes assessed in the context of a cognitive interview during scale development. For example, in the previously mentioned assessment of a measure for women with Type 1 diabetes in transition to motherhood, Rasmussen et al. (2013) explored both content and face validity in cognitive debriefing sessions. Patients were asked such questions as: "Did you have any difficulty understanding this question?", "What does the question mean to you?", and "Is the question relevant to you?"

For PROs, aspects of good scale construction impinge on the face validity of a measure. For example, the items on a scale with good face validity will necessarily be unambiguous (e.g., only minimal amounts of missing data) and worded in a manner that takes the reading level of the target population into account.

11.3 Designing and Reporting a Content/Face Validity Study

This section offers some guidance on the design of a content or face validity assessment, including advice about sampling and reporting.

11.3.a Study Design for Content/Face Validation

As noted earlier in this chapter, the more evidence regarding content or face validity that can be generated, the greater one's confidence in the measure, especially for PROs. Thus, we suggest a design that incorporates multiple data collection strategies and multiple types of reviewer. In many cases, a *mixed methods approach*, involving the collection of both qualitative and quantitative data, is likely to be appropriate. This suggests the need for a team that is knowledgeable about both types of methodologic approaches as well as data collection staff with appropriate training.

A comprehensive strategy for assessing content validity is likely to involve one-on-one or focus-group interviews with experts and patients as well as cognitive questioning of people from the target population. For interviews with patients, face-to-face (in person) interviewing is preferable, using interviewers with skills in probing and *listening*. With experts, however, other communication methods (e.g., telephone, mail, Internet) increase the likelihood that regional or national experts, and not just local ones, get invited to participate. Interviews with patients or experts typically do not involve a formal interview schedule (i.e., with a specific ordering and wording of questions and fixed response options). Rather, the *semi-structured interviews* are informed by a **topic guide** that indicates the important topics that interviewers must cover.

There is no single ideal strategy for sequencing activities in a content validity effort. Consultation with experts to refine a conceptual framework is typically undertaken at the outset, usually before items are developed. Personal and focus group interviews with patients, including cognitive interviews, are likely to occur early in the instrument development process. Two rounds of data collection may be desirable. For example, two phases of content validity work were undertaken in developing the previously mentioned Reflux Symptom Questionnaire (Vakil et al., 2012). In the exploratory phase, the researchers conducted 48 individual interviews and four focus group interviews and also consulted with two experts. In the confirmatory content validity phase, cognitive interviews were conducted with 42 patients, who were asked about the relevance of symptoms on the draft measure. As mentioned earlier, two phases of CVI assessment are also likely to be profitable if the first phase suggests the need for extensive modification.

For complex multidimensional constructs that are relatively abstract, a formal quantitative assessment using the CVI is likely to help enhance decision making about item revisions and can provide valuable information to potential users of the measure. A formal questionnaire, such as the partial example shown in Table 11.1, is used as the data collection tool. It might be noted that when experts are consulted regarding the content validity of an instrument, it can be useful to solicit their advice about other issues that impinge on instrument quality. For example, as experts in the construct, they are likely to have informed opinions about an appropriate test–retest interval for undertaking a retest reliability study. The experts could also be asked about their views on the stability of individual items, the degree to which each item might be responsive to intervention, and the suitability of a proposed "gold standard" if a criterion validity study is anticipated.

11.3.b The Sampling Plan for Content/Face Validation

For interviews with members of the target population, it is important to ensure that key subgroups within the population are included in the content/face validity sample. This could mean the recruitment of patients based on clinical criteria (e.g., those at different cancer stages) or based on demographic characteristics, such as age, sex, ethnicity, cultural background, and regional residence. The aim is not to achieve a sample that is truly "representative" of the target population but to ensure that important subgroups are not omitted from the sample altogether. This is a **purposive sampling** strategy, sometimes called *maximum variation sampling*, which is common in qualitative research (Patton, 2002). Sometimes it is useful to recruit a sample from more than one site to enhance coverage of diverse groups. For example, Notte and colleagues (2012) developed the Patient Perception of Intensity of Urgency Scale to measure the intensity of urgency for urinary incontinence episodes. In their work to assess the scale's content validity, cognitive interviews were conducted in two geographically diverse sites.

In terms of sample size, the number of participants in qualitative research is typically small, and sample size is seldom preestablished. Qualitative researchers use the principle of data **saturation** to inform their sample size decisions. Saturation involves sampling to the point at which redundant information is achieved and no new information is likely to be obtained by further interviewing. Redundancy can be affected by information quality, so the recruitment of people who are thoughtful and candid, and who have good communication skills, can reduce the number of people needed in the sample (Morse, 2000).

With respect to sampling for a formal content validity assessment using the CVI, the recruitment of experts from different (but relevant) specialty areas and disciplines is recommended to avoid a myopic perspective on a construct. Grant and Davis (1997) have offered advice on selecting and "training" content validity experts. The size of the expert panel is usually between 3 and 12. If two rounds of CVI assessment are envisioned, it is useful to start with a fairly large sample in the first round (e.g., 8 to 12 experts). By including a large sample of experts in the first round, researchers can assess the performance of the experts and select the most capable judges to participate in the second round. For example, researchers can use first-round data to identify judges who are consistently lenient (e.g., who gave a rating of 4 to most items) or harsh (e.g., who gave a rating of 1 or 2 to most items) or who gave ratings that are incongruent with those of the other experts. Also, if some experts offer no thoughtful qualitative feedback, this might suggest that they have not made a strong commitment to the project. Second-round CVI panels, then, might be composed of four to six of the most skillful judges.

11.3.c Reporting a Content/Face Validity Study

When preparing a paper or a report to describe content or face validity efforts, researchers should share important details, including design decisions, recruitment methods, characteristics of the target population and the sample, sample size, data collection methods, data analysis procedures, key findings, and the effect of the findings on the final instrument. For qualitative work, a statement about data saturation should be made to assure readers that efforts to improve content validity were exhaustive.

Because there is some overlap in methods used for item generation and refinement on the one hand and content and face validity inquiries on the other, the paper should indicate what specific criteria were used to draw conclusions about satisfactory levels of content and face validity. If the validation involved a series of activities completed in a sequence, a flow chart such as the one shown in Figure 11.2 can help readers to visualize the work that was undertaken.

When qualitative work informs the development of a conceptual model, the findings are reported by explicating the model and identifying the contribution made by the experts or patients. Content validity findings that contributed to instrument improvements, or that confirmed early conceptualizations, are typically reported in summary form. Here is an example from Vakil et al.'s (2012) confirmatory content validity interviews for the Reflux Symptom Questionnaire: "Individual interviews confirmed the relevance of the symptom items of the RESQ-eD. Patients collectively reported all symptoms included in the RESQ-eD, and endorsed all items as being relevant to their experience of GERD" (p. 4).

When reporting the results of a study in which CVI values were calculated, researchers should report both I-CVI and S-CVI values for the final set of items. I-CVI values can be shown in a table for each item (as Takasaki et al. [2012] did with their Neck Pain Driving Index) or as a range of values (e.g., "The I-CVI values for the final scale ranged from .87 to 1.00"). Inasmuch as there are two ways to calculate the S-CVI, researchers should be explicit about which method was used (Polit & Beck, 2006).

The COSMIN group has developed a set of evaluative questions relating to content validity (Terwee et al., 2012). Box D of the COSMIN checklists has five assessment questions that can serve as a guide to evaluating reports on content validation and as a self-assessment guide in preparing a paper on content validity efforts.

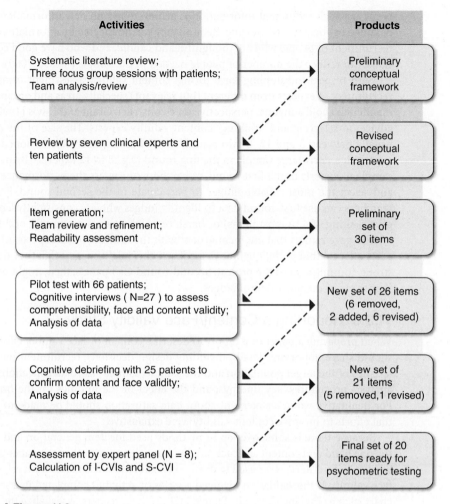

Figure 11.2
Example of a flow chart illustrating an instrument development process.

References

Beck, C. T., & Gable, R. K. (2000). Postpartum Depression Screening Scale: Development and psychometric testing. *Nursing Research, 49*, 272–282.

Beck, C. T., & Gable, R. K. (2001). Ensuring content validity: An illustration of the process. *Journal of Nursing Measurement, 9*, 201–215.

Brod, M., Tesler, L., & Christensen, T. (2009). Qualitative research and content validity: Developing best practices based on science and experience. *Quality of Life Research, 18*, 1263–1278.

Cicchetti, D. V., & Feinstein, A. R. (1990). High agreement but low kappa: II. Resolving the paradoxes. *Journal of Clinical Epidemiology, 43*(6), 551–558.

Crawford, B., Stanford, R. H., Wong, A., Dalal, A., & Bayliss, M. (2011). Development of a questionnaire to assess experience and preference of intranasal corticosteroids in patients with allergic rhinitis. *Patient Related Outcome Measures, 2*, 119–126.

Fleiss, J. L. (1981). *Statistical methods for rates and proportions* (2nd ed.). New York, NY: John Wiley & Sons.

Grant, J. S., & Davis, L. L. (1997). Selection and use of content experts in instrument development. *Research in Nursing & Health, 20*, 269–274.

Haynes, S., Richard, D., & Jubany, E. (1995). Content validity in psychological assessment: A functional approach to concepts and methods. *Psychological Assessment, 7*, 238–247.

Howell, E. A., & Concato, J. (2004). Obstetric patient satisfaction: Asking patients what they like. *American Journal of Obstetrics and Gynecology, 190*, 175–182.

Lang, A., Goulet, C., & Amsel, R. (2003). Lang and Goulet Hardiness Scale: Development and testing on bereaved parents following the death of their fetus/infant. *Death Studies, 27*, 851–880.

Lawshe, C. H. (1975). A quantitative approach to content validity. *Personnel Psychology, 28*, 563–575.

Lindell, M. K., & Brandt, C. J. (1999). Assessing interrater agreement on the job relevance of a test: A comparison of the CVI, T, rWG(J), and r'WG(J) indexes. *Journal of Applied Psychology, 84*, 640–647.

Martuza, V. R. (1977). *Applying norm-referenced and criterion-referenced measurement in education.* Boston, MA: Allyn & Bacon.

Merriam, S. B. (2009). *Qualitative research: A guide to design and implementation* (3rd ed.). San Francisco, CA: Jossey–Bass.

Mokkink, L. B., Terwee, C., Patrick, D., Alonso, J., Stratford, P., Knol, D. L., . . . DeVet, H. C. W. (2010). The COSMIN study reached international consensus on taxonomy, terminology, and definitions of measurement properties for health-related patient-reported outcomes. *Journal of Clinical Epidemiology, 63*, 737–745.

Morse, J. M. (2000). Determining sample size. *Qualitative Health Research, 10*, 3–5.

Notte, S. M., Marshall, T. S., Lee, M., Hakimi, Z., Odeyemi, I., Chen, W., & Revicki, D. (2012). Content validity and test-retest reliability of Patient Perception of Intensity of Urgency Scale (PPIUS) for overactive bladder. *BMC Urology, 12*, 26.

Park, T., Reilly-Spong, M., & Gross, C. (2013). Mindfulness: A systematic review of instruments to measure an emergent patient-reported outcome (PRO). *Quality of Life Research, 22*(10), 2639–2659.

Patton, M. Q. (2002). *Qualitative research and evaluation methods.* Thousand Oaks, CA: Sage.

Pilkonis, P. A., Choi, S., Reise, S., Stover, A., Riley, W., & Cella, D. (2011). Item banks for measuring emotional distress from the Patient-Reported Outcomes Measurement Information System (PROMIS®): Depression, anxiety, and anger. *Assessment, 18*, 263–283.

Polit, D. F., & Beck, C. T. (2006). The content validity index: Are you sure you know what is being reported? *Research in Nursing & Health, 29*, 489–497.

Polit, D. F., Beck, C. T., & Owen, S. V. (2007). Is the CVI an acceptable indicator of content validity? Appraisal and recommendations. *Research in Nursing & Health, 30*, 459–467.

Rasmussen, B., Dunning, T., Hendrieck, C., Botti, M., & Speight, J. (2013). Transition to motherhood in type 1 diabetes: Design of the pregnancy and postnatal well-being in transition questionnaires. *BMC Pregnancy and Childbirth, 13*, 54.

Remijn, L., Speyer, R., Groen, B., Holtus, P., van Limbeek, J., & Nijhuis-van der Sanden, M. (2013). Assessment of mastication in healthy children and children with cerebral palsy: A validity and consistency study. *Journal of Oral Rehabilitation, 40*, 336–347.

Riley, W. T., Rothrock, N., Bruce, B., Christodolou, C., Cook, K., Hahn, E., & Cella, D. (2010). Patient-reported outcomes measurement information system (PROMIS) domain names and definitions revisions: Further evaluation of content validity in IRT-derived item banks. *Quality of Life Research, 19*, 1311–1321.

Rodgers, B., & Knafl, J. (Eds.) (2000). *Concept development in nursing: Foundations, techniques and applications.* Philadelphia, PA: W.B. Saunders.

Rothman, M., Burke, L., Erickson, P., Kline Leidy, N., Patrick, D., & Petrie, C. (2009). Use of existing patient-reported outcome (PRO) instruments and their modification: The ISPOR Good Research Practices for evaluation and documenting content validity for the use of existing instruments and their modification PRO Task Force report. *Value Health, 8*, 1075–1083.

Sarmugam, R., Worsley, A., & Flood, V. (2013). Development and validation of a salt knowledge questionnaire. *Public Health Nutrition, 18*, 1–8.

Strauss, M. E., & Smith, G. T. (2009). Construct validity: Advances in theory and methodology. *Annual Review of Clinical Psychology, 5*, 1–25.

Takasaki, H., Johnston, V., Treleaven, J. M., & Jull, G. A. (2012). The Neck Pain Driving Index (NPDI) for chronic whiplash-associated disorders: Development, reliability, and validity assessment. *The Spine Journal, 12*, 912–920.

Terwee, C. B., Mokkink, L. B., Knol, D. L., Ostelo, R., Bouter, L. M., & DeVet, H. C. W. (2012). Rating the methodological quality in systematic reviews of studies on measurement properties: A scoring system for the COSMIN checklist. *Quality of Life Research, 21*, 651–657.

Tracy, S. J. (2013). *Qualitative research methods: Collecting evidence.* Malden, MA: John Wiley & Sons.

U.S. Food and Drug Administration. (2009). *Guidance for industry patient-reported outcome measures: Use in medical product development to support labeling claims.* Washington, DC: U.S. Department of Health and Human Services.

Vakil, N., Björck, K., Denison, H., Halling, K., Karlsson, M., Paty, J., . . . Rydén, A. (2012). Validation of the Reflex Symptom Questionnaire Electronic Diary in partial responders to proton pump inhibitor therapy. *Clinical and Translational Gastroenterology, 2*, e7.

Vogt, D. S., King, D., & King, L. (2004). Focus groups in psychological assessment: enhancing content validity by consulting members of the target population. *Psychological Assessment, 16*, 231–243.

Wagnild, G. M., & Young, H. M. (1993). Development and psychometric evaluation of the Resilience Scale. *Journal of Nursing Measurement, 1*, 165–178.

Wilson, J. (1963). *Thinking with concepts.* London, United Kingdom: Cambridge University Press.

Wynd, C. A., Schmidt, B., & Schaefer, M. A. (2003). Two quantitative approaches for estimating content validity. *Western Journal of Nursing Research, 25*, 508–518.

12

Criterion Validity

Chapter Outline

In this chapter, we discuss a type of validity called criterion validity. Consensus-based Standards for the selection of health Measurement Instruments (COSMIN) defined **criterion validity** as "the degree to which the scores of a measurement instrument are an adequate reflection of a gold standard" (Mokkink et al., 2010, p. 743). This definition implies that to undertake a validation from a criterion perspective, it is essential to identify an appropriate *gold standard* measure of the same construct and to compare scores on the gold standard with scores on the focal measure.

This chapter explains types of criterion validity and methods used to assess it. Different approaches and parameters are needed based on the measurement properties of both the focal measure and the criterion, and we illustrate several that are especially common.

12.1 Basics of Criterion Validity

We begin by describing some basic issues in criterion validation, including the underlying rationale.

12.1.a Rationale for Criterion Validity

Not all measures can be validated using a criterion approach because there is not always a "gold standard" measurement to use as the criterion. In the next section, we provide some examples of possible gold standards for various types of measures. Here, we consider the following question: If there is a criterion measurement, why would we need the focal measure at all, why not simply use the gold standard? The reasons for creating a new measure fall primarily into five categories.

- *Expense.* A new measure that is an "adequate reflection" of a criterion is often desired because the gold standard is too expensive to administer routinely. If a measurement made by means of a self-administered patient scale yields comparable information to a lengthy assessment by a physician, the instrument might be desirable in certain contexts. For example, self-reported measures of physical function are a less costly means of obtaining information than a battery of physical performance tests.

- *Efficiency.* A related reason for instrument development is to create a measure that is more efficient than the gold standard. Efficiency can be judged in terms of time required by professionals and also time required of patients themselves. For instance, if a 2-minute walk test yields comparable information to the 6-minute walk test, then in some situations, the 2-minute walk test might be preferred.

- *Risk and discomfort.* Sometimes the criterion involves a measurement that puts people at risk or is invasive, and a substitute is desired to lower the risk. A good example is invasive blood pressure monitoring (the gold standard) and noninvasive measurements using a sphygmomanometer. In other cases, the gold standard is not necessarily risky, but an alternative measure that causes less pain or discomfort is desired.

- *Criterion unavailable.* In some cases, a measure is needed because criterion measures are simply difficult or impossible to obtain routinely in clinical settings. For example, for an instrument measuring children's aggressiveness, the criterion might be conduct problems as recorded in school or police records. Such records might be inaccessible to researchers and are not routinely available to clinicians either.

- *Prediction.* One other reason for developing an instrument that can be validated against a criterion is that the criterion involves a measurement at a future point in time. In such situations, the measure is designed to predict the occurrence of the criterion.

12.1.b The "Gold Standard" Criterion

Sometimes a criterion that is problematic (e.g., too costly or too burdensome) is the impetus for developing a new measure, in which case a researcher does not have to "select" a gold standard. Often, however, instruments are developed for other reasons, and yet it still might be useful to assess criterion validity. In either case, the criterion must possess certain attributes. In particular, *the criterion measure must itself be capable of yielding valid and reliable scores.* There is little point in validating a new measure against a criterion measure that is itself of questionable quality.

A criterion is not available for all constructs, in which case researchers must use other validation approaches to persuade potential users that scores on the measure validly reflect the attribute of interest. For example, it might be difficult to identify a valid and reliable external criterion for such attributes as patients' satisfaction with care, quality of life, or self-efficacy. When this is the case, researchers typically rely on hypothesis-testing construct validation (Chapter 13).

DeVet, Terwee, Mokkink, and Knol (2011) have stated that patient-reported outcomes (PROs) "almost always lack a gold standard" (p. 161), but we respectfully disagree. A criterion may not be readily available for PROs that capture a totally subjective state, but many PROs involve asking patients to report on conditions, symptoms, or statuses that can be verified through other means and those "other means" could be suitable criteria. For example, consider the following two items:

1. I can climb a flight of stairs.
2. I feel exhausted when I climb a flight of stairs.

The first item can be objectively verified, and so there are possibilities for a "gold standard" with scales comprised of such items. Item 2, however, concerns patients' *feelings*, for which there is no external criterion; the patient's report *is* the gold standard. Identifying a criterion for some PROs is thus possible, although it may take some ingenuity and requires a clear conceptualization of the construct being measured.

Table 12.1	Examples of Measures and Gold Standards Used in Criterion Validation		
	Focal Measure	**Gold Standard**	**Citation**
PRO Measures			
	1. Cigarette Dependence Questionnaire	Salivary cotinine levels	Huang, Lin, and Wang (2010)
	2. Harvard Trauma Questionnaire	Structured clinical *DSM* interview	de Fouchier et al. (2012)
	3. Motivation rulers for assessing importance, readiness, and confidence in smoking cessation	Smoking behavior change (self-report)	Boudreaux et al. (2012)
	4. Ecologic Momentary Assessment of current physical activity (signal contingent self-report by mobile phone)	Time-matched measurements of physical activity by accelerometer	Dunton, Liao, Kawabata, and Intile (2012)
	5. Adolescent Stress Questionnaire	Wake-up salivary free cortisol levels	De Vriendt et al. (2011)
	6. TB Medication Adherence Scale	15-week pharmacy refill records	Yin et al. (2012)
	7. Athens Insomnia Scale	Sleep efficiency via Actiwatch parameters	Sun, Chiou, and Lin (2011)
Non-PRO Measures			
	8. Knee joint alignment via caliper measurement of distance between medial femoral condyles or medial malleoli	Frontal plane knee alignment via full-leg radiography	Navali, Bahari, and Nazari (2012)
	9. ActivPAL for activity count, as measure of sedentary behavior	Actigraph accelerometer	Dowd, Harrington, and Donnelly (2012)
	10. Measures of multimorbidity (e.g., the Charlson index)	3-year mortality	Brilleman and Salisbury (2013)
	11. Phipps Aggression Screening Tool	Documented acts of aggression in inpatient psychiatric setting	Jayaram, Samuels, and Konrad (2012)
	12. Postural control assessment using Midot Posture Scale Analyzer	Postural control assessment using the AccuGait force plate	Golriz, Hebert, Foreman, and Walker (2012)

Some PROs can be tested against expert clinical opinion as the gold standard. For example, an assessment by an expert using a *Diagnostic and Statistical Manual of Mental Disorders*, 5th edition (*DSM-V*) guided diagnostic interview can serve as the gold standard for measures of many psychiatric problems, such as neuroticism, suicidal ideation, or eating disorders. As another example, PROs that measure patient intentions can be tested against subsequent patient behaviors. Short-form versions of PROs are often validated against reliable and valid long-form PROs of the same construct. And sometimes physiologic or other clinical measures can be used as a gold standard for a PRO (e.g., for a measure of self-reported stress).

Although we cannot offer explicit guidance on selecting a suitable gold standard for criterion validation, we offer some examples from the literature in the hope that this will inspire creative thought about gold standards. These examples, from various health fields and using different types of assessment approaches, are shown in Table 12.1, separately for PROs and other types of health measures.

12.1.c Types of Criterion Validity

Although hypotheses are seldom formally stated in criterion validations, there is always an implicit hypothesis. The hypothesis is that the focal measure yields information that is as good as that obtained from the criterion. This in turn implies that scores on the two are hypothesized to be correlated or consistent with each other. When such a hypothesis is upheld through formal testing, users gain some assurance that the measure will support appropriate inferences regarding the attribute in question when used with the target population in a similar context.

Implicit hypotheses are associated with two types of criterion validity. **Concurrent validity** is the type of criterion validity that is assessed when the measurements of the criterion and the new instrument occur at the same time. In such a situation, the implicit hypothesis is that the new measure is an adequate substitute for a contemporaneous criterion.

Earlier, we mentioned that one reason for creating a measure that requires criterion validation is that the criterion has not yet occurred. In **predictive validity**, the focal measure is tested against a criterion that is measured in the future. Here, the hypothesis is that the new measure is a good predictor of the criterion. Screening scales are often tested against some future criterion, namely the occurrence of the phenomenon for which a screening tool is sought. As discussed in the next section, there is overlap in the methods and statistical parameters relevant for concurrent and predictive validity.

12.2 Statistical Approaches to Criterion Validity

Because criterion validation involves an inquiry into the *relationship* between the focal measure and the criterion, a wide variety of standard statistical methods can be used to scrutinize the relationship. Like any other inquiry that tests relationships, the appropriate statistic depends on the level of measurement of the two measures. Table 12.2 summarizes validity parameters frequently used in criterion validity studies, according to the level of measurement of the criterion and the focal measure. The bolded parameters are used most extensively. We organize this section in terms of three particularly common scenarios.

12.2.a Criterion Validity: Continuous Measure, Continuous Criterion

Often, both the focal instrument and the criterion are measured on a continuous scale. The two measures are administered independently, to the validity sample either at about the same time (concurrent validity) or at an interval sufficient to allow variation on the criterion (predictive validity).

| Table 12.2 | Parameters for Criterion Validity by Measurement Levels of the Focal Measure and the Gold Standard | | | | | | |

Measurement Level: Focal Measure			Measurement Level: Gold Standard			Measurements on Same Level	Validity Parameter[a]
Nominal	Ordinal	Continuous	Nominal	Ordinal	Continuous		
X			X				**Sensitivity/specificity**; predictive values; phi coefficient; kappa
	X		X				**Area under the curve** (AUC), ROC analysis; Mann–Whitney test
		X	X				**Area under the curve** (AUC), ROC analysis; t tests; logistic regression
	X			X			**Spearman's rho**
	X			X		X	**Spearman's rho**; weighted kappa or ICC
		X			X		**Pearson's r**; multiple regression
		X			X	X	ICC; paired t tests; Bland–Altman plots and Limits of Agreement (LOA)

[a]Bolded parameters are used with greatest frequency.

The most widely used approach is to compute a Pearson correlation coefficient between the two measures. For example, Andersson and colleagues (2011) assessed the reliability and validity of a 30-meter walk test as a measure of walking speed and physical function in patients with chronic obstructive pulmonary disease (COPD). The criterion was the 6-minute walk test (6MWT). The researchers concluded, on the basis of a Pearson's r of .78, that the 30-meter walk test had adequate concurrent validity.

Sometimes, especially in predictive validity studies, multiple regression is used. Indeed, the *Standards* published jointly by three professional organizations in psychology and education (AERA, APA, NCME, 2014) recommend multiple regression over Pearson's r. In such situations, the focal measure and other predictors or covariates are used to predict the criterion, and R or R^2 is the validity coefficient. As an example, Nasuti, Stuart-Hill, and Temple (2013) assessed the concurrent validity of a modified 6MWT for use with adults with intellectual disabilities. The criterion was peak oxygen uptake (VO_2 peak). Walk-test values entered first in the stepwise regression, and no other potential confounders (e.g., age, weight, height) were significantly predictive of VO_2 peak. With $R = .84$, the researchers concluded that the modified 6MWT was valid for adults with intellectual disabilities. This study illustrates that even "gold standards" like the 6MWT need validation if they are used with different populations or if they are modified.

When the focal measure and the criterion are measured on the exact same scale (same units of measurement), criterion validity can be assessed using intraclass correlation coefficients (ICCs), paired t tests, and Bland–Altman plots (see Chapter 10). For example, Golriz and colleagues (2012) compared two methods of assessing postural control concurrently.

The measure being tested was a portable clinical force plate measure (the Midot Posture Scale Analyzer), and the criterion was the standard force plate measure (AccuGait). Both yielded measurements on the same scale: center of pressure average velocity (mm/sec) and sway area (the area of an ellipse enclosing 95% of movements in mm^2). The ICC values were unacceptably low for both variables, and the paired t tests indicated significant differences. The Bland–Altman plots revealed that the greater the average velocity and sway area, the greater the difference in the values obtained from the two force plates. The researchers concluded that the portable clinical force plate should not be considered a substitute for the criterion.

12.2.b Criterion Validity: Nominal Measure, Nominal Criterion

When both measures are nominal (typically, dichotomous) measurements, standard statistical tools for assessing relationships (e.g., the phi coefficient) or agreement (kappa) can be used. Most often, however, methods of assessing **diagnostic accuracy** are applied. **Sensitivity** (the measure's ability to identify "cases" correctly, according to the gold standard) and **specificity** (its ability to classify noncases correctly) are important validity parameters, and highly useful to potential users of the measure.

To illustrate with a simple (if contrived) example, consider assessing the criterion validity of positron emission tomography (PET scan) to classify melanomas as malignant against the gold standard classification using sentinel lymph node biopsy (SLNB). Fictitious data for this example for a sample of 100 patients are shown in Table 12.3. Calculations for the sensitivity and specificity of the PET scan are shown at the bottom of the table, together with calculations for other widely used diagnostic accuracy statistics. In our example, the PET scans were moderate for sensitivity, the proportion of true positives (.750), but good for specificity, the proportion of true negatives (.917). Sometimes predictive values are more informative to clinicians. The **positive predictive value (PPV)** of .857 indicates the proportion of patients with a positive PET scan result who have malignant melanoma according to the SLNB. The **negative predictive value (NPV)** of .846 is the proportion of patients with a negative PET scan who have a negative result on the gold standard. The **likelihood ratio-positive (LR+)** of 9.036 indicates that we are about nine times as likely to find that a positive PET scan really *is* for a patient with a malignancy than for one without a malignancy. The

Table 12.3	Fictitious Data for Diagnosing Malignant Melanoma Using Positive Emission Tomography (PET) against the Gold Standard, Sentinel Lymph Node Biopsy

PET Scan	Sentinel Lymph Node Biopsy (Criterion)		
	Positive	Negative	Total
Positive	Cell A: True positives 30	Cell B: False positives 5	35 (A + B)
Negative	Cell C: False negatives 10	Cell D: True negatives 55	65 (C + D)
Total	40 (A + C)	60 (B + D)	100 (A + B+ C + D)

Sensitivity: A/(A + C) = .750
Specificity: D/(B + D) = .917
Positive predictive value (PPV):   A/(A + B) = .857
Negative predictive value (NPV): D/(C + D) = .846
Likelihood ratio-positive (LR+): Sensitivity/(1 − Specificity) = 9.036
Likelihood ratio-negative (LR−): (1 − Sensitivity)/Specificity = .273

likelihood ratio is attractive to clinicians because it summarizes the relationship between specificity and sensitivity in a single number.

These criterion validity parameters are often used when a **cutpoint** on a continuous focal measure is used to classify patients into two categories, which we discuss in the next section.

12.2.c Criterion Validity: Continuous Measure, Nominal Criterion

When the measure being assessed is continuous and the criterion is dichotomous, sometimes a simple *t* test can be used to compare mean score values on the measure for the two groups (e.g., *cases* vs. *noncases*). Another approach is to use logistic regression to predict the criterion using the continuous scores being evaluated as a predictor. For example, Boudreaux and colleagues (2012) used logistic regression to assess the predictive validity of different self-reported "motivation rulers" for smoking cessation (importance, readiness, and confidence in quitting) against the criterion of changed smoking behavior.

Most often, the analysis involves construction of a **receiver operating characteristic (ROC) curve** that plots each score on the index measure against its specificity and sensitivity for correct classification on the basis of the dichotomous criterion. As an example, Beck and Gable (2001) developed the Postpartum Depression Screening Scale (PDSS), as described in Chapter 11. In their concurrent validation, they used as their gold standard a diagnostic interview conducted by an expert clinician to classify mothers as having or not having postpartum depression (PPD). Then the researchers plotted the PDSS scores for women in the validation sample as potential cutpoints against the rate of true positives and false negatives. The resulting ROC curve is presented in Figure 12.1. To illustrate, a cutoff score of 95 on the PDSS was associated with a specificity of 1.00 (no false positives), but sensitivity was only .41, meaning only 41% of women actually diagnosed with PPD would be identified using such a high threshold. At the other extreme, a cutoff score of 45 would yield a sensitivity of 1.00 (all women with PPD would be identified), but there would be many false positives, over 70%. An appropriate cutoff point that balances sensitivity and specificity is usually near the shoulder of ROC curve. Beck and Gable used 60 as the cutpoint for screening positive for the risk of PPD.

In ROC analyses, the **area under the curve (AUC)** can be used as a validity parameter. AUC values close to 1.00 are desirable and are indicated when the curve hugs close to the upper left corner. When the curve is close to the diagonal, the AUC value is .50, indicating that the measure cannot differentiate between those who are positive and negative on the criterion. In Figure 12.1, the AUC value was an excellent .91.

When an ROC curve is used to establish the measure's cutpoint for defining caseness on the target attribute, then other diagnostic information discussed in the previous section is also reported as validity results. For example, once Beck and Gable's (2001) analysis indicated the desirable balance achieved with a cutpoint of 60 on the PDSS, they were able to state that sensitivity was .91, specificity was .72, PPV was .62, and NPV was .95.

It should be noted that the methods we have described for assessing criterion validity are applicable to all types of measures, including ones developed using item response theory methods. For example, LaPorta and colleagues (2011) created a Rasch-based measure of balance, the Unified Balance Scale (UBS), by merging items from three existing balance scales. Predictive validity was supported in a sample of patients in rehabilitation by confirming that scores at a UBS cutpoint predicted nursing home admission and a length of stay in a hospital rehabilitation unit of 6 weeks or more.

12.3   Designing a Criterion Validity Study

As noted earlier, criterion validity is not always possible because of the lack of a rational and psychometrically sound criterion. However, because information from many criterion

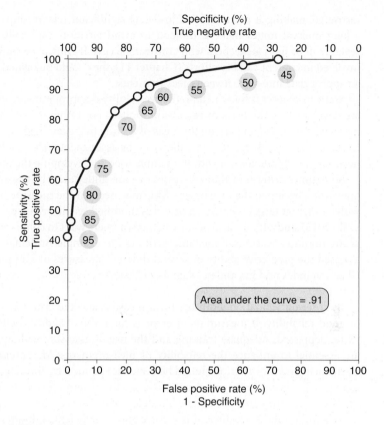

Figure 12.1

ROC curve for Postpartum Depression Screening Scale scores.
(From Figure 3 in Beck and Gable [2001].)

validity studies is so valuable to potential users—especially information about diagnostic accuracy—criterion validation is attractive. In this section, we offer some tips on planning and reporting a criterion validity study.

12.3.a Study Design in Criterion Validation

Concurrent validity efforts are often undertaken when instruments are in a state of completion or near-completion, especially in the case of PROs. For example, many researchers using a classical test theory (CTT) framework gather data for final item selection by means of item analysis and exploratory factor analysis (Chapter 5) at the same time they are measuring the criterion for a concurrent validity assessment. Such a design is efficient and has the additional advantage that the sample for such studies is typically large. However, if the measure needs to be modified on the basis of the item analyses or internal consistency results, then a new study would be needed. Concurrent validation may also be undertaken at a later point in a separate study using a finalized instrument and a different study sample—for example, in conjunction with an assessment of hypothesis-testing construct validity (Chapter 13) or structural validity (Chapter 14).

For predictive validity, at least two points of data collection are needed: the first for measuring the attribute with the focal measure and the second for measuring the criterion that the instrument is designed to predict. As with retest reliability, the interval between measurements is critical. A short interval might mean that variability on the criterion is restricted, making it more difficult to detect significant relationships. On the other hand, a long interval might make it difficult to avoid attrition, especially if the population is severely ill or has gatekeepers who constrain access. If clinical or substantive experts were involved in content validity efforts (Chapter 11), they could be invited to offer advice about an appropriate interval between measurements.

Some instruments for which predictive validity is appropriate are formative indexes that are developed on the basis of regression models. For example, a fall risk assessment scale might be developed, in part, on the basis of a study that examined factors that predict a fall. In such situations, the predictive validity of the assessment scale should be evaluated with a new sample of patients, not with the sample used in developing the measure.

Sometimes criterion validity assessments are undertaken by researchers other than the ones who developed the instrument. This may occur if the measure is being tested for use with a different target population or if it is modified, as illustrated previously in the Nasuti et al. (2013) study. It may also occur when researchers want to compare the criterion validity of two or more measures of the same attribute. For example, Brilleman and Salisbury (2013) assessed the predictive ability of several different measures of multimorbidity, such as the Charlson index and Expanded Diagnosis Clusters count, using 3-year mortality rates as the criterion.

In criterion validation, both the focal measure and the criterion should have evidence of good reliability. If measurement error is high, then validity coefficients will necessarily be depressed. Adequate training and the use of assessors with appropriate experience are essential to enhance the reliability of measurements. Measurements using the focal instrument and the criterion should be done independently. Blinding is often essential. For example, if expert clinical judgment is used as the criterion (as in Beck and Gamble's study on PPD), then the expert should be blinded to the scores on the focal measure.

When the validity coefficient is a correlation coefficient, a disattenuation correction to r (Chapter 9) might be deemed appropriate to take the unreliability of the measures into account. Disattenuation corrections are applied fairly often among nutrition researchers in their validation of food frequency questionnaires. For example, Jaceldo-Siegl and colleagues (2010) did a criterion validation of a Food Frequency Questionnaire (FFQ) against the gold standard 24-hour dietary recall method. Validity correlation coefficients were corrected for attenuation.

12.3.b Sampling in Criterion Validation

The sample for a criterion validity study should be selected to represent the target population. Heterogeneity on the focal attribute is essential because range restrictions can dampen estimates of criterion validity. Multisite assessment is advantageous, especially if there are regional variations with regard to the focal attribute.

Ideally, the sample should be fairly large to enhance the precision of validity coefficient estimates and to lessen the risk of Type II errors. In the COSMIN rating scales, it is stipulated that the sample size for criterion validation should be at least 100 to be graded as excellent (Terwee et al., 2012). However, it might be safer to base decisions about minimum sample size on a formal power analysis using widely available software. In estimating the size of the validity coefficient (e.g., Pearson's r) in the power analysis, it is prudent to be conservative rather than optimistic. The estimate of what the coefficient will be should ideally be based on evidence from earlier research and will not necessarily be the same as the standard for acceptability, discussed next.

With regard to ROC analyses, one approach to sample size is to estimate the number of cases needed for an AUC value to be significantly greater than .50, which is equivalent to the null hypothesis. If the estimate is that the AUC value will be .70, then a sample of 28 is needed. However, using .60 as a more conservative estimate of the results (while hoping, of course, for a value in excess of .70), the needed sample to achieve significance would be 104 (Streiner & Cairney, 2007).

12.3.c Standards for Criterion Validity

Ideally, researchers should decide prior to undertaking a validation study what their minimum standard for validity coefficients will be. In the absence of a standard, the risk is that almost any coefficient will be interpreted as adequate after the fact. If predesignated standards are not met, the researchers should consider how to improve their measure or their study design. For example, a better criterion might be needed, the validation sample might need to be more heterogeneous, or the measure's reliability might need to be improved.

It is not, unfortunately, possible to offer firm recommendations for acceptable validity values because in many situations, there are too many other factors to consider. This is especially true for sensitivity and specificity because the consequences of "getting it wrong" might be greater for false positives than for false negatives, or vice versa. Fischer, Bachman, and Jaeschke (2003) have suggested as a rough guide that AUCs between .50 and .70 be considered low, between .70 and .90 be considered moderate, and those greater than .90 be viewed as high. DeVet et al. (2011) from the COSMIN groups have suggested that a minimum value for an AUC statistic should be .70, and the same standard has been suggested for validity coefficients in the form of Pearson's r.

12.3.d Reporting a Criterion Validation Study

In the vast majority of cases, criterion validity is reported as part of a larger paper on the psychometric properties of a measure rather than as a stand-alone report. Guidance on reporting information about the study design and sampling in psychometric reports has been offered in earlier chapters, especially in Chapter 8.

When reporting on a criterion validation, the criterion should be fully described, including information on its suitability as a criterion and its psychometric properties. Procedures used to gather data on the criterion should be explained. For predictive validity, the time between measurements should be stated, and a rationale for the interval provided. If relevant, confidence intervals around validity estimates should be reported. The *a priori* standard of acceptability should be stated and used as a basis for interpreting the obtained validity estimates. If a disattenuation correction has been applied, both corrected and uncorrected values should be reported.

12.3.e Evaluating a Criterion Validation Study

The COSMIN group has offered guidelines and a scoring system for evaluating criterion validity evidence (Terwee et al., 2012). The website (www.cosmin.nl) lists seven questions in Box H to evaluate how the study was conducted. For example, there are items about missing values and sample size. The questions primarily concern the quality of the study rather than whether the results support an interpretation of adequate criterion validity of the measure in question.

The gold standard is an especially critical concern in evaluating a criterion validation. The researchers must persuade reviewers (and potential users) that the gold standard was appropriate and that it was reliably measured. Interpretation of the results is easiest if the researchers have stated their standards, but reviewers need to also consider whether those standards were appropriate. If the researchers establish .75 as an acceptable value for specificity and sensitivity, is this standard appropriate?

When criterion validity is tested together with other types of validity (e.g., construct validity), the entire body of validity evidence needs to be considered. However, it is also important to take into account which type of validity is most important for the types of applications envisioned for the instrument and to weigh the evidence for that type most heavily in an overall assessment.

References

American Educational Research Association, American Psychological Association, & National Council on Measurement in Education Joint Committee. (2014). *Standards for educational and psychological testing.* Washington, DC: American Psychological Association.

Andersson, M., Moberg, L., Svantesson, U., Sundbom, A., Johansson, H., & Emtner, M. (2011). Measuring walking speed in COPD: Test–retest reliability of the 30-metre walk test and comparison with the 6-minute walk test. *Primary Care Respiratory Journal, 20,* 434–440.

Beck, C. T., & Gable, R. K. (2001). Further validation of the Postpartum Depression Screening Scale. *Nursing Research, 50,* 155–164.

Boudreaux, E. D., Sullivan, A., Abar, B., Bernstein, S., Ginde, A., & Carmago, C. (2012). Motivation rulers for smoking cessation: A prospective observational examination of construct and predictive validity. *Addiction Science & Clinical Practice, 7,* 8.

Brilleman, S. L., & Salisbury, C. (2013). Comparing measures of multimorbidity outcomes in primary care. *Family Practice, 30,* 172–178.

de Fouchier, C., Blanchet, A., Hopkins, W., Bui, E., Ait-Aoudia, M., & Jehel, L. (2012). Validation of a French adaptation of the Harvard Trauma Questionnaire among torture survivors from sub-Saharan African countries. *European Journal of Psychotraumatology, 3.*

De Vriendt, T., Clays, E., Moreno, L. A., Bergman, P., Vicente-Rodriguez, G., Nagy, E., . . . De Henauw, S. (2011). Reliability and validity of the Adolescent Stress Questionnaire in a sample of European adolescents—The HELENA study. *BMC Public Health, 11,* 717.

DeVet, H. C. W., Terwee, C., Mokkink, L. B., & Knol, D. L. (2011). *Measurement in medicine: A practical guide.* Cambridge, MA: Cambridge University Press.

Dowd, K. P., Harrington, D. M., & Donnelly, A. (2012). Criterion and concurrent validity of the activPAL professional physical activity monitor in adolescent females. *PloS One, 7,* 247633.

Dunton, G. F., Liao, Y., Kawabata, K., & Intile, S. (2012). Momentary assessment of adults' physical activity and sedentary behavior: Feasibility and validity. *Frontiers in Psychology, 3,* 260.

Fischer, J. E., Bachman, L. M., & Jaeschke, R. (2003). A readers' guide to the interpretation of diagnostic test properties: Clinical example of sepsis. *Intensive Care Medicine, 29,* 1043–1051.

Golriz, S., Hebert, J. J., Foreman, K., & Walker, B. (2012). The validity of a portable clinical force plate in assessment of static postural control: Concurrent validity study. *Chiropractic & Manual Therapies, 20,* 15.

Huang, C. L., Lin, H. H., & Wang, H. H. (2010). Cigarette Dependence Questionnaire: Development and psychometric testing with male smokers, *Journal of Advanced Nursing, 66,* 2341–2349.

Jaceldo-Siegl, K., Knutsen, S., Sabate, J., Beeson, W., Chan, J., Herring, R., . . . Fraser, G. (2010). Validation of nutrient intake using an FFQ and repeated 24 h recalls in black and white subjects of the Adventist Health Study-2 (AHS-2). *Public Health Nutrition, 13,* 812–819.

Jayaram, G., Samuels, J., & Konrad, S. S. (2012). Prediction and prevention of aggression and seclusion by early screening and comprehensive seclusion documentation. *Innovations in Clinical Neuroscience, 9,* 30–38.

LaPorta, F., Frabceschini, M., Caselli, S., Susassi, Cavallini, P., & Tennant, A. (2011). Unified Balance Scale: Classic psychometric and clinical properties. *Journal of Rehabilitation Medicine, 43,* 445–453.

Mokkink, L. B., Terwee, C., Patrick, D., Alonso, J., Stratford, P., Knol, D. L., . . . DeVet, H. C. W. (2010). The COSMIN study reached international consensus on taxonomy, terminology, and definitions of measurement properties for health-related patient-reported outcomes. *Journal of Clinical Epidemiology, 63,* 737–745.

Nasuti, G., Stuart-Hill, L., & Temple, V. (2013). The Six-Minute Walk Test for adults with intellectual disability: A study of validity and reliability. *Journal of Intellectual and Developmental Disability, 38,* 31–38.

Navali, A., Bahari, L., & Nazari, B. (2012). A comparative assessment of alternatives to the full-leg radiograph for determining knee joint alignment. *Sports Medicine, Arthroscopy, Rehabilitation, Therapy, & Technology, 4,* 40.

Streiner, D. L. & Cairney, J. (2007). What's under the ROC? An introduction to receiver operating characteristic curves. *Canadian Journal of Psychiatry, 52,* 121–128.

Sun, J. L., Chiou, J. F., & Lin, C. C. (2011). Validation of the Taiwanese version of the Athens Insomnia Scale and assessment of insomnia in Taiwanese cancer patients. *Journal of Pain and Symptom Management, 41,* 904–914.

Terwee, C. B., Mokkink, L. B., Knol, D. L., Ostelo, R., Bouter, L. M., & DeVet, H. C. W. (2012). Rating the methodological quality in systematic reviews of studies on measurement properties: A scoring system for the COSMIN checklist. *Quality of Life Research, 21,* 651–657.

Yin, X., Tu, X., Tong, Y., Yang, R., Wang, Y., Cao, S., & Lu, Z. (2012). Development and validation of a tuberculosis medication adherence scale. *PloS One, 7,* e50328.

13

Construct Validity: Hypothesis Testing

Chapter Outline

Not all health measures can be assessed for criterion validity. For many abstract, unobservable human attributes (constructs), no gold standard criterion exists. For example, a construct such as somatosensory amplification—the tendency of a person to experience a somatic sensation as especially intense or noxious—does not have an obvious gold standard against which a self-report of this attribute could be tested. When there is no appropriate or reliable criterion for an attribute, researchers typically assess a measure's construct validity.

The construct validity question is basically this: What attribute is *really* being measured? In the Consensus-based Standards for the selection of health Measurement Instruments (COSMIN) taxonomy, construct validity is defined as the degree to which scores of a measurement instrument are consistent with hypotheses (Mokkink et al., 2010). Borrowing from the writings of esteemed methodologists Cook and Campbell (Cook & Campbell, 1979; Shadish, Cook, & Campbell, 2002), **construct validity** may be defined as the degree to which evidence about a measure's scores in relation to other scores supports the inference that the construct has been appropriately represented.

Evidence for construct validity comes from tests of hypotheses about the nature of the abstract construct and the scores on the measure. The researcher must speculate: If this instrument is, in fact, measuring Construct X, then how would we expect the scores to perform?

Construct validity within COSMIN encompasses three distinct aspects: hypothesis-testing validity, structural validity, and cross-cultural validity. In fact, all three types involve hypothesis tests. We maintain COSMIN's typology and discuss these three types of construct validity separately. This chapter focuses on the kind of **hypothesis-testing validity** that concerns the extent to which it is possible to corroborate hypotheses regarding how scores on a measure function in relation to scores for other variables or scores on other measures of the same variable. Hypothesis-testing validity is relevant for most health measures, including scales created in either the classical test theory (CTT) or item response theory (IRT) framework, formative indexes, observational measures, and performance measures.

13.1 Basics of Construct Validity

In this section, we discuss some basic issues of relevance to construct validity and, in some cases, of relevance to measurement validity in a broader sense.

13.1.a Construct Validity and Other Types of Validity

Health care researchers and psychometricians differ in their views of construct validity, especially with regard to its position in a validity hierarchy. In health care, criterion validity is held in high esteem. DeVet, Terwee, Mokkink, and Knol (2011) have stated that "Construct validation is often considered to be less powerful than criterion validity" (p. 169). Psychometricians, on the other hand, often see all other types of measurement validity as aspects of construct validity: Their view is that construct validity *is* validity (e.g., Strauss & Smith, 2009). This position is certainly understandable for psychological constructs, for which there is seldom a good criterion. Health constructs, by contrast, often have a highly reliable gold standard, as we discussed in Chapter 12.

Yet, there is some merit to the view that all types of measurement validity are connected to construct validity. Content validation, as we discussed in Chapter 11, is an early attempt to ensure that a construct is well represented by the subparts of a multicomponent instrument. Criterion validation can be construed as a hypothesis-testing effort: It involves an implicit test of the hypothesis that scores on the focal measure and the criterion are correlated or consistent with each other.

All types of validity share other features as well, including the following:

- *Validity efforts require a clear understanding of what and who are being measured and how measurements will be used.* It is not possible to design a strong validation study of any type without having a firm grasp of what it is that is being measured (the construct), with which population it will be applied, and what its intended use is.

- *Validity is not an "all-or-nothing" characteristic.* In their seminal early paper on construct validity, Cronbach and Meehl (1955) wrote: "The problem is not to conclude that the test 'is valid' for measuring the construct," but rather the challenge is to "state as definitively as possible the *degree* [emphasis added] of validity" (p. 13). This applies to all types of validity.

- *Validity is not a fixed property of a measure.* As is true for other measurement properties described thus far, validity is not "determined" but rather "assessed." One gathers evidence to support an inference that the instrument is a valid measure of the construct, for a particular population and a particular use of an instrument. New populations and novel uses require new validation efforts.

Construct validity does, however, differ from content and criterion validity in certain crucial respects. In a construct validation, the instrument developer must have not only a firm conceptualization of the construct itself (this is also true in content validation) but also a conceptualization of how the construct is related to other constructs. In other words, there needs to be an overarching conceptual model of different processes and traits of relevance to the construct. We discuss this in the next section.

Another distinction is that content and criterion validation typically involves only the team of researchers who develop the instrument or those who revise it, shorten it, or translate it for other cultures or languages. Construct validity, by contrast, is a never-ending evidence-building enterprise. Inferences for a measure's construct validity are strengthened as evidence accumulates. Instrument developers provide preliminary evidence that may persuade other researchers to adopt it. When the measure is used by others, and their hypotheses are confirmed, this increases confidence in the measure's validity.

Finally, construct validation typically involves more than a test of the validity of the measure. The findings can have implications for the validity of the conceptual model (Strauss & Smith, 2009). Of course, because study designs for construct validation may be flawed (e.g., insufficient sample size), failure to confirm construct validity hypotheses cannot be construed as evidence that the theory lacks validity.

13.1.b Construct Validity and Conceptual Models

A central concern of construct validity is to link the realm of the theoretical and abstract with the realm of the observable. To make this linkage, researchers need to have a strong conceptualization of the construct of interest. In Chapter 11, we illustrated a conceptual model that focused on the dimensionality of a multidimensional construct. Figure 11.1 illustrated seven dimensions of the construct *postpartum depression* (PPD). For construct validation, a broader conceptual model is often developed to depict hypothesized relationships among constructs. These hypothesized relationships are the basis for construct validation.

Sometimes the conceptual model embodies a well-developed formal theory. For example, social cognitive theory (Bandura, 2001), which is sometimes called *self-efficacy theory*, has been used as the basis for developing many health instruments. As one example, Latimer, Walker, Kim, Pasch, and Sterling (2011) developed a Physical Activity and Nutrition Self-Efficacy Scale for self-efficacy in weight loss in postpartum women. More often, however, a conceptual model is not based on a full-blown formal theory but rather on a thorough understanding of the construct and factors that predict its manifestation or severity as well as outcomes that the construct affects. A detailed literature review can suggest how to "map" a construct in relation to other constructs. Such a conceptual model should be evidence-based and not developed on the basis of "hunches" or personal experience alone.

As an example, Figure 13.1 presents a possible model for generating hypotheses to test the construct validity of a measure of PPD. This model includes factors that are hypothesized to affect levels of maternal depression (e.g., predelivery depression, social isolation) as well as factors hypothesized to be affected by PPD (e.g., maternal responsiveness). This model is incomplete in that not all factors relating to PPD are included, but it provides a basis for testing the construct validity of a measure of PPD. If, for example, socially isolated mothers do not have higher PPD scores than other mothers on the measure, then (assuming a well-designed study with an appropriate population) either the model is flawed or the measure may have construct validity problems.

Constructs with multiple dimensions may require separate models for different dimensions. For example, Figure 11.1 showed that one dimension of PPD is the contemplation of self-harm. For this dimension, predictive factors may include prior suicide attempts, prenatal scores on a suicide ideation scale, or a history of domestic violence.

A successful construct validation effort requires in-depth understanding of the construct, and it also requires insight and creativity. Researchers must challenge themselves to develop diverse and complementary ways of testing whether their measure is, indeed, measuring the construct of interest. As pointed out by Streiner and Norman (2008), those who seek to validate their measures are "limited only by their imagination in devising studies to test their hypotheses" (p. 252).

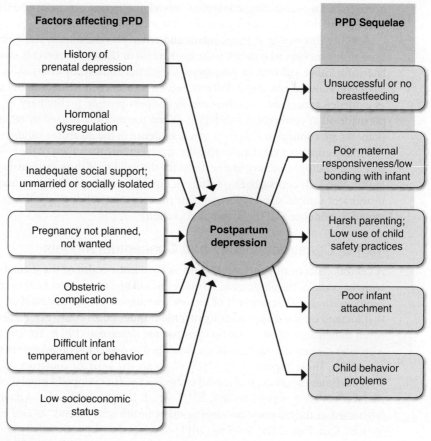

Figure 13.1
A conceptual model of postpartum depression (PPD).

13.1.c Reliability and Validity

An assertion often made in the psychometric literature is that a measure that is not reliable cannot be valid. Another way to state this is that reliability is a necessary (but insufficient) condition for validity. The case is made that if a person's score fluctuates from one measurement to another (i.e., if there is poor test–retest or interrater reliability), then the measure would be too erratic to validly measure the construct it purports to measure. One problem, however, is that reliability coefficients are strongly affected by a sample's homogeneity (Chapter 8). If a population whose weight ranged from 159 to 161 pounds were measured to the nearest pound, the retest reliability of the weight measurements would be low. This does not mean that the weighing scale is not valid for measuring people's weight. It does, however, mean that in this population, validation will be difficult because the small score range constrains both reliability and validity coefficients. Thus, if early assessments of reliability indicate poor reliability performance of a measure, validity will also be low within that population.

13.2 Types of Hypothesis-Testing Construct Validity

All of hypothesis-testing construct validation follows a similar path: A hypothesis is developed regarding a relationship between scores on the focal measures and scores on another construct, data are collected to test the hypothesis with a sample from a specified population, and then conclusions are reached on the basis of the hypothesis test. Different types of evidence can be brought to bear on construct validity, however, leading to approaches that have been given different names. Unfortunately, there are inconsistencies in the measurement literature with regard to what some of those names are. Because the names of different validation approaches are often confusing and misidentified in the literature, Table 13.1 presents a quick summary chart, which includes validity terms from other chapters as well.

13.2.a Convergent Validity

Convergent validity is the degree to which scores on the focal measure are correlated with scores on measures of constructs with which there is a hypothesized correlation—that is, the degree to which there is conceptual convergence. Sometimes, the other measure is a different measure of the same construct (but not a measure that could be construed as a "gold standard"). For example, if we were developing a new and improved patient-reported outcome (PRO) measure of fatigue in patients with cancer, we might predict that scores on

Table 13.1	Types of Measurement-Related Validity	
Type of Validity	**Notes**	**Chapter[a]**
Content validity	Concerns the adequacy of content for multicomponent measures; especially important for formative measures	11
Face validity	Concerns whether a measure "looks" as though it is measuring the relevant construct; especially important in clinimetric measures	11
Criterion validity		
Concurrent validity	Tests whether a measure is consistent with a criterion (gold standard), measured at the same time	12
Predictive validity	Tests whether a measure is consistent with a criterion (gold standard), measured at a future point in time	12
Construct validity (hypothesis testing)		
Convergent validity	In the absence of a gold standard, tests the correlation between the focal measure and a measure of a construct with which conceptual convergence is expected	13
Divergent (discriminant) validity	Tests that the focal measure is not a measure of a different construct other than the one intended	13
Known groups (discriminative) validity	Tests the degree to which a measure can discriminate between groups known to differ with regard to the focal construct	13
Structural validity	Tests whether a measure captures the hypothesized dimensionality of a construct	14
Cross-cultural validity	Concerns the extent to which a translated or adapted measure is equivalent to the original	15

[a]For full definitions, see relevant chapters.
Bolded terms are components in the Validity Domain of the measurement taxonomy (Figure 3.1, page 25).

our new scale would correlate fairly strongly and positively with patients' scores on another fatigue scale, such as the Piper Fatigue Scale (Piper et al., 1998).

From a broader perspective, convergent validity concerns the extent to which the focal measure correlates with variables in a manner consistent with an underlying theory or conceptual model. So, for example, some evidence of convergent validity for a PPD scale would be obtained, based on the model in Figure 13.1, if scores on the PPD scale correlated negatively with scores on the Duke–UNC Functional Social Support Questionnaire (Broadhead, Gehlbach, de Gruy, & Kaplan, 1988) because social support is hypothesized to be associated with a lower risk of PPD.

A psychometric evaluation of the Activities-specific Balance Confidence Scale (ABC) in people with multiple sclerosis (Nilsagård, Carling, & Forsberg, 2012) provides an actual example of a convergent validity assessment. These researchers hypothesized that scores on the ABC would correlate positively with patients' scores on several performance tests, such as the Timed Up and Go Test, the Dynamic Gait Index, and the Four Square Step Test. Significant correlations in the hypothesized direction ($-.61$, $.62$, and $-.59$, respectively) were obtained, leading the researchers to conclude that the convergent validity of the ABC scale for use with people with mild-to-moderate multiple sclerosis was supported.

With convergent validity, the validity parameter is typically the correlation coefficient between two measures, most often Pearson's r. More advanced statistical techniques can be used to test more complex hypotheses. For example, using our PPD model, multiple regression could be used to test the hypothesis that scores on the PPD measure predicted maternal responsiveness, over and above the effects of background factors such as maternal education and marital status. If the conceptual model was a hypothesized causal model, then structural equation modeling could be used. In short, the usual menu of hypothesis-testing statistical methods can be used to shed light on a measure's convergent validity.

It might be noted that sometimes there is confusion between convergent validity and concurrent validity. As we saw in Chapter 11, concurrent validity requires that a "gold standard" criterion be measured at the same time as the focal measure. Researchers sometimes use the term *concurrent* validity, when in fact the second measure is not truly a criterion, and they sometimes use the term *convergent* when the second measure could easily be construed as a gold standard.

13.2.b Known-Groups (Discriminative) Validity

A method that is strongly related to convergent validity is *known-groups validity*, which has also been called *discriminative validity* and *contrast validity*. **Known-groups validity** relies on hypotheses concerning a measure's ability to discriminate between two or more groups known (or expected) to differ with regard to the construct of interest. For example, using our model in Figure 13.1, we might hypothesize that women who had planned their pregnancy would have more favorable scores on a PPD scale than women whose pregnancy was unwanted. If the scores on the PPD measure do not differ for the two groups, one might question the scale's validity, given the existing evidence that women whose pregnancies are planned and wanted are less susceptible than other women to PPD. The known-groups approach is one of the most widely used methods of testing construct validity.

Researchers often use the known-groups validation method by comparing scores for people known to have a clinical problem or clinical condition with people who do not. For example, Meltzer and colleagues (2012) developed the Children's Report of Sleep Patterns-Sleepiness Scale (CRSP-S) for children aged 8 to 12 years. In their validation study for the CRSP, the researchers compared children in pediatric sleep clinics or sleep labs with children from a general school population and found significantly greater sleepiness in the clinical group ($t[214] = 3.45, p < .001$).

Often, researchers set up multiple "known-group" comparisons to test a series of discriminative hypotheses. For example, Khagram, Martin, Davies, and Speight (2013) undertook a validation study for the Self-Care Inventory-Revised (SCI-R), which assesses the self-care behaviors of adults with Type 2 diabetes. The researchers tested hypotheses that compared SCI-R scores for subgroups with high and low levels of HbA_{1c} (cutpoint of 58 mmol/mol, 7.5%), long and short diabetes duration (cutpoint of 16 years), and presence or absence of complications. The first two hypotheses were supported.

This example illustrates that a primary difference between convergent validity and known-groups validity concerns the measurement level of the validation variable. Continuous scores can be used to create "known" groups for discriminative purposes by dividing the sample into subgroups (known-groups validity), but continuous variables can be correlated directly with scores on the focal measure (convergent validity). It is best to use a well-established cutpoint for "caseness" to divide sample members into distinct subgroups based on continuous scores.

With known-groups validity, the statistical method used is typically a t test, or a non-parametric equivalent (e.g., a Mann–Whitney U test). More complex methods such as analysis of covariance or receiver operating characteristic (ROC) analysis are alternatives. Sometimes researchers calculate an effect size (such as *Cohen's d*, the *standardized mean difference*) to document the magnitude of group differences in a standardized fashion because effect size values are widely understood. For example, St. Clare and colleagues (2009) used a known-groups approach to validate their Unhelpful Thoughts and Beliefs about Stuttering Scale. The scale discriminated well between groups of stuttering and non-stuttering participants, with a very large effect size ($d = 2.5$). As we shall see in Chapter 18, effect size indexes are widely used in connection with longitudinal construct validity (responsiveness).

13.2.c Divergent (Discriminant) Validity

Divergent validity (which is often called *discriminant validity*) concerns evidence that a measure is *not* a measure of a different construct, distinct from the focal construct. We use the term *divergent* because it is a good contrast with *con*vergent validity and also because of possible confusion between the terms discriminant and discriminative (known-groups) validity.

In a divergent validation, researchers typically measure both the focal attribute and a similar—but distinct—attribute as a means of ensuring that the two are not really measures of the same construct but with different labels. Thus, in a divergent validation, the hypothesis is that the two measures are only weakly correlated. For example, a team of researchers (Bergman, Reeve, Moser, Scholl, & Klein, 2011) developed a 74-item Heart Disease Knowledge Questionnaire. Scores on the test were moderately correlated with an existing heart knowledge test (convergent validity) but only weakly correlated with a general measure of health literacy (divergent validity).

Sometimes researchers want to demonstrate that their measure is not merely capturing socially desirable responses. In such cases, divergent validity is assessed by examining correlations between scores on the focal measure and scores on a measure of social desirability. As an example, Hildebrandt, Langenbucher, Lai, Loeb, and Hollander (2011) created a measure called the Appearance and Performance Enhancing Drug Use Schedule (APEDUS). Scores on subscales of the APEDUS correlated highly with convergent measures (e.g., eating disorder pathology, impulsivity) but were uncorrelated with scores on a social desirability scale.

This example illustrates the point that sometimes hypotheses are stated in relative rather than absolute terms, especially when there are both convergent and divergent hypotheses. For example, an absolute hypothesis for a new PPD scale might say that scores would correlate only modestly with scores on a measure of anxiety about maternal role performance to distinguish the PPD construct from maternal role anxiety. The researcher could also state relative hypotheses. For example, we could hypothesize that scores on a PPD scale would correlate more strongly with scores on an alternative measure of PPD (convergent validity) than with scores on the maternal role anxiety scale (divergent validity).

The primary approach to divergent validation is to compute correlation coefficients. The problem, however, is to reach a reasonable conclusion when, essentially, the actual hypothesis being tested is a null hypothesis. The absence of statistical significance is a poor basis for drawing conclusions about divergent validity. Researchers should stipulate in advance how "weak" a correlation would need to be as evidence of divergent validity.

13.2.d The Multitrait–Multimethod Matrix Approach

Psychometricians Donald Campbell and Donald Fiske (1959) introduced a construct validation procedure that brings together evidence of convergent and divergent validity. The **multitrait–multimethod (MTMM) matrix** method involves distinguishing two or more constructs ("multitrait") that are measured by two or more methods ("multimethod"). Divergence (discriminability) focuses on the ability to distinguish two similar but distinct constructs across multiple methods of measurement. Convergence is manifested when multiple methods of measuring the same construct are correlated: Different measurement approaches should converge on the construct.

Implicit in the MTMM procedure is the notion of *method effects* in measurement. Method effects occur when a feature of the instrument or the measurement process contributes variance to scores, over and above what is attributable to the construct of interest. If blood pressure is measured indirectly by sphygmomanometer and directly through invasive penetration of the arterial wall, differences in values within a sample of patients would reflect a method effect.

A full implementation of the MTMM requires a fully crossed design in which people are measured for two or more traits using two or more methods (i.e., a minimum of four scores per person). To illustrate an MTMM, suppose we wanted to assess the construct validity of a new scale to measure perceived autonomy among geriatric patients. We wish to distinguish autonomy from perceived control over daily life. Both autonomy and control are considered constructs relevant to quality of life in the elderly. We would expect that perceived control and perceived autonomy would be correlated, but not too highly. We administer our autonomy scale and a scale of perceived control to a sample of elders living in assisted living facilities. Additionally, family members are asked to rate the elders on both traits, based on their observations of the elders' behavior.

Fictitious data for this study are presented in Table 13.2. The numbers in parentheses on the diagonal represent the reliability (test–retest) coefficients for the four measures (two traits × two methods). These range from .89 for patient-reported autonomy to .70 for the observational rating of control. The remaining values in the table are correlation coefficients among scores on the four measures. For instance, the coefficient of .29 at the intersection of AUT_1–CON_1 is the correlation between the scores for the two patient-report scales (monomethod) measuring autonomy and control (heterotrait).

Various entries of the MTMM matrix shed light on construct validity. The most direct (convergent) evidence comes from correlations between two different methods (heteromethod) that measure the same trait (monotrait). In the case of AUT_1–AUT_2, the coefficient is .51, which is moderately high; in fact, it is the highest coefficient in the matrix other than reliability coefficients. Convergent validity should be large enough to encourage further scrutiny of the matrix. Second, the convergent validity entries should be higher, in absolute magnitude, than correlations between measures that have neither method nor trait in common (heterotrait, heteromethod coefficients). That is, AUT_1–AUT_2 (.51) should be greater than AUT_2–CON_1 (.14) or AUT_1–CON_2 (.05), as it is here. This requirement is a minimum one that, if failed, should cause researchers to have serious doubts about the validity of the measures. Third, convergent validity coefficients should be greater than coefficients between measures of different traits by a single method. Once again, the matrix in Table 13.1 fulfills this criterion: AUT_1–AUT_2 (.51) and CON_1–CON_2 (.49) are both higher

Table 13.2	**Fictitious Example of a Multitrait–Multimethod (MTMM) Matrix for a Construct Validation of a Scale Measuring Perceived Autonomy in an Elderly Population**

| | | Methods | | | |
| | | Patient Reports (1) | | Observational Ratings (2) | |
	Traits	AUT_1	CON_1	AUT_2	CON_2
Method 1[a]	AUT_1	(.89)			
	CON_1	.29	(.87)		
Method 2	AUT_2	.51	.14	(.72)	
	CON_2	.05	.49	.21	(.70)

[a]Method subscripts: 1 = Patient report; 2 = Family members' observational rating.
AUT, perceived autonomy trait; CON, perceived control over life trait.

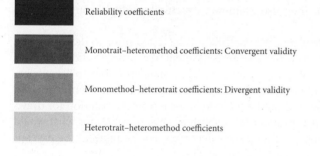

Reliability coefficients

Monotrait–heteromethod coefficients: Convergent validity

Monomethod–heterotrait coefficients: Divergent validity

Heterotrait–heteromethod coefficients

than AUT_1–CON_1 (.29) and AUT_2–CON_2 (.21). The last requirement provides evidence for divergent (discriminant) validity.

The evidence is seldom as clear cut as in this contrived example. Indeed, a common problem with MTMM concerns interpreting the pattern of coefficients. Another issue is that there are no clear-cut criteria for deciding whether MTMM requirements have been met. That is, there is no objective means of assessing the magnitude of similarities and differences within the matrix, and so different investigators can come to different conclusions with the same results. The MTMM is nevertheless a valuable tool for exploring construct validity, and methods for analyzing MTMM data using confirmatory factor analysis and structural equation modeling have been proposed (e.g., Eid et al., 2008; Kenny & Kashy, 1992).

An even bigger issue in health care research is that constructs are seldom deliberately measured with two or more distinct methods. In many construct validity studies, it is simply not feasible to make methods an explicit part of the study design. Nevertheless, the MTMM method has been used in several health measurement studies, most often when methodologic issues are at center stage. For example, Erhart, Wetzel, Krugel, and Ravens-Sieberer (2009) used the MTMM to examine telephone versus mail survey methods to measure health-related quality of life and mental health problems in German adolescents. The MTMM has also been used to assess the construct validity of proxy reports and self-reports. Thaler, Kazemi, and Wood (2010), for example, used the MTMM in their assessment of child versus parent reports on the Multidimensional Anxiety Scale for Children (MASC), designed for children with learning disabilities.

13.3 The Design of Hypothesis-Testing Construct Validation Studies

Construct validation is most often undertaken for complex and abstract measures that are based on patient reports or on observational assessments by clinicians. Psychometric scales and formative clinimetric indexes usually require construct validation, unless there are good gold standard measures for a criterion validation. This section describes some issues to consider in designing and reporting construct validity work.

13.3.a Explicit Hypotheses and Explicit Criteria

Most researchers identify multiple hypotheses for their construct validity efforts and often include several different types of validation approaches in a single study. For example, in the previously mentioned study to evaluate the Children's Report of Sleep Patterns-Sleepiness Scale (CRSP-S), Meltzer and coresearchers (2012) tested convergent hypotheses about correlations between CRSP-S scores and several other measures, including parent-reported measures of child sleep behavior and actiGraph measures of sleep time. They used known-groups methods to compare different groups of children (a clinical and school sample) as well as different subgroups (e.g., those with scores above and below a cutoff score on the Children's Sleep Hygiene Scale). They also examined structural validity through a confirmatory factor analysis.

It is clearly important to articulate the hypotheses to be tested prior to designing and implementing a validation study. And, because an assessment of construct validity involves interpretation and judgment, it is also important to establish standards prior to data collection to avoid overinterpretation of modest results. Statistical significance is strongly affected by sample size, so significance should not be the sole or even primary criterion for drawing conclusions about validity. It is prudent to establish a range of values for what would be considered moderate or strong correlations or effect sizes. For example, in the psychometric evaluation of the Lymphoedema Functioning, Disability, and Health Questionnaire (Lymph-ICF), the researchers specified that validity correlation coefficients would be interpreted as follows: $<.40$ was weak, .40 to .74 was moderate, .75 to .90 was strong, and $>.90$ was very strong (Devoogdt, Van Kampen, Geraerts, Coremans, & Christiaens, 2011).

When many hypotheses are tested, it is also useful to have a criterion for how many of them need to be supported to be considered strong evidence of construct validity. Again the validation of the Lymph-ICF provides a good example. Altogether, the researchers articulated 45 hypotheses (some were for items and subscales) that were summarized in a table: five hypotheses for convergent validity, five for divergent validity, and the remainder for known-groups validity. The researchers stipulated that construct validity would be considered very good if 90% of all hypotheses were supported, good if 75% to 90% were supported, and moderate if 40% to 74% of the hypotheses were supported. The results indicated that 89% (40 out of 45) of the hypotheses were confirmed.

13.3.b Study Design in Construct Validation

Researchers typically undertake construct validation (including hypothesis-testing validity and structural validity) with a finalized measure that has been assessed for reliability. The design is usually cross-sectional, with all validation data collected at a single point in time. A longitudinal design might, however, be needed if the validation sample will be used to assess responsiveness (Chapter 18) or if some of the hypotheses require two rounds of data collection. For example, if we wanted to test the hypothesis from Figure 13.1 that women with prenatal depression are more susceptible to PPD, then we would need to administer a depression scale to sample members during their pregnancy. If two or more rounds of data collection are needed, it is important to devise strategies to minimize attrition.

When known-groups validation is the primary strategy, thought should be given to en-suring that the groups being compared are similar with regard to potentially confounding variables. For the validity evidence to be persuasive, differences in scores on the focal measure should reflect differences in the validating variable and not merely differences in, say, age or ill-ness severity. Thus, sometimes matching or balancing of the comparison groups might be de-sirable. Another alternative is to remove the effect of any confounders in the statistical analysis.

The data collection plan is a particularly crucial part of a validation study design. Multiple validation variables are typically identified in the hypotheses, and methods of measuring each variable are needed. If multivariate analyses are planned, then covariates may need to be identified and measured as well. Care needs to be taken to ensure that each measure included in the study is itself reliable and valid, and appropriate for the population.

As mentioned in the previous chapter, when validity results are reported as correlation coefficients, researchers can decide whether to correct for the attenuated values stemming from imperfect reliability of the measures. In health research, disattenuation corrections (Chapter 9) are more likely to be applied for criterion validity than for construct validity. In the field of psychology, however, corrections are sometimes used to better understand the upper limits of construct validity correlation coefficients (Muchinsky, 1996).

13.3.c Sampling in Construct Validation

Our advice about sampling for construct validation is similar to the advice we gave about criterion validation in the previous chapter. The sample should be drawn from a heteroge-neous population, and multisite validation is especially desirable.

We noted in Chapter 8 that it is not appropriate to estimate the reliability of a measure with a sample that includes members of a different population than the one for whom the measure is designed. For example, in developing a PRO measure of chronic pain for patients with fibromy-algia, it would be inappropriate to do a test–retest analysis with a sample that included members of a population without chronic pain. Such a study would not tell us how reliably we could de-tect variation in pain levels among patients with fibromyalgia. However, in validating a measure, supporting evidence can come from a known-groups comparison of patients from the target population with people from a population presumed to have different levels of the construct under study. The previously mentioned study that compared stutterers and nonstutterers on the Unhelpful Thoughts and Beliefs about Stuttering scale (St. Clare et al., 2009) is an example.

As is true in most quantitative health care research, large samples are preferred to small ones. There is no single number that can be recommended, although the COSMIN group's scoring system gives a rating of "excellent" for samples of 100 or more for construct valid-ity studies (Terwee et al., 2012). Sample size needs vary by the expected size of the effects. For example, if the effect size for a known group comparison is anticipated to be .35, then a sample of about 130 would be needed for the group difference to be significant with $\alpha = .05$ at power $= .80$. We noted earlier that statistical significance yields incomplete evidence for construct validity, but it is worth striving for, nonetheless. With a small sample size, a non-significant finding will likely result in doubts about the validity estimate. And, with a small sample, confidence intervals around the validity estimate will be so large that doubts may remain even when results are significant.

13.3.d Interpretation of Construct Validity Results

Drawing conclusions about a measure's construct validity is typically far more complex than interpreting results for other measurement properties, such as reliability or measure-ment error. One major difference is that for many measurement parameters, only a single number needs to be interpreted. For example, an intraclass correlation coefficient (ICC) is computed with test–retest data, and that value *is* the estimated reliability coefficient. For criterion validity, there is typically a single statistic that summarizes the observed degree of consistency between the measure and the gold standard. There is seldom a single "validity coefficient" in construct validation because many parameters are estimated in the course of testing multiple hypotheses. Indeed, the more supporting evidence there is, the greater the confidence one can have about the measure's validity. However, results are often "mixed": Some hypotheses are supported and others are not. This fact underscores the desirability of establishing a priori standards for how much confirmatory evidence is considered sufficient.

When the evidence supporting a measure's construct validity is reasonably strong, one interpretive issue concerns the possibility of "rival hypotheses." In other words, could the observed correlations or effect size estimates be the result of some extraneous influence, rather than the performance of the measure per se? If rival hypotheses can be discredited or ruled out, then confidence in the measure's construct validity is enhanced. Another interpretive issue to consider is what the findings mean for the conceptual model. Both the model and the measure gain credibility with an abundance of construct validity evidence.

When the validity results are ambiguous or discouraging, researchers need to dig deeper to unravel what they might mean. Perhaps the theory is wrong—that is, maybe the hypotheses were not reasonable or realistic. Or, perhaps there is a design flaw, as might happen with un-matched groups in a known-groups validation. The psychometric properties of the validation measures also merit careful scrutiny. Poor reliability of either the focal measure or the validation measures will reduce the validity coefficients. Range restrictions on any of the measures will also depress validity estimates. Thus, when results are negative, researchers should carefully inspect the distributions of all variables. In essence, making sense of "negative" construct validity results is similar to coming to conclusions about negative results (retention of the null hypothesis) in any health care study. One must "get to the bottom" of what the results mean by looking for interpretive clues in the conceptual model, the research design, sampling plan, data collection strategy, or the analytic approach. If one comes to the conclusion that the focal measure was not given a fair test in the construct validation, then a more rigorous study needs to be planned.

13.3.e Reporting a Construct Validation Study

Construct validity efforts are typically described in papers summarizing the major measurement properties of a new measure, although structural validity work, as described in the next chapter, may be reported in a separate paper because of its complexity. In describing the construct validity portion of a project, researchers need to clarify their conceptual framework or the basis for hypotheses that were tested. Hypotheses, and criteria for their confirmation, should be explicitly stated and the appropriate term should be used to identify the type of validity being assessed (i.e., convergent, known groups, and so on). The comparator validating measures need to be explained in some detail, including what constructs they measure, why they were selected, their suitability for the target population, and how valid and reliable they are. A rationale for the sample size should be offered, including the results of a power analysis, if one was undertaken.

The validity coefficients for convergent and divergent validity are often presented in a correlation matrix. Table 13.3 presents an example from a study in which Cane, Nielson, McCarthy, and Mazmanian (2013) developed the Patterns of Activity Measure-Pain (POAM-P) to measure activity patterns for people with chronic pain. Three 10-item sub-scales measured Avoidance (avoidance of pain-associated activities); Overdoing (persevering with activity despite increasing pain); and Pacing (alternating activity and rest on a time-contingent rather than pain-contingent basis). Table 13.3 shows that the correlations between scores on the three subscales of the POAM-P were moderate and in expected directions. Participants in the study also completed two other scales. The obtained pattern of results provides some support for convergent validity; for example, scores on the Pacing subscale had a correlation of .62 with subscale scores for pacing on the Chronic Pain Coping Inventory. By contrast, Pacing subscale scores were not correlated with scores on the Tampa Scale of Kinesiophobia ($r = .00$), supporting divergent validity.

Table 13.3 Table Showing Convergent and Divergent Validity Results: The Patterns of Activity Measure-Pain (POAM-P)			
	POAM-P Subscales		
Scale or Subscale	Avoidance	Overdoing	Pacing
POAM-P Avoidance	—	$-.31^a$	$.25^a$
POAM-P Overdoing	—	—	$-.48^a$
Chronic Pain Coping Inventory-Pacing Scale	$-.02$	$-.22$	$.62^a$
Tampa Scale of Kinesiophobia	$.42^a$	$-.26^a$	$.00$

N = 393 patients.
[a]$p < .01$
Adapted from Cane, D., Nielson, W. R., McCarthy, M., & Mazmanian, D. (2013). Pain-related activity patterns: Measurement, interrelationships, and association with psychosocial functioning. *Clinical Journal of Pain, 29,* 435–442. Table 4, "POAM-P Interscale Correlations and Correlations With Existing Measures"

When known-groups validation is tested and there are multiple comparisons, the results can be summarized in a table. An attractive way of reporting multiple known-groups tests is to show them simultaneously in a series of box plots. Some fictitious results are shown in Figure 13.2 for two hypothesis tests for scores on Beck and Gable's (2001) Postpartum Depression Screening Scale (PDSS), based on hypotheses suggested in Figure 13.1. The box plots show the median PDSS score for various subgroups (e.g., married vs. unmarried mothers), the interquartile range, the subgroup size, and the significance of groups differences.

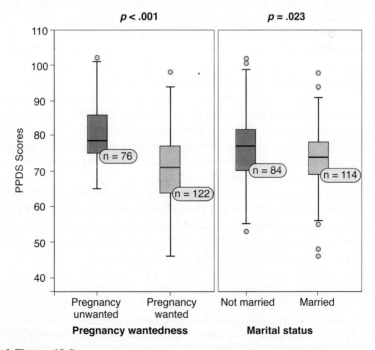

Figure 13.2

Fictitious box plots showing results of two hypothesis tests regarding postpartum depression scale scores (PPDS).

In reporting their results, many researchers use language that is inconsistent with the nature of the validation effort. It is not appropriate to state that the instrument's validity was "confirmed," "proved," "determined," or "established." Evidence from validation work helps to "support" a certain degree of confidence that a measure is measuring the focal construct—and the better the evidence, the stronger the level of confidence.

13.3.f Evaluating a Construct Validation Study

The COSMIN workgroup has offered some guidelines for evaluating construct validity evidence (Terwee et al., 2012). Their scoring system, shown in the Box F checklist on the COSMIN website, provides specific ratings for such issues as how missing values were handled, whether the design was flawed, and so on. We expand on issues covered in their ratings.

For those evaluating construct validations, there is an abundance of issues to consider, starting with the adequacy of the conceptual framework and the reasonableness of the hypotheses. One should consider not only whether the hypotheses presented make sense but also whether important relevant hypotheses were *not* tested. In other words, a key consideration is whether the researchers have been sufficiently thoughtful and creative in devising multiple hypothesis tests in an effort to triangulate evidence about the measure's construct validity. If the researchers only examined convergent validity, for example, the evidence may not be sufficiently persuasive.

If the researchers stated their a priori standards for the construct validity evidence, it is appropriate to consider whether those standards were defensible. If the researchers did not state any criteria, one needs to pay special attention to how the results were interpreted. In particular, did the researchers come to the conclusion that the construct validity of their measure was supported, despite results that were modest or equivocal?

Aspects of the study design also need to be evaluated in interpreting the results. For example, if the sample size was too small, are the study findings ambiguous? And if the sample was large, how did the authors make sense of statistically significant but modest correlations or effect sizes? If a known-groups method was used, one should consider whether the groups being compared were similar in terms of confounding variables known to be correlated with the focal construct. In other words, can significant differences really be interpreted as evidence of construct validity, or do the findings potentially reflect sample peculiarities or the effects of confounding factors?

A particularly important issue is to assess how the validating constructs were measured. The report should include information about the reliability, validity, and population-appropriateness of all comparator measures. Also, if the known-groups approach was used to assess validity by dichotomizing a continuous variable, one should evaluate whether the cutpoint used to divide the sample was reasonable or whether the researchers should have simply computed a correlation coefficient.

An evaluation of a construct validity paper takes many things into consideration but boils down to two key issues. The first is whether the quality of the evidence was strong as a result of good design, measurement, and sampling decisions. A rigorous study is a necessary but insufficient condition for the second issue: whether the evidence supports an interpretation of adequate validity for the measure in question.

References

Bandura, A. (2001). Social cognitive theory: An agentic perspective. *Annual Review of Psychology, 52,* 1–26.

Beck, C. T., & Gable, R. K. (2001). Further validation of the Postpartum Depression Screening Scale. *Nursing Research, 50,* 155–164.

Bergman, H. E., Reeve, B., Moser, R., Scholl, S., & Klein, W. (2011). Development of a comprehensive heart disease knowledge questionnaire. *American Journal of Health Education, 42,* 74–87.

Broadhead, W. E., Gehlbach, S., de Gruy, F., & Kaplan, B. (1988). The Duke–UNC Functional Support Questionnaire: Measurement of social support in family medicine patients. *Medical Care, 26*, 709–723.

Campbell, D. T., & Fiske, D. W. (1959). Convergent and discriminant validation by the multitrait-multimethod matrix. *Psychological Bulletin, 56*, 81–105.

Cane, D., Nielson, W. R., McCarthy, M., & Mazmanian, D. (2013). Pain-related activity patterns: Measurement, interrelationships, and association with psychosocial functioning. *Clinical Journal of Pain, 29*, 435–442.

Cook, T. D., & Campbell, D. T. (1979). *Quasi-experimentation: Design and analysis issues for field settings.* Chicago, IL: Rand McNally.

Cronbach, L. J., & Meehl, P. E. (1955). Construct validity in psychological tests. *Psychological Bulletin, 5*, 281–302.

DeVet, H. C. W., Terwee, C., Mokkink, L. B., & Knol, D. L. (2011). *Measurement in medicine: A practical guide.* Cambridge, MA: Cambridge University Press.

Devoogdt, N., Van Kampen, M., Geraerts, I., Coremans, T., & Christiaens, M. (2011). Lymphoedema Functioning, Disability and Health Questionnaire (Lymph-ICF): Reliability and validity. *Physical Therapy, 91*, 944–957.

Eid, M., Nussbeck, F. W., Geiser, C., Cole, D., Gollweizer, M., & Lischetzke, T. (2008). Structural equation modeling of multitrait-multimethod data: Different models for different types of methods. *Psychological Methods, 13*, 230–253.

Erhart, M., Wetzel, R. M., Krugel, A., & Ravens-Sieberer, U. (2009). Effects of phone versus mail survey methods on the measurement of health-related quality of life and emotional and behavioural problems in adolescents. *BMC Public Health, 9*, 491.

Hildebrandt, T., Langenbucher, J., Lai, J. K., Loeb, K., & Hollander, E. (2011). Development and validation of the Appearance-and-Performance Enhancing Drug Use Schedule. *Addictive Behaviors, 36*, 949–958.

Kenny, D. A., & Kashy, D. A. (1992). Analysis of the multitrait-multimethod matrix by confirmatory factor analysis. *Psychological Bulletin, 112*, 165–172.

Khagram, L., Martin, C., Davies, M., & Speight, J. (2013). Psychometric validation of the Self-Care Inventory-Revised (SCI-R) in UK adults with type 2 diabetes using data from the AT.LANTUS follow-on study. *Health and Quality of Life Outcomes, 11*, 24.

Latimer, L., Walker, L. O., Kim, S., Pasch, K., & Sterling, B. (2011). Self-efficacy for weight loss among multi-ethnic women of lower income: A psychometric evaluation. *Journal of Nutrition Education and Behavior, 43*, 279–283.

Meltzer, L. J., Biggs, S., Reynolds, A., Avis, K., Crabtree, V. M., & Bevans, K. (2012). The Children's Report of Sleep Patterns-Sleepiness Scale: A self-report measure for school-aged children. *Sleep Medicine, 13*, 385–389.

Mokkink, L. B., Terwee, C., Patrick, D., Alonso, J., Stratford, P., Knol, D. L., . . . DeVet, H. C. W. (2010). The COSMIN study reached international consensus on taxonomy, terminology, and definitions of measurement properties for health-related patient-reported outcomes. *Journal of Clinical Epidemiology, 63*, 737–745.

Muchinsky, P. M. (1996). The correction for attenuation. *Educational and Psychological Measurement, 56*, 63–75.

Nilsagård, Y., Carling, A., & Forsberg, A. (2012). Activities-specific balance confidence in people with multiple sclerosis. *Multiple Sclerosis International, 2012*, 613925.

Piper, B. F., Dibble, S. L., Dodd, M. J., Weiss, M. C., Slaughter, R. E., & Paul, S. M. (1998). The Piper Fatigue Scale: Psychometric evaluation in women with breast cancer. *Oncology Nursing Forum, 25*, 677–684.

Shadish, W. R., Cook, T. D., & Campbell, D. T. (2002). *Experimental and quasi-experimental designs for generalized causal inference.* Boston, MA: Houghton Mifflin.

St. Clare, T., Menzies, R., Onslow, M., Packman, A., Thompson, R., & Block, S. (2009). Unhelpful thoughts and beliefs linked to social anxiety in stuttering: Development of a measure. *International Journal of Language & Communication Disorders, 44*, 338–351.

Strauss, M. E., & Smith, G. T. (2009). Construct validity: Advances in theory and methodology. *Annual Review of Clinical Psychology, 5*, 1–25.

Streiner, D. L., & Norman, G. R. (2008). *Health measurement scales: A practical guide to their development and use* (4th ed.). Oxford: Oxford University Press.

Terwee, C. B., Mokkink, L. B., Knol, D. L., Ostelo, R., Bouter, L. M., & DeVet, H. C. W. (2012). Rating the methodological quality in systematic reviews of studies on measurement properties: A scoring system for the COSMIN checklist. *Quality of Life Research, 21*, 651–657.

Thaler, N. S., Kazemi, E., & Wood, J. J. (2010). Measuring anxiety in youth with learning disabilities: Reliability and validity of the Multidimensional Anxiety Scale for Children (MASC). *Child Psychiatry and Human Development, 41*, 501–514.

14

Construct Validity: Structural Validity

Chapter Outline

Structural validity is one type of construct validity, as shown in the taxonomy in Figure 3.1. Like validation efforts described in the previous chapter, structural validation involves tests of hypotheses about the nature of the construct being measured. Structural validity is, however, only relevant for multicomponent measures of complex constructs, notably multi-item scales.

Similar to the Consensus-based Standards for the selection of health Measurement Instruments (COSMIN) group, we define **structural validity** as the extent to which the structure of a multi-item instrument adequately reflects the hypothesized dimensionality of the construct being measured. Structural validity concerns which dimensions of a broader construct are captured by the instrument and whether the dimensions are consistent with theory.

Structural validity is best evaluated using a technique called **confirmatory factor analysis (CFA)**. CFA is a method for examining covariances among variables based on *structural equation modeling* (SEM). This chapter describes some basic features of CFA, but it is beyond the scope of this book to elaborate on the statistical basis of CFA or to provide detailed guidance on conducting a CFA. Readers interested in learning more about CFA should consult Brown (2006), Kline (2011), or Tabachnick and Fidell (2013).

14.1 Basics of Structural Validity and Confirmatory Factor Analysis

In this section, we discuss some basic structural validity issues, with emphasis on how it can be evaluated using CFA.

14.1.a Structural Validity and Other Types of Validity

Like other types of validity, structural validity requires researchers to have a strong conceptualization of the construct. A conceptual model of the focal construct, based either on theory or on a preliminary understanding of the construct's dimensionality from an exploratory factor analysis, forms the basis for structural validity hypotheses.

Like most measurement properties, structural validity is not a "fixed" attribute of an instrument. The dimensionality, and hence the structural validity, of a measure can vary from one population to another and often does. The Center for Epidemiologic Studies Depression Scale (CES-D; Radloff, 1977) provides a good example. The full 20-item CES-D and various short forms of the CES-D have been subjected to dozens of exploratory and confirmatory factor analyses with different populations, and numerous different factor solutions have been derived, ranging from one to four factors (Carleton et al., 2013). In this chapter, we will illustrate some features of CFA with the CES-D, using the data set of 1,000 low-income women we used in Chapter 5 for an exploratory factor analysis (EFA).

Evidence from a structural validity study alone should not be considered adequate evidence of a measure's construct validity because the analyses do not in and of themselves address the central construct validity question: Does this instrument really measure the construct it purports to measure? For example, if we imagined that the CES-D measured two aspects of anxiety (rather than depression), and a CFA yielded two dimensions that we decided to name as anxiety dimensions, nothing in the analysis itself would correct our flawed thinking. Moreover, if the global construct of depression encompassed four dimensions, but there were no items in the analysis to tap two of the four dimensions, then those two dimensions would not be revealed in the factor analysis. Thus, although some researchers make claims of construct validity when they have only examined a measure's structural validity, supplemental evidence of construct (and content) validity is always needed.

14.1.b Exploratory Factor Analysis Versus Confirmatory Factor Analysis: Advantages and Disadvantages

Both EFA and CFA are complex statistical methods that can be used to illuminate shared variance among measured variables. Many writers who compare EFA and CFA note that the purpose of EFA is to explore the structure and dimensionality of an instrument in the absence of a priori hypotheses, whereas the purpose of CFA is to test explicit hypotheses about the measure's dimensionality. Although such descriptions are true to a certain extent, they do not totally reflect the reality of modern-day scale construction efforts. Many EFAs are undertaken with measures for which a fully elaborated conceptual model has been developed and affirmed by a panel of content experts (Chapter 11). In other words, an EFA can "confirm" a preliminary conceptual model, although it can result in some surprises. And with CFA, even though an explicit hypothesized model is necessary, a lot of tinkering may occur during the analysis to modify the model. Thus, there is an "exploratory" side to some CFAs.

To be sure, there are important differences between the two. With EFA, preliminary notions about an instrument's dimensionality can only vaguely be communicated to the computer program. For example, a researcher could force most programs to rotate four factors for the CES-D items to correspond to a four-factor conceptual model (for example) but could not designate which items would load on the factors. An EFA can be very illuminating, however, so it is usually better not to impose constraints on the number of factors initially. EFA is particularly useful for identifying problematic items and so is a useful tool during scale development.

A clear advantage of CFA for structural validation, relative to EFA, is that it provides more statistical indexes that indicate the extent to which the data fit the hypothesized factor structure. Thus, a CFA that confirms a hypothesized structure is more compelling evidence of structural validity than results from an EFA. CFA also makes it possible to formally test whether a proposed model is a better fit to the data than alternative models. CFA is used widely to test a hypothesized unidimensional structure for a set of items used in the development of an item response theory (IRT) scale (Chapter 6).[1]

Another advantage of CFA is that it can be used to formally test whether a factor structure is comparable for different groups of people (e.g., men and women), for different populations (e.g., the general population vs. a population with a particular disease or condition), and for different versions of an instrument. This is an especially important application with instruments that have been translated or culturally adapted. We discuss the use of CFA for assessing measurement equivalence of translated measures in Chapter 15. CFA has also been used to compare factor structures for instruments that have been shortened. For example, Cole, Rabin, Smith, and Kaufman (2004) confirmed that their CES-D short form had a factor structure comparable to the 20-item version using CFA. Finally, CFA has been used to assess *response shift*, a phenomenon in which people responding to an instrument may alter their responses even when the amount of the underlying construct has not changed because they reconceptualize the questions (e.g., following a change in health). Response shift is discussed in Chapter 17.

Some advantages of CFA are practical ones. For example, some software programs include procedures for imputing missing values, including sophisticated imputation methods such as *expectation maximization* (EM).

CFA, as a method within SEM, benefits from extreme flexibility. For example, some of the assumptions associated with EFA (e.g., the independence of the item error terms) can be altered to some extent in a CFA. As another example, a CFA can test a conceptual model with both correlated and uncorrelated factors. Also, CFA can accommodate reflective scales and, unlike EFA, formative[2] indexes. Although the flexibility of CFA offers advantages for model refinement, it has been pointed out that such flexibility can "create more opportunities for making poor decisions" (DeVellis, 2012, p. 152).

The flexibility of CFA methods also makes it more complex and daunting than many other statistical procedures. Moreover, CFA is not included in most general-purpose statistical software packages, such as SPSS or SAS. The most widely used software for SEM includes AMOS, Mplus, LISREL, and EQS.

Sometimes researchers with a conceptual model that has been affirmed by content experts directly subject their model to a CFA rather than starting with an EFA. This is not necessarily the best approach if there is a possibility that items would need to be revised or eliminated because there is less item diagnostic information in a CFA than in an EFA (Yang et al., 2011; Yang & Jones, 2008; Yang, Tommet, & Jones, 2009). Even when a hypothesized model has a good fit to the data in a CFA, this does not guarantee that a different model or different set of items would not yield an even better fit. When a CFA results in a poor-fitting model, some have argued that an EFA is a reasonable follow-up (Schmitt, 2011).

14.2 The Confirmatory Factor Analysis Process

In CFA, researchers are required to hypothesize, in advance, the number of factors a measure has, which items load on the factors, and whether or not the factors are correlated. The process

---

[1]Moreover, results indicating a good fit in an IRT analysis further supports a hypothesized unidimensional structure.
[2]For further information on fitting models with formative indicators, readers can consult Brown (2006) or Roberts and Thatcher (2009).

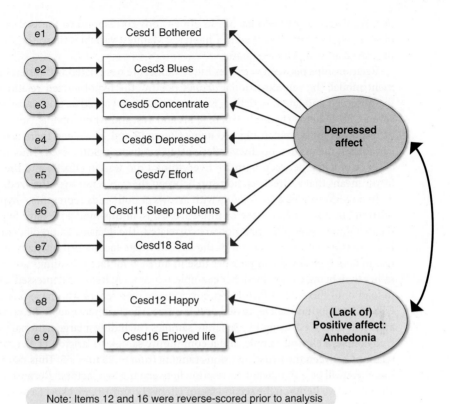

Note: Items 12 and 16 were reverse-scored prior to analysis

Figure 14.1
Measurement model for nine CES-D items.

can be described as having five basic steps: specifying the model to be tested, attending to identification, developing parameter estimates, testing the model fit, and modifying or re-specifying the model as necessary. This section provides a very brief overview of the process.

14.2.a Measurement Models in Confirmatory Factor Analysis

In a CFA, the hypotheses to be tested are embodied in a **measurement model** that is subjected to formal testing. The model stipulates the hypothesized relationships among the **latent variables** (the factors that are not directly measured) and the **manifest variables** (the measured variables which in our examples are items). The researcher uses the hypothesized measurement model to estimate a population covariance matrix that is compared to the actual covariance matrix.

Our measurement model for the nine CES-D items that we factor analyzed in Chapter 5 is presented in Figure 14.1. We note that CFA works best when there are at least three manifest variables for each latent variable, but we opted for a small number of items in our original factor analysis to simplify the presentation, so we are pursuing the CFA with the structure that resulted from the EFA.

Our measurement model uses several conventions that help to communicate our hypotheses.[3] In a CFA (or any structural model), an *oval* (or circle) is used to designate a latent variable. In our model, there are two latent traits hypothesized as the major dimensions of depression on our nine-item CES-D short form: (1) Depressed Affect, and (2) (Lack of)

---

[3]Our model shows a horizontal arrangement with items on the left and latent traits on the right. Sometimes the traits are displayed on the left, and sometimes a vertical arrangement is used to portray the model, usually with latent traits on the top of the figure.

Positive Affect or Anhedonia. These dimensions correspond to the two factors that were observed in the EFA described in Chapter 5. Manifest variables (here, the CES-D items) are portrayed as *rectangles* or squares.

Relationships between variables in the model are designated with lines. In our measurement model, the one-directional *arrows* portray the hypothesized relationships between the observed and latent variables. Depressed affect is viewed as the "cause" of responses to seven CES-D items (Items 1, 3, 5, 6, 7, 11, and 18), and Anhedonia is viewed as the "cause" of responses to the remaining two items (Items 12 and 16). When there is no line between variables, it means that no direct relationship has been hypothesized. Thus, for example, the absence of a line between Item 7 ("Everything I did was an effort") and the Positive Affect factor means that a direct relationship between the two is not hypothesized.

In an SEM model, a *curved line* with arrows at both ends represents a hypothesized correlation but not a direct cause or influence. Thus, in this model we have hypothesized that the two dimensions of Depression are correlated. The decision to predict correlated factors is in contrast with our decision in the EFA to rotate factors orthogonally, and this is what researchers typically do, in part because in an EFA, all factor loadings are freely estimated rather than being constrained. For example, in our CFA, Item 6 ("depressed") will not be free to load onto the second factor. Moreover, many researchers who have factor analyzed the CES-D have found the Depressed and Positive Affect dimensions to be correlated. For example, in their CFA using five separate samples (including a large nationally representative U.S. sample, a clinical sample, and a community sample), Carleton et al. (2013) found correlations between the two dimensions ranging from −.23 to −.65. Thus, our model predicts that there will be a significant correlation between the two factors.[4] Because we have reverse scored the two items on the second factor (Items 12 and 16), we expect a positive correlation.

The last elements in the measurement model are the small *circles* on the left, which designate **error terms** (sometimes called *disturbance terms*). Each of the nine measured variables has an error term (*e*) associated with it. The error term incorporates both measurement error and anything other than the latent trait that affects item responses, such as response bias. In measurement models, every *endogenous variable* (a variable hypothesized to have a cause within the model, as designated by an arrow pointing to it) must have an error term. (In the literature, the measurement model sometimes shows the error terms and latent traits with a double-headed curved arrow starting and returning to them, representing the variance of that variable).

Thus, the model in Figure 14.1 summarizes our two principal hypotheses: (1) that there is a two-factor model with a simple structure (each item loading on one and only one latent trait) for the nine CES-D Items and (2) that the two latent traits are positively correlated. A CFA will be undertaken to test these hypotheses (i.e., to test the extent to which our data fit the specified model). It might be noted that in some CFA software, measurement models can be created and used directly as input for the analysis (e.g., AMOS).

Although we do not present a figure to illustrate this, some measurement models include a *second-order factor*. We might, for example, hypothesize that Depressed Affect and Anhedonia are two aspects of a broader latent trait, Depressive Symptoms. Such a model would show an oval to the right of the existing two ovals in Figure 14.1, with one-directional arrows going from this third oval (Depressive Symptoms) to the other two latent traits. Such models, if there is a good fit to the data, provide a justification for combining subscale scores into one total score, which is usually what occurs with the CES-D. Several researchers have confirmed a second-order factor with the CES-D (e.g., Cole et al., 2004; Zhang et al., 2011).

The model presented in Figure 14.1 is the model that we hypothesize based on our EFA results, but we will test several alternative models to illustrate how results are often

---

[4]On a more technical note, a model with correlated factors was needed in our example because a model with uncorrelated factors could result in identification problems as a result of having only two items for the second factor. For an uncomplicated explanation of why this is so, see Babyak and Green (2010).

examined in a comparative context. Indeed, some CFA experts advocate testing alternative theoretically defensible models because a model with a good fit does not necessary mean that it is the best model. By testing multiple models that are consistent with prevailing research or theory, analysts can compare their relative fit. In our CFA, we will test our model with four others. The first is the most parsimonious possibility, a one-factor model with all nine items loading on a single factor. Second, we look at a two-factor model with uncorrelated factors. Third, we test a model with a second-order factor, as described in the previous paragraph. Finally, we examine the fit of a two-factor model after removing Item 7. As noted in several earlier chapters, Item 7 ("I felt that everything I did was an effort") has some potential problems within our sample of low-income urban women.

14.2.b Identification in Confirmatory Factor Analysis

A concept referred to as **identification** (or *identifiability*) has relevance to model testing in CFA. A statistical model can be described as *identified* if the known information available implies that there is one best value for each model parameter whose value is unknown. In a CFA, only models that are identified can be estimated. Although a detailed description of the issue of identification will not be presented here, we note that some measurement models cannot be tested because too many parameters are estimated relative to the number of *observations*. Observations in our CFA context does not refer to sample size but rather concerns the number of measured variables. The formula for calculating observations is:

$$\text{Observations} = \frac{k \times (k + 1)}{2}$$

where k is the number of items or variables. In our model, the number of observations is $(9 \times 10)/2 = 45$.

Thus, the number of parameters (e.g., variances, covariances, disturbances, path coefficients) that can be estimated with our nine measured variables cannot exceed 45. Models are most likely to run into identification problems if they are overly complex, which is not the case in our model in Figure 14.1. Models can be simplified by "fixing" or constraining some of the parameters.

In a CFA, there are three types of parameters. *Free parameters* can assume any value and are the ones that are estimated in the analysis. *Fixed parameters*, by contrast, are assigned specific values ahead of time. For example, the unstandardized regression coefficients from the error terms to the measured variables are often fixed to be 1. Another common practice is to set one regression coefficient between a latent trait and a measured variable (item) equal to 1.[5] The SEM software can select one measured variable per latent trait automatically, although it may be advantageous to designate a specific item—the one believed to have the strongest relationship with the latent trait. In some models, there are *constrained parameters,* which are unknown (like free parameters) but which are constrained to be the same value as another parameter.

In the model shown in Figure 14.1, we would estimate 19 free parameters. Seven of them would be the regression weights between the latent traits and the items (two others would be fixed at 1). We would also estimate the covariance between the two latent traits. The final 11 parameters are the variances for the nine error terms, plus variances for the two latent traits. With 45 observations and 19 parameter estimates, there would be 26 degrees of freedom $(45 - 19)$. Although the proposed model suggests no identification issues, the conditions for identification are complex and so cannot be fully assessed until the estimation procedure is undertaken. If there are problems, the output from the analysis provides a warning message. (For our measurement model in Figure 14.1, no identification problems were observed when we ran the analyses).

---

[5]Alternatively, the variance of the latent traits could be fixed to 1.

14.2.c Parameter Estimation for Confirmatory Factor Analysis

Once a measurement model with no apparent identification problems has been developed, the next step is to estimate the free parameters. There are many different estimation procedures from which to choose, and unfortunately, there is no one approach that can claim clear superiority over all the others. The default for many SEM programs, and the estimation method most often used, is *maximum likelihood* (ML) estimation. ML estimation works best (yields the least biased parameter estimates) when the assumption of multivariate normality holds and when the variables are interval- or ratio-level measures. Items such as those in the CES-D are ordinal and are often skewed, thus creating potential problems when ML estimation is used. A correction procedure known as the Bollen–Stine bootstraps (Bollen & Stine, 1992) is sometimes used to address nonnormality violations, including in CFAs of the CES-D (e.g., Cole et al., 2004). Another adjustment for nonnormality in ML estimation is the Satorra–Bentler correction (Satorra & Bentler, 2001). Several simulation studies that have examined the robustness of ML estimates in nonnormality situations have found that parameter estimates remain valid, but standard errors in the presence of excessive skewness do not (McDonald & Ho, 2002).

Other estimation methods include the *unweighted least squares* (ULS) and *weighted least squares* (WLS) methods, neither of which make assumptions about the distributions of the variables. These methods do, however, have other requirements. For example, the WLS estimation requires a large sample size to work well. The WLS method was used, for example, in the CFA of the 20-item CES-D with 976 patients with scleroderma (Kwakkenbos et al., 2013). Another estimation procedure that deals with nonnormality is the *asymptotically distribution-free* (ADF) estimator, which also requires a large sample size. Cole and colleagues (2004) originally attempted to use ADF in their CFA of the CES-D with a sample of 410 community-dwelling people. They found that ADF "did not yield a viable solution" (p. 365), so used ML estimation with the Bollen–Stine bootstraps. Several other estimation procedures have also been developed, and each has pros and cons in relation to sample size and violations of assumptions of normality, independence of errors, and item scaling (for a further discussion see, for example, Tabachnick & Fidell, 2013).

With measurement models based on ordinal-level items, the LISREL program has a procedure (PRELIS) that will calculate an appropriate covariance matrix from noninterval data. Norman and Streiner (2008) recommend that if a program other than LISREL is used, one approach is to test the model with more than one estimation method and inspect to see whether the results are consistent. If there are serious inconsistencies, it might be possible to undertake data transformations that will result in better estimation.

14.2.d Indexes of Model Fit in Confirmatory Factor Analysis

After the specified measurement model has been estimated, the key question is whether the model is a good fit to the data (i.e., whether the hypothesized model accounts for the correlations among variables in the data set). Before looking at formal indexes of model fit, it is important to look at the parameters themselves. For example, are the path coefficients (standardized regression weights) between latent variables and items sizeable and in the predicted direction? The path coefficients can be interpreted much as factor loadings in EFA, so we would expect the coefficients to be large, statistically significant, and in the "right" direction.

Figure 14.2 presents a diagram showing the major parameter estimates for our measurement model.[6] The coefficients over the arrows are the path coefficients. For example, the coefficient between Depressed Affect and Item 1 ("I was bothered by things that don't usually bother me") was .674. This coefficient suggests a strong relationship in the expected

---

[6]For simplicity, maximum likelihood estimation results are shown.

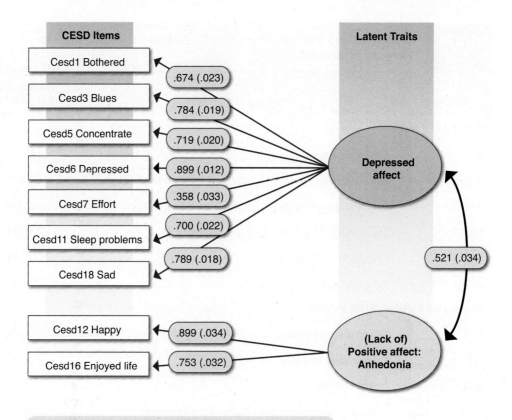

Note: Items 12 and 16 were reverse-scored prior to analysis

Figure 14.2
CFA results for nine CES-D items with parameter estimates.

direction (greater amounts of depressive affect correspond to greater frequency of occurrence of being bothered), and it was statistically significant (significance tests are not shown). A very strong path coefficient (.899) was observed for Item 6 ("I felt depressed") on the Depressed Affect factor, which is analogous to results obtained in the EFA (Table 5.6). The weakest coefficient (.358) was for Item 7 ("Everything I did was an effort"), which we identified as a potentially problematic item in the EFA described in Chapter 5. For the second factor, both items had high coefficients (e.g., .899 for Item 12, "I was happy"). Figure 14.2 also shows that the two latent traits of Depressed Affect and (Lack of) Positive Affect are positively correlated (.521); this correlation is statistically significant. Thus, parameter estimates are consistent with our hypotheses.

Many indexes are available in SEM programs to shed light on the goodness of fit of the overall model. Table 14.1 summarizes a few of the most widely used indexes and offers guidelines for cutoff values for concluding that the model has an adequate fit. As noted earlier, a good fit does not mean that the model is "ideal" or that it accounts for a large proportion of variation in the data. Indexes confirming an adequate model fit are merely evidence that the model is plausible.

The most basic index is an overall **chi-square goodness of fit** statistic, which we designate as χ^2_{GOF}. What one hopes for as indicative of a good fit is a chi-square value that is *not* significant (i.e., $p > .05$). This is because we are not testing observations against a null hypothesis of no relationship, as is usually the case with hypothesis tests, but rather against a hypothesized model with which we want the results to be congruent. Unfortunately, the χ^2_{GOF} is sensitive to sample size and to departures from normality and thus is seldom used

Table 14.1	Confirmatory Factor Analysis: Selected Fit Indexes and Threshold Guidelines	
Acronym	**Fit Index: Full Name**	**Threshold for Acceptance**[a]
Absolute Fit Indexes		
χ^2_{GoF}	Chi-square goodness of fit	$p > .05$
χ^2_{GoF}/df	Chi-square goodness of fit, divided by degrees of freedom	<2
RMSEA	Root mean square error of approximation	$\leq.06$
SRMR	Standardized root mean square residual	$\leq.08$
GFI	Goodness of fit index	$\geq.90$
AGFI	Adjusted goodness of fit index	$\geq.90$
Comparative (Relative) Fit Indexes		
CFI	Comparative fit index	$\geq.95$
IFI	Incremental fit index	$\geq.95$
NFI	Normed fit index	$\geq.95$
NNFI (or TLI)	Nonnormed fit index (aka Tucker–Lewis index)	$\geq.95$

[a]The thresholds suggested in this table are derived from the work of Hu and Bentler (1999); from Schreiber, Stage, King, Nora, and Barlow (2006); or from Tabachnick and Fidell (2013).

as the sole criterion for model fit. When the sample is small, the desired nonsignificant result can occur because of inadequate power, even with a poor-fitting model. Conversely, when the sample is large, a model with decent fit can be statistically significant, and this often turns out to be the case. As another rule of thumb using the chi-square statistic, it is desirable to have the value of χ^2_{GOF}/df be less than two; some suggest that less than three is adequate.

Because the chi-square test is not always a dependable fit index as a result of sample size issues, other fit indexes have been developed, none of which has an associated test of statistical significance and none of which is considered a "gold standard." The various indexes take different aspects of the analysis into account—for example, the amount of variance explained, the parsimoniousness of the model, or the size of the residuals. Cutoffs for acceptable values of these indexes have been proposed and tested in simulations, but again, there is not total consensus about the values or the merits of having cutoffs.

Absolute fit indexes estimate how well the a priori model reproduces (fits) the data. The χ^2_{GOF} test is one such index. Others include the *root mean square error of approximation* (**RMSEA**), *the standardized root mean square residual* (**SRMR**), the *goodness of fit index* (**GFI**), and the *adjusted goodness of fit index* (**AGFI**). The first two (RMSEA and SRMR) are indexes that indicate better fitting models when the values approach zero. Based on simulations, Hu and Bentler (1999) concluded that an RMSEA of $\leq.06$ indicates a good fit, whereas an SRMR of $<.08$ is desirable. Hu and Bentler found that RMSEA erred most in rejecting a true model when the sample size was small. The other absolute fit indexes (GFI and AGFI) are scaled to range from .00 (indicating no fit) to 1.0 (indicating a perfect fit). Usually, a value greater than .90 for these indexes is considered adequate and .95 or greater is considered good. Some simulations suggest, however, that the GFI and AGFI are not pre-ferred indexes of fit (Schreiber et al., 2006).

Another class of indexes is called indexes of *comparative fit* (or "relative fit"). These in-dexes compare the chi-square value for the hypothesized model with that from a "baseline" or null model in which all of the variables are uncorrelated and so have a large chi-square value indicative of poor fit. Indexes in this grouping include the *comparative fit index* (**CFI**), the *incremental fit index* (**IFI**), the *normed fit index* (**NFI**), and the *nonnormed fit index* (**NNFI**), which is sometimes referred to as the *Tucker Lewis Index*, or **TLI**. For all of these indexes, values greater than .95 offer good evidence of model fit.

Models that have a good fit tend to produce consistent results on many different indexes. Decisions about which indexes are best for interpretation and reporting purposes may rely on the personal preferences of the research team (or a journal editor or reviewer). Hu and Bentler (1999) recommend the SRMR and a CFI. Schreiber and colleagues (2006) prefer the NNFI, CFI, and RMSEA. Kline (2011) recommends the χ^2_{GOF}, CFI, RMSEA, and SRMR.

When the indexes provide contradictory indications about model fit, it is usually neces-sary to carefully reexamine the model. If the χ^2_{GOF} is significant but all other indexes indi-cate good fit, it likely reflects a sample size issue, in which case it is probably safe to conclude that the model has adequate fit. If the hypothesized model has a poor fit, the estimated parameters should not be interpreted because their values may well be incorrect.

As noted earlier, we tested several alternative models for the nine CES-D items, in addition to the hypothesized model depicted in Figure 14.1. Table 14.2 presents val-ues for χ^2_{GOF}, CFI, and RMSEA for each model. Because of our large sample, all the χ^2_{GOF} values are statistically significant, so we will rely primarily on the other fit statis-tics. The fit statistics for the one-factor model (Model a) support our conclusion in Chapter 5 that the nine items do not form a unidimensional scale: The CFI was too low (.893) and RMSEA was too high (.163) for an adequately fitting model. The two-factor model with orthogonal factors (Model b) had fit statistics that were even less desirable, which is not surprising given that the two factors had a reasonably high correlation (.521). Our hypothesized model (Model c) had the best CFI value (.988) and the best RMSEA value (.056), but the model with a second-order factor for overall Depression (Model d) was nearly identical. Omitting Item 7 from the "Depressed Affect" subscale did not im-prove model fit. Thus, we conclude that both Models c and d are especially plausible for these data.

Table 14.2   Confirmatory Factor Analysis: Selected Fit Indexes for Five Models for Nine- CES-D Items

Model	χ^2_{GoF} (*df*)	*p*	CFI	RMSEA
(a) 1 Factor	732.553 (27)	<.001	.893	.163
(b) 2 Factor, orthogonal	1224.071 (29)	<.001	.818	.205
(c) 2 Factor, correlated factors	105.172 (26)	<.001	.988	.056
(d) Hierarchical (second order for Depression)	109.321 (27)	<.001	.987	.056
(e) 2 Factor, correlated, Item 7 omitted	532.476 (27)	<.001	.923	.138

Note: The nine items were those used in the exploratory factor analysis in Chapter 5: Items 1, 3, 5, 6, 7, 11, and 18 for Factor 1 and Items 12 and 16 for Factor 2 (see Table 5.2 for item wording).
CFI, comparative fit index; RMSEA, root mean square error of approximation.

14.2.e Model Modification

Models can be modified to improve model fit or to develop a more parsimonious model. Most SEM programs provide modification indexes that can offer guidance for minor modifications. For example, the *Lagrange multiplier test* is a statistical test used to evaluate improvements from freeing parameters that were initially fixed. The *Wald statistic* is used to evaluate improvements resulting from dropping parameters from the model (i.e., setting them to zero). Of course, modifications should be theoretically justifiable and not done purely on the basis of statistical criteria. The risk with model modifications is that they can be abused and result in a more exploratory than confirmatory effort. It is usually inadvisable to pursue modifications if the initial hypothesized model has good fit, barring legitimate substantive arguments to do so.

We do not present model modifications for our analysis but offer an example from a published study of a two-factor CFA model for the CES-D, with factors similar to our own (Kwakkenbos et al., 2013). These researchers used modification indexes to identify pairs of items which, if error terms were free to covary rather than being fixed, would result in improved model fit. They accepted such modifications if there were "theoretically justifiable shared method effects" (p. 3), such as similar item wording. As an example, their respecified model allowed correlated error terms for Items 17 ("I had crying spells") and 18 ("I felt sad"), which they concluded had "clearly recognizable overlap in the items' content" (p. 4).

14.3 The Design of Structural Validation Studies

This section discusses some issues to consider in designing and reporting structural validity studies and evaluating confirmatory factor analyses reported by others.

14.3.a Study Design in Structural Validation

As noted in Chapter 13, construct validations, including structural validations, are typically undertaken after a measure has been finalized (except when CFA is used to test the unidimensionality assumption in an IRT analysis). This usually means that the measure has already been subjected to an EFA and an internal consistency analysis, has been revised as necessary based on the results, and has yielded good test–retest reliability estimates.

Typically, a CFA occurs within the context of a fully elaborated construct validity study involving (for example) efforts to gather evidence about convergent or known-groups validity, although structural validity results may be reported in a separate paper. Designs for CFAs are cross-sectional unless the goal of the CFA is to shed light on whether people have reconceptualized a construct (response shift), usually following a change in overall health (Chapter 17).

If a structural validation is conducted independently of other construct validity efforts, the only data that need to be collected are the responses for the instrument in question and data that can provide a good description of the sample. If a CFA is one aspect of a broader construct validation, data for additional corroborating measures would need to be gathered, as described in Chapter 13.

Although we do not offer explicit analytic advice with regard to model testing, we note that a good place to begin a CFA analysis is to examine the data set for potential problems. For example, researchers should examine the extent of missingness, the skewness and kurtosis of item distributions, the linearity of relationships among items, and the possibility of multicollinearity or multivariate outliers. The results of these preliminary analyses, and size of the sample, are likely to affect several analytic decisions, such as which estimation method to use and which fit indexes would be most suitable.

14.3.b Sampling for Confirmatory Factor Analysis

A CFA of a multidimensional instrument should be undertaken with a sample from the population for whom the measure is intended. The sample should be a different one from the sample used to finalize the instrument using EFA to ensure that the model does not reflect the idiosyncrasies of a single sample.[7] Another alternative, if the sample is very large, is to divide the sample in half at random and perform the EFA on one random half-sample and the CFA on the other.

When a previously validated instrument is under consideration for use with a new population, then its structural validity (and other types of validity) should be reassessed. One of the reasons that there are dozens of published CFAs of the CES-D is that the CES-D has been evaluated for use with diverse clinical and demographic populations.

Like EFA, CFA works best when the sample is large, so that parameter estimates are stable. Several complex procedures have been developed for estimating sample size requirements based on estimates of power and precision (see, for example, Schmitt, 2011). One widely cited rule of thumb is that there should be at least 10 cases for each parameter estimated, with a minimum of 200 cases in the analyses. Larger samples are, however, desirable when there are major violations of the normality assumption. In our example, we have a ratio of about 50 cases per parameter ($50 \times 19 = 950$), which is a favorable ratio.

Random sampling from the target population is desirable because population parameters are being estimated. Although random sampling is seldom feasible, researchers should strive to have a representative sample to the extent possible. This may involve recruitment from multiple sites to account for variation with regard to such demographic characteristics as race, ethnicity, and socioeconomic status.

14.3.c Reporting a Structural Validation

Because of the complexity of a CFA, and the many decisions that the analyst must make, researchers must juggle competing objectives in writing a paper on structural validity. They must balance the desire for thoroughness and transparency on the one hand with the journal page constraints on the other. For example, those who have offered guidance on reporting CFA results often state that it is desirable to report on the model conditions that will secure identification, but authors seldom mention identification (Schreiber et al., 2006). A useful strategy, when details about the analysis must be excluded because of space, is to indicate how any omitted information can be obtained from the research team or whether a more detailed technical report is available.

Certain features are, however, essential. Certainly, it is necessary to provide a good description of the hypothesized model and its theoretical foundations. If an EFA was the basis for the model, then the results need to be briefly summarized, but a more substantive or theoretical defense is also important. In terms of the model itself, some authors present both the initial model, as in Figure 14.1, and the final model with parameter estimates, as in Figure 14.2. When the initial model is confirmed, a single model is likely to suffice. If alternative models are being tested for comparative purposes, the theoretical basis for the alternatives should be summarized. And if the possibility of model modification is envisioned, the researchers should note in advance the nature and theoretical justification of the modifications.

The population for whom the model is relevant should be specified, together with a description of the sample used in the analysis. Sample size and sampling strategy should be reported together with a rationale for the size, especially if the size is marginal or risky with the chosen estimation method.

---

[7]We used the same sample for both the EFA and CFA, purely for illustrative purposes.

The results of analyses to examine the items' distributional characteristics should be reported, as well as information about any missing values and how they were handled. The chosen estimation method should be stated and, if standard assumptions are known to have been violated, the rationale for the decision about estimation method should be discussed. Readers should be able to understand the robustness of the researchers' conclusions about the final model. Also, the specific computer program used to do the analysis (both program and version number) should be stated.

The researchers should present the key parameter estimates (e.g., in a figure) and should discuss how the parameters match the hypotheses. The statistical significance of the parameters should be stated. Sometimes the unstandardized coefficients, the standard errors, and t or z values for individual items are reported in a table.

If only one model has been tested, the relevant indexes of overall model fit can be reported in the text, but if multiple models are being compared, a table is essential. Often, two or three indexes of model fit are reported. Any model modifications should be described and linked back to the theoretical rationale provided earlier in the paper. If modifications suggest the desirability of revising the instrument (e.g., deletion of an item), the implications of such revisions need to be spelled out, especially if the instrument is already in use. The discussion section of the paper should help readers to come to conclusions about the structural validity of the instrument or about what additional research with the measure is needed.

Many authors have written more detailed suggestions about how to present the results from SEM. Readers may wish to consult Boomsa (2000), McDonald and Ho (2002), or Schreiber et al. (2006).

14.3.d Evaluating a Structural Validation

The COSMIN workgroup has created some guidelines for evaluating structural validity assessments (Terwee et al., 2012). Given the complexity of CFA, however, the COSMIN scoring checklist, shown in Box E on the COSMIN website, may be incomplete. Suggestions in the previous section on what information should be included in a report on a CFA may help those reviewing a structural validation paper. Some elements are likely to prove much easier to critique than others. For example, if a CFA for a 20-item instrument was undertaken with a sample of 150, then it is probably safe to conclude that the ratio of sample points to parameters is too low to yield stable estimates. When information about certain aspects of the analyses is not provided (e.g., violation of assumptions), it will be difficult to evaluate some of the decisions, such as the appropriateness of the estimation method that was used.

Reviewers should be particularly alert to situations in which the model fit indexes are inconsistent. They should also be concerned if model modifications were made that appear to have primarily a statistical rather than a substantive rationale.

References

Babyak, M. A., & Green, S. B. (2010). Confirmatory factor analysis: An introduction for psychosomatic medicine researchers. *Psychosomatic Medicine, 72*, 587–597.

Bollen, K., & Stine, R. (1992). Bootstrapping goodness-of-fit measures in structural equation models. *Sociological Methods and Research, 21*, 205–229.

Boomsa, A. (2000). Reporting analyses of covariance structures. *Structural Equation Modeling, 7*, 461–483.

Brown, T. A. (2006). *Confirmatory factor analysis for applied research.* New York, NY: The Guilford Press.

Carleton, R. N., Thibodeau, M., Teale, M., Welch, P., Abrams, M., Robinson, T., & Asmundson, G. (2013). The Center for Epidemiologic Studies Depression Scale: A review with a theoretical and empirical examination of item content and factor structure. *PLoS One, 8*(3), e58067.

Cole, J. C., Rabin, A., Smith, T., & Kaufman, A. (2004). Development and validation of a Rasch-derived CES-D short form. *Psychological Assessment, 16*, 360–372.

De Vellis, R. F. (2012). *Scale development: Theory and application* (3rd ed.). Thousand Oaks, CA: Sage.

Hu, L. T., & Bentler, P. N. (1999). Cutoff criteria for fit indexes in covariance structure analysis: Conventional criteria versus new alternatives. *Structural Equation Modeling, 6,* 1–55.

Kline, R. B. (2011). *Principles and practice of structural equation modeling* (3rd ed.). New York, NY: The Guilford Press.

Kwakkenbos, L., Arthurs, E., van den Hoogen, F., Hudson, M., van Lankveld, W., Baron, M., . . . Thombs, B. (2013). Cross-language measurement equivalence of the Center for Epidemiologic Studies Depression (CES-D) Scale in systemic sclerosis. *PLoS One, 8*(1), e53923.

McDonald, R. P., & Ho, M. R. (2002). Principles and practice in reporting structural equation analyses. *Psychological Methods, 7,* 64–82.

Norman, G. R., & Streiner, D. L. (2008). *Biostatistics: The bare essentials* (3rd ed.). Shelton, CT: People's Medical Publishing House.

Radloff, L. S. (1977). The CES-D scale: A self-report depression scale for research in the general population. *Applied Psychological Measurement, 1,* 385–401.

Roberts, N., & Thatcher, J. (2009). Conceptualizing and testing formative constructs: Tutorial and annotated example. *ACMSIGMIS Database archive, 40,* 9–39.

Satorra, A., & Bentler, P. (2001). A scaled difference chi-square test statistic for moment structure analysis. *Psychometrika, 66,* 507–514.

Schmitt, T. A. (2011). Current methodological considerations in exploratory and confirmatory factor analysis. *Journal of Psychoeducational Assessment, 29,* 304–321.

Schreiber, J. B., Stage, F., King, J., Nora, A., & Barlow, E. (2006). Reporting structural equation modeling and confirmatory factor analysis results. *The Journal of Education Research, 99,* 323–337.

Tabachnick, B., & Fidell, L. (2013). *Using multivariate statistics* (6th ed.). Boston, MA: Pearson Education.

Terwee, C. B., Mokkink, L. B., Knol, D. L., Ostelo, R., Bouter, L. M., & DeVet, H. C. W. (2012). Rating the methodological quality in systematic reviews of studies on measurement properties: A scoring system for the COSMIN checklist. *Quality of Life Research, 21,* 651–657.

Yang, F. M., Heslin, K. C., Mehta, K. M., Yang, C. W., Ocepek-Welikson, K., Kleinman, M., . . . Mungas, D. (2011). A comparison of item response theory-based methods for examining differential item functioning in object naming test by language of assessment among older Latinos. *Psychological Test and Assessment Modeling, 53,* 440–460.

Yang, F. M., & Jones, R. N. (2008). Measurement differences in depression: Chronic health-related and sociodemographic effects in older Americans. *Psychosomatic Medicine, 70,* 993–1004.

Yang, F. M., Tommet, D., & Jones, R. N. (2009). Disparities in self-reported geriatric depressive symptoms due to sociodemographic differences: An extension of the bi-factor item response theory model for use in differential item functioning. *Journal of Psychiatric Research, 43,* 1025–1035.

Zhang, B., Fokkema, M., Ciujpers, P., Li, J., Smits, N., & Beekman, A. (2011). Measurement invariance of the Center for Epidemiological Studies Depression Scale (CES-D) among Chinese and Dutch elderly. *BMC Medical Research Methodology, 11,* 74.

Cross-Cultural Validity

Chapter Outline

Health research has increasingly become multicultural and international in scope. This, in turn, has sparked efforts to adapt and translate high-quality health measures for use in diverse cultures. Original instruments are often in English, created with the predominant cultural group in mind.

In the Consensus-based Standards for the selection of health Measurement Instruments (COSMIN) taxonomy, and in the taxonomy presented in Figure 3.1, cross-cultural valid-ity is one of three types of construct validity. Similar to COSMIN (Mokkink et al., 2010), we define **cross-cultural validity** as the degree to which the components (e.g., items) of a translated or culturally adapted measure perform adequately and equivalently, individually and collectively, relative to their performance on the original instrument. Although this chapter addresses cross-cultural validity, it differs from other chapters in Part IV in that the focus is not exclusively on validation procedures but also on the steps required to translate, adapt, and pilot test the measure.

15.1 Basics of Cross-Cultural Validity

Before describing actual steps in instrument adaptation and testing, we discuss some basic issues that are important to any undertaking in cross-cultural measurement. We note that although most cross-cultural efforts in health care measurement have been undertaken with patient-reported outcome (PRO) measures, observational instruments have undergone adaptation using similar procedures. For example, an English-language observational screening scale to measure delirium in intensive care unit (ICU) settings—the Intensive Care Delirium Screening Checklist, or ICDSC—was translated and adapted for use in Swedish ICUs (Neziraj, Sarac Kart, & Samuelson, 2011).

15.1.a Cross-Cultural Validation Scenarios

Developing a high-quality and cross-culturally valid instrument requires even more time and effort than starting from scratch with a new instrument. Yet, without such projects, it would be impossible to understand health outcomes globally. If, for example, we want to learn whether health-related quality of life differs across countries, comparisons cannot be made with disparate instruments. As another example, many drug trials are international in scope, and such trials benefit from the use of the same outcome measures. Several coordinated multinational efforts have been undertaken to adapt widely used English-language scales. For example, one major project involved translations of the SF-36 Health Survey (Ware & Sherbourne, 1992), as documented in an entire issue of the *Journal of Clinical Epidemiology* (volume 51, issue 11). And, as noted in Chapter 6, the Patient Reported Outcomes Measurement Information System (PROMIS®) initiative has involved the translation of many item banks for computerized adaptive testing.

Even within a single country, increased multiculturalism often necessitates the adaptation of well-validated instruments. For example, understanding health disparities in countries like the United States requires the use of measures with cross-cultural validity for different ethnic, racial, and language groups.

Beaton, Bombardier, Guillemin, and Bosi Ferraz (2000) noted four scenarios in which a cross-cultural adaptation is required. These include adaptations for use with (1) long-term immigrants residing in a "source" country (i.e., the country where the instrument was developed); (2) residents of another country where the language is the same as the source country but with different idioms and spellings; (3) residents in the source country who do not speak the same language, such as new immigrants; and (4) use in a different country by people who speak a different language. In all four scenarios, cultural adaptation is usually required, but translation is necessary only in the last two. To streamline our presentation, when we discuss translation processes in this chapter, we are referring to both linguistic and cultural "translations" unlike otherwise stated.

15.1.b Centered and Decentered Translations

Translations can be described as either centered or decentered. In a **centered** (or *asymmetric*) **translation**, the instrument is translated into another language, with no effect on the wording of the original instrument. In other words, loyalty to the wording on the original instrument is maintained, and the original version is the standard against which translations are compared. Such translations typically occur after the fact, that is, after the original measure has been validated and has been identified as a candidate for translation because it has desirable features, such as good reliability and validity, brevity, acceptability, and lack of noteworthy floor or ceiling effects.

By contrast, a **decentered** *(symmetric)* **translation** involves the possibility of modifications to items on the original instrument. Such decentered translations often reflect the goal of replacing culturally exclusive language with more universally understood language. This approach is often adopted when the developer knows in advance that the scale will be used in two languages, so translation activities are built into the scale development process. For example, in the United States, it may be prudent to anticipate the need for a Spanish translation during the instrument development phase and to pursue a decentered approach (Marin & Marin, 1991). As an example, Coffman (2008) translated the Diabetes Self-Efficacy Scale into Spanish using a decentered approach.

Even with well-developed and widely used measures, translations sometimes result in adaptations to the original instrument, so some decentering is possible even with established instruments. A good example is the SF-36, which is used in many countries and cultures. In a project called the *International Quality of Life Assessment* (IQOLA), the original SF-36 was translated into 10 languages and also adapted for use in other same-language countries, such as Australia. Wagner and other members of the IQOLA team (1998) described how the translation process unveiled some of the ambiguities and problems inherent in original SF-36 items. As a result, two items that were difficult to translate because of embedded colloquialisms were modified in version two of the SF-36 for use in the United States.

15.1.c The Issue of Equivalence

The goal of instrument adaptations and translations is to create an instrument that is *equivalent* to the original one. In cross-cultural measurement, equivalence is as important as reliability and construct validity. The concept of **equivalence** is, however, complex. Flaherty and colleagues (1988), for example, proposed a hierarchy of five different types of cross-cultural equivalence. Herdman, Fox-Rushby, and Badia (1997) defined 18 different types of equivalence mentioned in adaptations of quality of life measures. Most recently, Johnson (2006), in his article on cross-cultural measurement, listed 60 terms that characterized different types of equivalence.

It is beyond the scope of this book to define the various types of equivalencies in cross-cultural research, but several important types require explanation because they are often assessed in adaptation efforts. Johnson (2006) clustered the various types of equivalence into two broad groupings, what he called *interpretive* forms and *procedural* forms of equivalence. Interpretive equivalencies are those concerned with "similarities and differences in the meaning of concepts, constructs, questions, expressions, and words across cultural groups" (p. S17). Within this interpretive grouping, conceptual, content, and semantic equivalence (all of which have been defined in varying ways) are especially salient.

■ **Conceptual equivalence** concerns the extent to which the construct of interest exists in another culture and whether the construct has similar meaning. In other words, the question is whether there is a high degree of conceptual agreement across cultures regarding the focal construct. Herdman et al. (1997) found that conceptual equivalence was the most frequently mentioned type of equivalence in quality-of-life research. In the Flaherty et al. (1988) hierarchy, conceptual equivalence was at the pinnacle. Without conceptual equivalence, there may be little point in an instrument adaptation. For example, is the construct of *pleasure* meaningful in devastatingly poor societies in which daily survival entails struggle? Does the construct of *obesity* have the same meaning and connotations across cultures? Conceptual equivalence overlaps with another type of equivalence mentioned in the literature: *experiential equivalence.* If an activity, behavior, or feeling is not experienced in the target culture, then the construct is unlikely to have much meaning and an adaptation might not be feasible.

■ **Content equivalence** concerns the cultural relevance of individual items for the focal construct within the culture under consideration. For example, the SF-36 has an item that asks about the respondent's ability to do moderate activities such as "bowling" or "playing golf." These examples of moderate activity would have low relevance in many countries. Other activities that require a similar amount of exertion and that are appropriate for both men and women must be substituted as examples of moderate activity (e.g., "riding a bicycle" in Italy and the Netherlands [Wagner et al., 1998]).

■ **Semantic equivalence** is the extent to which the meaning of an item is the same in the target culture after the item is translated as it was in the original. Semantic equivalence, then, concerns the adequacy of the translation. Literal translations are never satisfactory. The translation needs to preserve the underlying meaning of the original wording rather than the exact wording. Rigorous translation procedures are discussed later in this chapter. There is considerable overlap between semantic equivalence and what some people refer to as *functional equivalence* (Herdman et al., 1997).

Procedural equivalence, the second broad grouping in Johnson's (2006) scheme, concerns technical problems of cross-cultural measurement. Two types of procedural equivalence are often examined, although, again, the terms are inconsistently defined.

■ **Technical** (or *operational*) **equivalence** concerns the equivalence of assumptions about the methods of instrument administration. A translated instrument may lack technical equivalence if the culture's norms differ from those in the original culture with respect to respondent burden, self-disclosure, privacy, and members' ability to understand the instrument response task. Method bias can occur when there are cultural differences in motivation to complete a scale, experience with closed-ended questions, or experience with any technology used in data gathering, such as computers (Hambleton, 2001).

■ **Measurement equivalence**, as we define it,[1] concerns the comparability of various measurement properties in the original and translated versions of a scale, such as comparability of reliability, internal consistency, construct validity, and so on. A particular type of measurement equivalence is **factorial equivalence** (or **factorial invariance**), one aspect of which concerns the extent to which the dimensionality of a construct is similar for an adapted measure and original measure. Measurement and factorial invariance are often associated with evidence that shows that the adapted measure places individuals who are similar on the attribute at the same point along a continuum of scores. In other words, a person's "true score" on a construct is the same on an adapted measure as it would be on the original.

We discuss methods of addressing and evaluating these forms of equivalence in this chapter. A rigorous, incremental approach is required, building into each step more evidence about equivalence on many fronts.

15.1.d The Process of Cross-Cultural Adaptation and Validation

An adaptation should never be considered a "shortcut" to creating a measure for a specific cultural or language group. Researchers who pursue an instrument adaptation project undertake a wide array of tasks that are even more demanding than the ones required for an original instrument development effort. Many diverse skills are required, and this is typically accomplished by assembling a multidisciplinary team of methodologic (qualitative and quantitative), statistical, substantive, linguistic, and cultural experts.

Once an instrument is selected for possible adaptation, the first task is to assess conceptual and technical equivalence, as described in the next section. If conceptual equivalence is considered adequate, the translation or adaptation is undertaken next. The end product in this phase, which in itself involves a sequence of tasks that may be iterative, is a fully translated

---

[1]Measurement equivalence is sometimes defined more broadly to include both interpretive and procedural equivalence (e.g., Meredith & Teresi, 2006) but also more technically to refer to complex assessment methods such as various differential item functioning (DIF) approaches.

draft measure deemed to have semantic equivalence to the original. Pretests of the adapted measure and assessments relating to content equivalence are undertaken in the next phase, which may lead to further revisions and improvements. Then the psychometric properties of the translated scale are assessed and efforts to understand measurement equivalence are pursued. Factorial equivalence is often explored as an important tool for cross-cultural validation.

Figure 15.1 presents a simplified flowchart that summarizes key activities in this process.

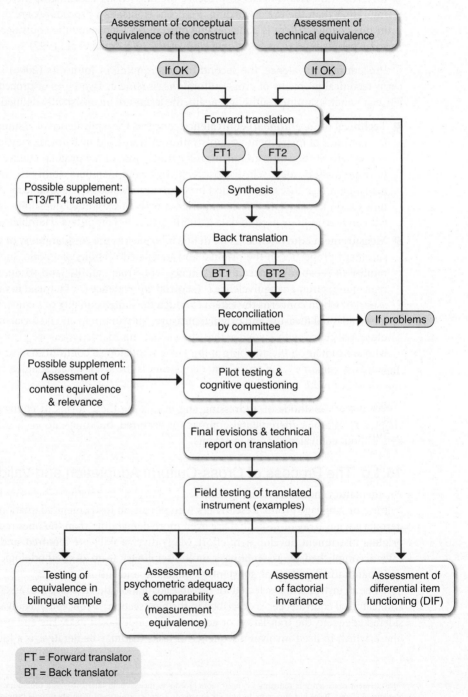

Figure 15.1
A model of processes in cross-cultural adaptation and validation.

15.2 Conceptual and Technical Equivalence

Several cross-cultural experts have advised that the first place to begin an adaptation project is to learn a lot about the culture and to ascertain that the construct being measured is meaningful in that culture—that is, to gain a preliminary understanding of the conceptual equivalence of the construct in the original and target cultures (e.g., Hui & Triandis, 1985; Sidani, Guruge, Miranda, Ford-Gilboe, & Varcoe 2010; Streiner & Norman, 2008). Herdman et al. (1997) pointed out that many investigators fail to do this upfront assessment, relying on evaluations of conceptual equivalence after the translation has been completed, if at all. He suggested that in cross-cultural quality-of-life research, the implicit assumption has typically been that constructs are largely invariant across cultures—a stance referred to as an *absolutist* approach. Ethnocentric attitudes inherent in absolutism can lead to measurements that are meaningless or impossible to interpret. Perspectives that are "universalist" accept that culture can have a significant impact on how constructs are construed and expressed.

Conceptual equivalence is not an "all-or-nothing" attribute; it is situated on a continuum. At one end of the continuum, people in the two cultures are in total agreement about the existence and meaning of the construct and on how the construct is manifested. At the other end, the focal construct does not even exist in the target culture. In health research, conceptual equivalence is often partial, in-between these two extremes. That is to say, the construct of interest exists in the other culture but is not identical in its nature; for example, it may be of greater (or lesser) cultural importance, it may have different dimensions or components, or it might be manifested in different behaviors, customs, or outlooks. Cross-cultural researchers need to attend to such nuanced differences.

As noted by Herdman et al. (1997), conceptual equivalence does not occur so much at the item level as at a higher and more abstract level. The degree of conceptual equivalence should be investigated before any translation work begins, although it can be further verified as part of the translation process. A good place to begin is to include one or more members of the target culture on the research team or on an advisory panel. For example, when Jones, Lee, Phillips, Zhang, and Jaceldo (2001) translated a coping scale into Chinese and Tagalog, they began by convening a meeting of cultural experts who were asked to assess the cultural relevance of the coping construct. Sidani and colleagues (2010) offered some explicit guidance regarding the work of an advisory board in assessing conceptual equivalence prior to translation. Various qualitative research methods with people from the target culture (e.g., in-depth or focus group interviews) can help researchers to understand how the construct is conceptualized (Nápoles-Springer & Stewart, 2006).

Reviewing the literature to explore conceptual equivalence is essential, and this should include a review of both quantitative and qualitative literature in multiple health disciplines. If one is fortunate, there may be existing cross-cultural evidence regarding conceptual equivalence. For example, Beck, Bernal, and Froman (2003) described their project to translate the Postpartum Depression Screening Scale or PDSS, described in Chapter 11, from English into Spanish. In the 1980s, postpartum depression (PPD) had been viewed as a culture-bound disorder found primarily in developed Western societies. Later studies, however, suggested that it was a more universal phenomenon. One mixed methods international study, in particular, provided evidence that there was consistency of mothers' experiences and symptoms of PPD across nine countries spanning five continents, including Spanish-speaking countries.

The assessment of conceptual equivalence may lead researchers to conclude that the construct is sufficiently similar to warrant moving on to a translation. The assessment might also uncover ways in which the instrument might need to be modified (e.g., removal of some items) or augmented.

Preliminary assessments of *technical* equivalence can employ similar methods of expert opinion, literature review, and feedback from the target population. The focus of such efforts is to assess whether the *methods* used in the measurement are congruent with cultural beliefs, values, and experiences. Such an inquiry is likely to be especially important for undeveloped non-Western cultures or in certain subcultures. The assessment of technical equivalence may lead researchers to abandon plans for a translation or may lead to creative solutions for alternative measurement strategies.

A special problem relating to technical equivalence concerns how different cultures use rating scales and how response biases differ. For example, in cultures where humility is valued, reduced variability in scores may be observed as a result of a moderacy bias (i.e., the tendency to select nonextreme items), whereas in cultures that value resoluteness, variability may be inflated as a result of an extreme response bias. Knowledge of the culture, and familiarity with prior translation work in that culture, can help to prepare the research team for such issues in technical equivalence.

One final note is that in large-scale item-banking projects using item response theory (IRT) models, the items in the initial item pool may be subjected to a *translatability assessment*. For example, in the PROMIS® project, item translations were envisioned from the start and so a preliminary review was undertaken. Forrest and colleagues (2012) described how, for the pediatric item banks, a translation expert reviewed items prior to any IRT analyses to identify complex sentences, difficult idiomatic expressions, and concepts that are not readily translated into other languages. The review led to the removal or revision of problematic items.

15.3 Semantic Equivalence: The Translation/Adaptation Process

Contemporary efforts to establish semantic equivalence date back to the pioneering work of Richard Brislin (1970, 1986), who introduced the procedure called *back translation* that is described in this section. Brislin's original methods have been adapted, expanded, and standardized to some degree, but they all involve back translations. Congruent with the literature in this field, we refer to the *source language* as the language of the original measure that is being translated, although in some cultural adaptations, the language does not change and so it would be considered a source *version*. The language into which the measure is being translated is called the *target language* (target version). The translation process is often described as unfolding in four phases: forward translation, synthesis, back translation, and reconciliation.

15.3.a Step 1: Forward Translation

The first step in the translation process is called the **forward translation**, in which the measure's items, response options, and instructions are translated from the source language into the target language. Current recommendations (e.g., Beaton et al., 2000; Mallinckrodt & Wang, 2004) call for a team of translators, not just one.

Often the translating team includes two bilingual individuals, whom we will designate as the FT1 and FT2 forward translators. Each translator, whose native tongue should be the target language, works independently to translate the measure from the source to the target language, blinded to the work of the other translator. If possible, the translators should be bicultural as well as bilingual, so as to better grasp subtleties and idiomatic expressions, and ideally they would have had prior translating experience.

Beaton et al. (2000) have recommended that one of the FT translators be familiar with the construct that is being measured (e.g., have some appropriate clinical knowledge). They recommend that FT2, however, be a "naïve" translator who is less influenced by academic concerns and is attuned to the language used by the target population. One difficulty,

items have phrases such as "down in the dumps" and "downhearted and blue" that required careful thought in translation (Wagner et al., 1998). Beck had created her PDSS based on several in-depth studies of women with PPD and sometimes used their words directly in the scale items. This worked very well in the original, but it meant that such conversational expressions as "I felt like I was jumping out of my skin" were difficult for the translators (Beck et al., 2003).

A particularly good example of problems that can arise when translating idioms comes from Spanish translations of the Mini-Mental State Examination (Folstein, Folstein, & McHugh, 1975), a widely used screening measure for cognitive impairment in adults. One of the items asks patients to repeat this common English expression: "No ifs, ands, or buts." Ramirez, Teresi, Holmes, Gurland, and Lantingua (2006) described the many different ways this item has been translated into Spanish, for Latinos living in the United States, and for patients living in Mexico, Spain, Puerto Rico, and Argentina. Examples of translations include "Buenos días niños" (Good morning children); "Tres perros en un trigal" (Three dogs in a wheatfield); "Ni si, ni no, ni peros" (Neither yes, nor no, nor buts); and "El flan tiene frutillas y frasbuesa" (The flan has fruits and raspberries). Translations of idioms require a full understanding of the intent of the item, which cannot always be inferred. In this example, Folstein et al. (1975) wanted to test dysarthria (difficulty in the repeated articulation of consecutive consonants) using a common idiom, which some of the Spanish translators probably did not realize. It may be noted that in the revised version of the measure (MMSE-2), the phrase has been replaced with another phrase, specifically to facilitate translation into other languages (Folstein, Folstein, White, & Messer, 2010).

15.3.f Types of Translation Errors

Research teams should be aware of some distinct types of translation errors that have been identified by several writers (e.g., Capitulo, Cornelio, & Lenz, 2001; Yu et al., 2004). Illustrations of often repeated errors can perhaps be incorporated into the training material for translators. Most of these errors are detected through back translations.

One type of error concerns adding words. The addition of adjectives or adverbs can often change the meaning of an item. Capitulo and colleagues (2001) found an instance of this in the translation of the Perinatal Grief Scale (PGS) into Spanish. The forward translator added the word *many* into the item "I have let (many) people down."

Deletions are another type of error. For example, in the PGS scale, translators made several deletions, such as "I feel (somewhat) apart and remote" and "I have adjusted (well) to the loss" (deleted words are in parentheses).

A more pervasive and challenging error concerns translations that alter words or phrases so that they no longer convey the same meaning. An example from the PGS was "I blame myself," which was translated as "Me siento culpable," and back-translated as "I feel guilty" (Capitulo et al., 2001). As another example, the original translation of the MOS-SSS item "Someone to help you understand a situation" into Chinese was back-translated as "Someone to enable you to have a better understanding of a situation." The translation added meaning that conveyed a greater level of understanding than implied in the original.

Another type of error is to translate items into words that require a higher reading level than is appropriate for the population of interest. It is important to emphasize the desired reading level to translators and to assess readability with the final translated items.

It is by undertaking the arduous process described earlier that such errors can be detected and fixed. If errors can be prevented or minimized through training or the selection of well-qualified translators, so much the better. Translation errors and equivalence problems can be further explored in the next phase of a translation project, the pilot testing of the "prefinal" translated instrument.

15.4 Pretesting the Prefinal Translated Version

Before a full field testing of the translated instrument, researchers typically conduct a pretest by administering the prefinal version to 30 to 50 monolingual people from the target culture or country. The pretest sample should reflect the kind of diversity expected in the population of interest, including those with the lowest levels of education. Frequency distribution information from the pretest is then examined for clues to potential problems, such as floor or ceiling effects and high rates of missing data on items, but qualitative information at this stage is also critical.

15.4.a Cognitive Questioning

The pretest of a translated instrument often incorporates cognitive questioning (Chapter 4) as a further means of examining semantic and conceptual equivalence (Nápoles-Springer et al., 2006). Cognitive questioning typically occurs after a respondent has completed the scale rather than as a think-aloud procedure during actual completion. Careful probes are used to shed light on how respondents interpreted each item.

Nápoles-Springer and colleagues (2006), whose system of coding interviewer and respondent behavior during cognitive interviewing was described in Chapter 4, used five types of probes in their development of a multicultural, decentered English–Spanish survey to examine the quality of interpersonal processes of health care. The scripted probes were designed to help the researchers understand (1) if Latino, Black, and non-Latino White respondents understood the intended meaning of specific words or phrases; (2) whether there were any perceived redundancies in questions; (3) what cognitive processes were used in responding to a question; (4) if any items were offensive; and (5) if items were culturally appropriate. As an example of the latter, respondents were asked to define the term *health belief* and also asked about its relevance to them. As another example of cognitive interviews used in translation research, Beck et al. (2003) asked respondents in the pretest of the translated PDSS to paraphrase each item and also to answer such questions as "What do you think that statement means?" and "Were there any words or phrases that were difficult to understand?" (p. 71). Such probing can lead to further item revisions.

15.4.b Content "Validation" of Cultural Relevance

Sometimes the prefinal version of the translated instrument is also subjected to a type of content validation that focuses specifically on content relevance. For example, Yu and colleagues (2004), in their translation of the MOS-SSS into Chinese, convened a panel of six experts to rate the cultural relevance of each item in measuring the construct of perceived social support in Chinese patients with a chronic illness. The ratings were used to compute a content validity index (CVI), as described in Chapter 11. A scale-level CVI of .82 was obtained, which lead the researchers to conclude that content equivalence was adequate.

15.4.c Final Review and Report

Prior to coming to a conclusion that the adapted instrument is ready to be field tested, the accumulated evidence should be compiled and subjected to a final review, preferably in a face-to-face meeting of a review committee. The team should include those who played a major role in the adaptation project and, if possible, the developer of the original instrument. When there are lingering concerns about conceptual or other types of equivalence, the committee could include additional cultural experts. Hambleton (2006) recommended that, prior to field testing, the adaptation researchers should undertake a formal cultural review and a "bias" review for items that could favor one group relative to another. He argued that many of the problems that can lead to an assessment of differential item functioning, discussed later in this chapter, can be identified by well-trained reviewers.

Findings from the translation process, the pretest, and final review are usually compiled into a technical report. The report should document the adaptation process as well as the rationale for all decisions made in the adaptation. Such a report is invaluable for subsequent translations of the same instrument into other languages (Wild et al., 2005).

15.5 | Field Testing of the Final Instrument for Measurement Equivalence

Once the translated scale has been finalized, it needs to be rigorously tested. During the testing phase, there are two goals: (1) to evaluate the extent to which the measurement properties of the new scale meet usual quality standards for the intended application, using methods described in this book for an original scale; and (2) to gather further evidence regarding the equivalence of the translated and original scale. In this section, we focus on the second of these goals, which can address equivalence at both the item and the scale level. We begin by discussing tests with a bilingual sample.

15.5.a Testing Equivalence Using a Bilingual Sample

Bilingual testing with parallel language forms has been recommended by a panel convened by the International Test Commission (Hambleton, 1994). Efforts to test various equivalencies by administering both the original and translated scale to a bilingual sample from the target population date back to Brislin (1970).

When bilingual samples are used to test parallel forms of a measure, the full versions of both scales are usually administered to everyone in the sample, in random order of presentation. For example, Lane, Jajoo, Taylor, Lip, and Jolly (2007) translated the Hospital Anxiety and Depression Scale (HADS) into Punjabi using a translation process similar to the one described earlier in this chapter. They administered both the English and Punjabi versions to a bilingual sample of 73 patients attending clinics in Birmingham, England, in counterbalanced order. In this study, the two scales were administered on the same day, but in other studies, such as in the translation of the Pittsburgh Sleep Quality Index into Brazilian Portuguese (Bertolazi et al., 2011), an interval of 1 to 2 weeks between administrations was adopted.

In such bilingual field tests, the focus is on the comparability of statistical results in the two versions. For example, the researchers typically compare sample means and standard deviations on the two versions and the scale's internal consistency. Parallel test reliability coefficients are sometimes computed (e.g., Beck et al., 2003). Some researchers use Bland–Altman plots to examine differences in the two versions. As an example, Lane and colleagues (2007), in their translation of the HADS into Punjabi, used paired t tests to compare item, subscale, and full scale scores on the English and Punjabi versions. Bland–Altman plots were used to assess agreement for the Anxiety and Depression subscales. They found that 93% and 95% of the scores for the two subscales, respectively, fell within the 95% confidence intervals. Item-subscale correlations were computed for each item in the two versions and then compared. All correlations were acceptably strong and for the most part similar in the two versions. Values of coefficient alpha were greater than .70 for the two subscales in both languages. Finally, the researchers used cutoff points to classify patients as cases or noncases for anxiety and depression. The degree of concordance, and kappa values, were high, although the Punjabi version tended to overestimate, relative to the English version, the number of borderline depressed patients.

Mallinckrodt and Wang (2004) have proposed a method for assessing semantic and measurement equivalence that they call the *dual-language, split-half* (DLSH) method. This approach involves creating two alternate forms for administration to a bilingual sample. Each form has half the items in the source language and half in the translated language, and none of the items on the two forms overlap. For example, Form A might have all the odd-numbered items in the source language and all the even-numbered items in the target language, and Form B would have the reverse. In other words, the DLSH method does not require respondents to complete the same item twice. All same-language items are grouped together, but the order of presentation of languages is alternated on different forms, thus yielding four versions.

In their illustration of the DLSH method, Mallinckrodt and Wang (2004) translated the Experiences in Close Relationships Scale or ECRS (a measure of adult attachment) into Chinese, using the forward-back translation and committee methods described earlier. Thirty bilingual Chinese university students (who were screened for English proficiency using a formal test) were randomly assigned to complete one of the four versions of the alternate forms. The 30 students in the bilingual sample completed the same scale twice, with an interval of about 10 days, so that retest reliability could be assessed. Paired t tests to test the difference of the means of the English and Chinese split-half subscales (Avoidance and Anxiety) were nonsignificant at both the first and retest administration. Internal consistency was comparable and retest reliability coefficients for the two subscales, for both the English and Chinese half-scales, were all in excess of .90. Mallinckrodt and Wang claimed that their method represents an improvement over the more usual bilingual testing approach involving full scales because it reduces respondent burden and avoids "the priming effect that occurs when a participant who does not understand a given item in one language can rely on the alternative language version of the item for assistance" (p. 375).

Testing parallel forms of translated instruments with a bilingual sample offers some obvious advantages for corroborating the equivalence of translated measures. Lane and colleagues (2007) declared that their bilingual testing approach overcame some of the criticisms that have been leveled at other translation efforts with the HADS. Similar claims about the value of bilingual testing were made by the researchers in a study involving the translation of the Quality of Recovery Scale for assessing postsurgical patients (Chan, Lo, Lok, Choi, & Gin, 2008). Jones et al. (2001) illustrated how pretesting their original translations of a coping scale with bilingual women (50 in English–Chinese and 50 in English–Tagalog) led to some further wording refinements. Nevertheless, there are some problems with bilingual testing, one of which is that it is often difficult to find participants who are sufficiently bilingual. This, in turn, means that sample sizes are typically small, so using statistical significance as a criterion for equivalence may be inappropriate, and statistical techniques requiring a large sample (e.g., factor analysis) cannot be used. Finally, a bilingual sample is almost assuredly not representative of the population of interest for most measures. Thus, bilingual testing is a useful strategy but should be supplemented with other efforts to assess cross-cultural validity.

15.5.b Comparing Basic Measurement Properties in Monolingual Samples

Most often, translated instruments are tested in monolingual samples. If the primary focus of the field test is on the psychometric adequacy (e.g., reliability, internal consistency, construct validity) of the translated scale then the study may not make explicit comparisons with the original scale. If the goal is to assess measurement and factorial equivalence and cross-cultural validity, then the study must have an actual or implicit comparison group.

In many cases, the "comparison group" is the group with whom the original version was validated, and the translation researchers rely on published information about the scale's measurement properties. Frequently, the translation researchers focus their analyses on the psychometric properties of the translated scale and use the Discussion section of the report to reflect on similarities and differences between the properties of the translated and original measure. In other words, for many cross-cultural validations, the researchers do not actually have access to comparative data from the field test of the original instrument.

For example, Torres and colleagues (2009) assessed the Brazilian version of the Child Perceptions Questionnaire (CPQ_{11-14}), a scale used to assess health-related quality of life. Their analyses focused on the translated scale's retest reliability, internal consistency, convergent validity, and known-groups validity. For all of these properties, the researchers used the Discussion section to make specific comparisons to the properties of the original English-language version of the scale and other scale adaptations, as reported in separate articles by different researchers.

When items from an IRT-derived item bank are translated, IRT analyses are essentially replicated with the field test sample for the adapted or translated version. In such situations, the unidimensionality assumption is evaluated and, if the assumption is upheld, IRT parameters are estimated (e.g., Paz, Spritzer, Morales, & Hays, 2013). Comparisons can then be made between the two versions for item difficulty (location), item discrimination (in 2-PL models), and item and test information. It is particularly useful to be able to compare item location and discrimination for items that required major alterations to accommodate idiomatic expressions. The application of differential item functioning in translation studies is discussed in a later section.

15.5.c Assessing Factorial Equivalence

Factor analysis, especially confirmatory factor analysis (CFA), is often used to further examine the measurement equivalence of adapted and original measures. Building on the work of Meredith (1993), Gregorich (2006) provided a framework for thinking about the ways in which factorial equivalence can be examined. In his nested hierarchy, five types of factorial invariance can be assessed.

Dimensional invariance requires that a multi-item instrument represent the same number of latent traits in the original and adapted instrument. Figure 15.2 illustrates a hypothetical measure with dimensional invariance, as depicted for illustrative purposes in a factor analysis of a four-item scale with two groups (samples). For both groups of respondents, the measure has a two-factor structure. Dimensional invariance can be examined using exploratory factor analysis (EFA), but CFA is preferred.

Next in Gregorich's (2006) hierarchy is *configural invariance*, which concerns whether the same items are configured on the same factors in the original and adapted versions. In Figure 15.2, the hypothesis of configural variation is supported—in both groups, Items 1 and 2 cluster onto the first latent trait, and Items 3 and 4 cluster onto the second latent trait. It is possible to subjectively assess configural invariance in an EFA, but a formal test of this type of invariance is possible using CFA, using tests of model fit described in Chapter 14.

Dimensional and configural invariance are the most commonly tested forms of factorial equivalence. These tests of invariance are typically undertaken using data from only one sample (i.e., the sample for field testing the adapted/translated scale). The goal is to assess whether the CFA model for the adapted instrument can replicate the model confirmed with the original measure in the primary field test. For example, Scorza and colleagues (2013) undertook a cross-cultural validation of the World Health Organization's Disability Assessment Schedule for children in Rwanda and confirmed the hypothesized six-factor structure and item-to-factor distribution supported in previous CFAs of the instrument.

Gregorich (2006) argued that both dimensional and configural invariance are desirable but are insufficient for the purposes of directly comparing the two groups. In his hierarchy, comparisons across groups rely on evidence of other types of invariance. These include metric, scalar, and residual equivalence, which correspond to Meredith's (1993) hierarchy of weak, strong, and strict invariance. *Metric invariance* requires the comparability of factor loadings of items onto common factors (latent traits) across groups. In Figure 15.2, factor loadings are shown as λ, so metric invariance requires that λ_{11} equal λ_{12}, λ_{21} equal λ_{22}, and so on. CFA allows tests of the equal-loadings hypothesis. However, unlike dimensional and configural invariance, such tests require raw data from the two groups being compared to

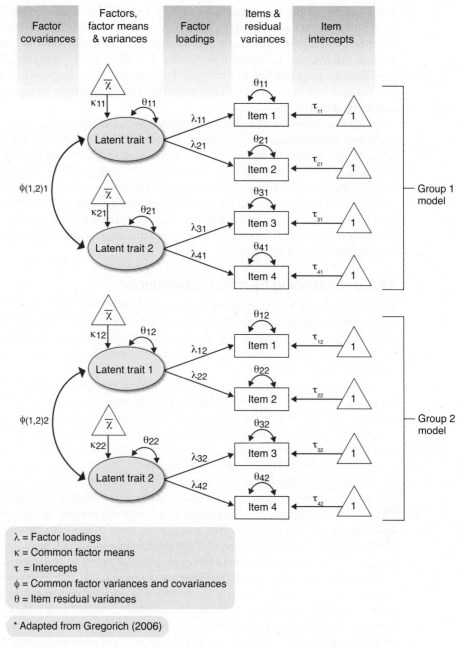

Figure 15.2

Testing factorial invariance in two groups.

perform statistical tests of difference. When metric invariance is supported, group comparisons of estimated factor variances and covariances are defensible because any group differences are uncontaminated by possible group differences in residual variation.

Gregorich (2006) noted that if metric invariance is not supported, there could be two explanations. First, the latent traits may not have the same meaning in the two groups (i.e., the items are not capturing latent traits in the same way across groups). A second possibility is that the factor loading estimates could be biased in a systematic way as a result of differences in response sets (Chapter 4). For example, in one culture, there may be a tendency to select extreme responses, independent of the item content (extreme response bias), whereas in others, there may be a tendency to avoid extreme responses (a moderacy bias). Differences in response set tendencies can affect score variation and thus can affect item loadings.

Next in Gregorich's (2006) hierarchy is *scalar invariance*, or what is also called *strong factorial invariance*. Scalar invariance requires equality of the item intercepts, which are shown as τ in Figure 15.2. For scalar invariance, τ_{11} must equal τ_{12}, τ_{21} must equal τ_{22}, and so on. The hypothesis of scalar invariance may not hold because of other response set biases that reflect cultural norms. For example, acquiescence response bias has an additive effect that can inflate observed means. If such a bias is more prevalent in one culture than in another, the group means may be different even when average true scores for the focal trait are not. Gregorich's paper explains how to rescale CFA parameters to test for scalar invariance using item-level data from the two groups being compared. When the hypothesis of scalar invariance is upheld, group differences in mean scale scores are unbiased estimates of group differences on the latent trait. Thus, to legitimately compare group means, Gregorich argued that evidence of the four types of invariance discussed thus far is needed.

The fifth type of factorial equivalence in the hierarchy is *strict factorial invariance*, which concerns equality of the residuals (the θs in Figure 15.2). Gregorich stated that residual invariance is of limited practical value but worth assessing when comparisons of both means and variances across groups are of interest. Meredith and Teresi (2006) argued that when the aim of studying factorial invariance "is to ensure fairness and equity, strict factorial invariance is required" (p. S69).

Many of the studies that have examined weak, strong, or strict factorial invariance are not translation studies but rather are based on a single version of an instrument. Studies of factorial equivalence often are designed to test for invariance in different racial/ethnic, age, or gender groups. For example, Lix and associates (2012) assessed dimensional, configural, metric, and scalar invariance of the SF-36 in Caucasian and non-Caucasian male and female subgroups living in Canada. One multicultural, dual-language study that examined all five types of factorial invariance also involved a CFA of the SF-36. Sudano and colleagues (2011) tested the eight-factor structure of the SF-36 identified in the 10-country IQOLA project to assess increasingly stringent criteria for factorial equivalence in four racial/ethnic and language groups in the United States.

15.5.d Testing Equivalence Using Differential Item Functioning

As explained in Chapter 6, **differential item functioning (DIF)** signifies that an item functions differently for one subgroup or culture than another. When there is evidence of DIF, it means that there are items on a scale for which two groups of people *who are equivalent with respect to the latent trait* have score differences on the item. Interest in DIF began with concerns about biases in standardized tests when used to assess competencies in different cultural or racial groups (e.g., use of the Scholastic Assessment Test for college admission in the United States) but has expanded to assessments of health-related rating scales and screening tests.

An analysis of DIF is not focused on whether one group is different from another in terms of performance on an item (e.g., whether item means are similar) because true differences might, in fact, exist. Rather, DIF analysis is designed to detect whether people from different groups with the same amount of an attribute have different probabilities of giving a certain response.

As noted in Chapter 6, several different procedures for assessing DIF have been developed. The main approaches are the Mantel–Haenszel procedure, logistic regression, and methods based on IRT (for an overview, see Teresi, 2006). These methods vary in complexity, assumptions, the use of modeling, availability of software, handling of missing values, the criterion for diagnosing DIF, and the method of matching groups. Even within a given approach, many different decisions are required, and so DIF analyses and results can vary across studies. Some approaches, such as logistic regression or the Mantel–Haenszel procedure, can rely on general-purpose statistical software packages such as SPSS or SAS. Examples of software for IRT-based models and DIF detection were discussed in Chapter 6. Readers interested in more technical detail about DIF can consult one of several books that explain statistical approaches in detail (e.g., Holland & Wainer, 1993; Osterlind & Everson, 2009).

In DIF studies, it is essential to match the groups being compared with regard to the attribute being measured. In IRT-based analyses of DIF, item performance is compared for groups matched on the latent trait (θ), but in other approaches, the matching criterion is scores on the overall test. If substantial DIF is present and all in a consistent direction (e.g., showing a consistent bias toward one of the groups), then matching might be problematic. For example, if the cumulative effect of DIF is to lower the scores of one group by an average of two points on the overall scale, then the matching will also be biased. Hambleton (2006) and others recommend a two-stage approach to the DIF analyses. The first stage looks for evidence of DIF when matching on the overall score. Then, if DIF is found to be substantial, the analyst removes the biased items from the calculation of the total score in the second stage (a process referred to as *purification*), and then reruns the DIF analysis.

Although DIF procedures are powerful means of assessing measurement equivalence at the item level, one interesting project made clear some of the problems with DIF analyses. In this project, undertaken for a special issue of the journal *Medical Care* (2006, volume 44, number 11, Supp 3, "Measurement in a Multi-Ethnic Society"), several researchers described results using different DIF approaches with the same dataset. The sample consisted of 913 English speaking and 665 Spanish-speaking U.S. patients with potential dementia, who were administered the original or a translated version of the MMSE. The special issue included papers in which the analysis was based on the Mantel–Haenszel approach (Dorans & Kulick, 2006), an IRT approach (Edelen Orlando, Thissen, Teresi, Kleinman, & Ocepek-Welikson, 2006), IRT using the MIMIC (multiple indicators, multiple causes) model (R. Jones, 2006), and ordinal logistic regression (Crane, Gibbons, Jolley, & vanBelle, 2006) as well as several others. Evidence for DIF between the two language groups was found in every analysis—but the same items were not always flagged as being nonequivalent across studies.

The various analyses were consistent in their diagnosis of DIF for only 9 out of 21 items. For 5 items (e.g., "What is the year?") the analyses uniformly indicated the absence of DIF, whereas item bias was universally detected for four others. All analyses found that certain items gave English speakers an advantage ("What state are we in?"), and that other items favored those responding to the Spanish translation (Repeating the phrase "No ifs, and, or buts"). Figure 15.3 shows item characteristic curves for these two items, as presented in the paper by Jones (2006). For example, English-speaking people with a cognitive impairment level of 0.0 had about 0.10 probability of getting Item 6 wrong, compared to a nearly 0.50 probability of error among those with the same trait level in the Spanish language group. With regard to the other 12 items analyzed in this project, there was no uniform agreement on DIF. Borsboom (2006) concluded that the likely cause of the variation among researchers is that different criteria were used to define DIF. Hambleton (2006) argued that these disparate results suggest the desirability of using multiple approaches to DIF analyses and triangulating the evidence.

Because there are various approaches to DIF, interpretation of the results is not always straightforward. Hambleton (2006) recommended an interpretive approach that involves looking for *patterns* in the DIF results rather than interpreting on an item-by-item basis. One strategy is to list the DIF items, in rank order of the strength of the evidence, and then compare the list to a list of non-DIF items to see if any general explanations emerge (analogous to interpreting an EFA). Hambleton (2006) also recommended using a team or committee to interpret DIF results, and others have suggested having an external blind

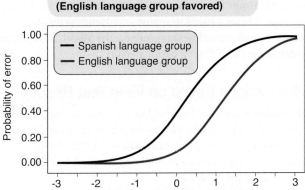

Item 6: Able to name the correct state (English language group favored)

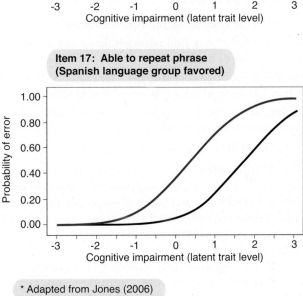

Item 17: Able to repeat phrase (Spanish language group favored)

* Adapted from Jones (2006)

Figure 15.3

Item characteristic curves for two items with DIF from the Mini-Mental State Examination.

review (Scott et al., 2010). Sometimes it is easy to discern the underlying problem contributing to DIF, but sometimes DIF may be indicated when no clear explanation can be inferred. Common sense, a theoretical grounding in the construct, and understanding of the cultures or groups are often needed to make sense of DIF results.

Studies of DIF are especially common for assessing item equivalence for subgroups within a population or country (e.g., English-speaking and Spanish-speaking Americans), but cross-national DIF studies also exist. For example, DIF analyses were undertaken in the IQOLA project to compare differences in item functioning for the Danish version of the SF-36 compared to the English version administered to an American sample (Bjorner, Kreiner, Ware, Damsgaard, & Bech, 1998). DIF was identified for 12 items. In this study, interpretation was aided by the availability of translators' item-level ratings of translation difficulty and conceptual equivalence, as discussed earlier in this chapter. For some items, interpretation of the DIF diagnosis was easy because the items had previously been identified as problematic. For example, the item "Lifting or carrying groceries" had been judged to be low on conceptual equivalence because the word *groceries* has no exact equivalent in

Danish. On the other hand, DIF was difficult to interpret for several items that had been given high ratings for the quality of the translation. One example is the item "Felt down in the dumps." Danes tended to report experiencing this less frequently than Americans with the same overall mental health score on the SF-36, but matched Danes were also less likely to endorse the item "Been a happy person."

15.5.e Actions Based on Field Test Results

Field tests such as those discussed in this section may confirm measurement equivalence at the item and scale level, in which case it is usually concluded that the adaptation or translation has been a success and is ready for use. Often, however, there is some evidence that full measurement equivalence has not been attained. Decisions on how to proceed may include actions such as the following:

1. Accepting the evidence on nonequivalence without taking any further steps
2. Accepting the evidence on nonequivalence and maintaining the scale, but establishing new cutpoints or norms
3. Modifying the original instrument—for example, dropping an item that proved difficult to translate, or scoring an item on a different subscale than was true originally
4. "Going back to the drawing board" to make further revisions to the translated (or even the original) instrument, followed by a new field test
5. Abandoning the translation effort altogether

Several factors affect which course of action is most appropriate. These include the nature and amount of nonequivalence, how the nonequivalence is interpreted, what the purpose of the adaptation is, and how well established the original measure is. If the measure is one with a strong reputation and extensive evidence of excellent measurement properties, the modification option (Option 3) may be unattractive, for example.

Some evidence of nonequivalence requires strong action, such as revising the translation (Option 4) or giving up entirely (Option 5). For example, if the field test indicates that the new measure has low reliability or construct validity, minor modifications are unlikely to solve the problem (Option 3), and the evidence cannot simply be ignored (Options 1 or 2).

In a typical situation, there is some evidence of measurement invariance (e.g., in a DIF or CFA). Before making decisions about how to move forward, the degree of nonequivalence usually has to be considered. Several writers on DIF analysis have urged that researchers look at the *practical* impact of measurement invariance. Within some DIF procedures, it is possible to identify how many items with DIF in the same direction are needed to amount to a one-point difference in a person's total score (Hambleton, 2006). When there is DIF in different directions, the decision about how to proceed may be based on how DIF affects overall scale performance. For example, in the Danish translation of the SF-36, Bjorner et al. (1998) reported that when the DIF items were included in the SF-36 scales, they had minor impact on conclusions about the health in the general population for cross-national comparisons. The investigators rejected the idea of removing items with DIF from the Danish version of the SF-36 scale because of the small number of items on certain subscales. They also worried that any revisions to items with DIF might worsen other item characteristics, such as readability. They decided to maintain the translated version despite evidence of DIF.

A major factor in decisions about "next steps" concerns the reason for creating the adaptation and the applications to which the instrument are expected to be put. Stricter equivalence is necessary in certain circumstances. Sometimes an instrument is translated without an explicit goal of comparisons across cultures. If the goal is to create a good instrument for use *within* a new culture or country, then minor divergencies are unlikely to require drastic action. For example, one of the reasons that Bjorner et al. (1998) did not recommend further revisions to the Danish version of the SF-36 was that the IQOLA translation had yielded "a scale that is well functioning within the Danish language" (p. 1200). Also, if an instrument is translated for use in multinational clinical trials, the central concern is testing for treatment and control group differences. In such situations, it might not matter that the mean scores on a PRO are two points higher in Germany than in Sweden, for example, if it holds true in both the experimental and control groups. Borsboom (2006) also noted that nonequivalence may be irrelevant when the instrument will be used primarily in research to examine correlations among variables. For example, if one is interested in examining whether alcohol consumption is related to cognitive decline in both English-speaking and Spanish-speaking subgroups of American adults, then the lack of evidence for item-level measurement invariance in the MMSE is unlikely to affect the conclusions.

Two applications require fairly strong evidence of equivalence. The first concerns direct comparison of mean scores or percentages for the purpose of describing the amount or prevalence of an attribute in different groups. For example, if an instrument is used to describe the prevalence of drug abuse in different cultural subgroups of adolescents based on a self-report measure, the adapted and original instruments must demonstrate conceptual, semantic, and measurement equivalence for the comparisons to be justifiable. A second application requiring stricter equivalence is the use of an instrument for making clinical decisions or for allocating scarce resources. For example, if further testing or a particular course of therapy is recommended for people whose MMSE scores are above a certain cutpoint, then it is imperative that the cutpoint indicate the same level of cognitive impairment in different cultural groups. For translated instruments, this may mean undertaking a new norming or criterion validity study to establish appropriate cutpoints, but it could also mean working harder to get an adaptation with a higher degree of equivalence to the original.

15.6 The Design and Evaluation of Cross-Cultural Validation Studies

This final section briefly discusses some design issues and offers some suggestions for reporting and evaluating cross-cultural validity work.

15.6.a Study Design and Sampling in Cross-Cultural Validation

It is difficult to give generic advice about design and sampling for cross-validation work because there are so many different components and phases. Earlier chapters have provided guidance with regard to design and sample size for many aspects of such a project, such as pilot testing and cognitive questioning, and the assessment of reliability, internal consistency, and construct validity.

When direct comparisons of language or cultural groups are undertaken during the field testing of an adapted instrument, such as in testing equivalence in a monolingual sample (Section 15.5.b); assessing weak, strong, or strict factorial invariance in multigroup samples (Section 15.5.c); or analyzing for DIF (Section 15.5.d), an effort should be made to match the groups being compared as carefully as possible on key demographic or clinical characteristics. The extensive work with DIF has demonstrated that many items are sensitive to education, ethnicity, age, and/or gender. Thus, the groups being compared in cross-cultural validations would ideally be similar with regard to such characteristics, differing only in terms of the culture or language that is the central focus of the research.

In terms of sample size, large samples are needed for CFA (Chapter 14) and especially for comparative CFAs. In DIF studies, the power to detect DIF increases with sample size. Very large sample sizes are usually recommended, especially for IRT-based DIF procedures. Indeed, DIF statistics can be unstable even with large samples (Hambleton, 2006).

However, it should also be noted that a large sample size in DIF analyses might result in a diagnosis of DIF when in fact the degree of bias is insubstantial (Borsboom, 2006). Therefore, good judgment is needed in interpreting DIF results.

As we have urged with regard to other measurement properties, the careful researcher should articulate a priori criteria for acceptable levels of equivalence in every phase of the project. For example, when comparing reliability or internal consistency coefficients for the original and adapted versions, what is an acceptable level of difference? Statistical significance alone should not be used to make final decisions, especially with very large (or very small) samples.

15.6.b Reporting a Cross-Cultural Validation Study

Cross-cultural validity work is often too extensive to describe in a single journal article. Sometimes the translation and pilot testing results are published in one paper and the field test results are presented in another. It is useful to include in one of the papers a flow chart such as Figure 15.1 so that readers can evaluate the researchers' thoroughness. The project may also result in one or more methodological paper. If DIF analyses have been performed, a separate paper is typically devoted to these findings. A comprehensive technical report (or *User's manual)* summarizing all major activities and results can be of immense help to other researchers.

It is difficult to give advice on how to present results from a DIF analysis because there are so many different approaches. Table 15.2 shows an example of DIF results using the Mantel–Haenszel procedure for nine MMSE items for English- and Spanish-speaking adults with potential dementia (Dorans & Kulick, 2006). Two of the items shown in the

Table 15.2	**Example of Mantel–Haenszel DIF Results for Selected Mini-Mental State Examination Items**				
	Mantel–Haenszel		**Proportion Correct**		
Item	**Delta Difference**[a]	**Standard Error**	**English (n = 891)**	**Spanish (n = 655)**	**Total (n = 1546)**
1. What is the year?	−.39	.40	.71	.74	.72
2. What is the season?	**−3.11**	**.35**	**.73**	**.58**	**.66**
3. What is the date?	1.31	.31	.51	.64	.56
4. What is the day?	−.05	.39	.73	.77	.75
5. What is the month?	−.58	.38	.73	.75	.74
6. Where are we—what state?	**−4.34**	**.38**	**.81**	**.58**	**.71**
7. What country?	**−3.50**	**.59**	**.88**	**.84**	**.86**
8. What town or city?	−1.09	.40	.74	.74	.74
17. Repeat phrase ("No ifs, ands, or buts")	**5.09**	**.46**	**.61**	**.89**	**.73**

[a]Delta is an index of item difficulty; large values of delta correspond to difficult items. Bolded entries show Mantel–Haenszel delta difference values for the two groups greater than an absolute value of 1.5.

Adapted from Dorans, N. J., & Kulick, E. (2006). Differential item functioning on the Mini-Mental State Examination: An applicaof the Mantel-Haenszel and standardization procedures. *Medical Care, 44*(Suppl 3), S78–S94, Table 3, with permission.

table are the ones whose item characteristic curves are shown in Figure 15.3, Items 6 and 17. This table shows items with DIF in bold, which is a device that is frequently used in DIF reports.

15.6.c Evaluating a Cross-Cultural Validation Study

Equivalence is the key issue in cross-cultural validations. Thus, in evaluating a cross-cultural measurement study, reviewers should focus on the quality of evidence for various kinds of equivalence. For example, for conceptual equivalence, was there an upfront assessment that the construct had meaning and relevance in the focal culture or group? Was conceptual equivalence addressed at the item level through cognitive questioning? For semantic equivalence, was a rigorous forward–backward translation process used with well-trained and appropriately qualified translators? Was a committee used to integrate the results and reconcile any problems? If the problems could not readily be resolved, was a second round of forward–backward translation initiated?

An evaluation of the field test of the new instrument needs to take into consideration the study's design and sample size. If a single monolingual sample was used in the field test, was the evidence adequate for assessing the measurement equivalence of the adaptation and the original? Many single-group field tests focus more on the measurement properties of the adapted scale (e.g., reliability or item difficulty) than on the issue of measurement equivalence. For any comparisons to be meaningful, the researchers should have selected a sample with characteristics similar to those in the sample used in field testing the original measure. Similarly, in a multigroup or bilingual sample, either the design should maximize demographic similarity of the groups or appropriate statistical adjustments should be made. Throughout the evaluation, a reviewer should consider the rigor of the steps that *were* taken as well as the damage done by steps that were not taken. Careful attention needs to be paid to the researchers' interpretation of their results. Additional guidance for evaluating cross-cultural validity studies has been developed by the COSMIN workgroup (Terwee et al., 2012) and is presented in the Box G checklist on the COSMIN website.

References

Beaton, D. E., Bombardier, C., Guillemin, F., & Bosi Ferraz, M. (2000). Guidelines for the process of cross-cultural adaptation of self-report measures. *Spine*, *25*, 3186–3191.

Beck, C. T., Bernal, H., & Froman, R. D. (2003). Methods to document semantic equivalence of a translated scale. *Research in Nursing & Health*, *26*, 64–73.

Bertolazi, A. N., Fagondes, S. C., Hoff, L. S., Dartora, E. G., Miozzo, I., de Barba, M., & Barreto, S. (2011). Validation of the Brazilian Portuguese version of the Pittsburgh Sleep Quality Index. *Sleep Medicine*, *12*, 70–75.

Bjorner, J. B., Kreiner, S., Ware, J. E., Damsgaard, M., & Bech, P. (1998). Differential item functioning in the Danish translation of the SF-36. *Journal of Clinical Epidemiology*, *51*, 1189–1202.

Borsboom, D. (2006). When does measurement invariance matter? *Medical Care*, *44*(Suppl. 3), S176–S181.

Brislin, R. W. (1970). Back-translation for cross-cultural research. *Journal of Cross-Cultural Psychology*, *1*, 185–216.

Brislin, R. W. (1986). The wording and translation of research instruments. In W. J. Lonner & J. W. Berry (Eds.), *Field methods in cross-cultural research*. Beverly Hills, CA: Sage.

Bullinger, M., Alonso, J., Apolone, G., Leplege, A., Sullivan, M., Wood-Dauphinee, S., … Ware, J. E. (1998). Translating health status questionnaires and evaluating their quality: The IQOLA project approach. *Journal of Clinical Epidemiology*, *51*, 913–923.

Capitulo, K. L., Cornelio, M., & Lenz, E. (2001). Translating the short version of the Perinatal Grief Scale: Process and challenges. *Applied Nursing Research*, *14*, 165–170.

Chan, M., Lo, C., Lok, C., Choi, K., & Gin, T. (2008). Psychometric testing the Chinese Quality of Recovery score. *Anesthesia & Analgesia*, *107*, 1189–1195.

Coffman, M. J. (2008). Translation of a Diabetes Self-Efficacy Instrument: Assuring content and semantic equivalence. *The Journal of Theory Construction & Testing*, *12*, 58–62.

Crane, P. K., Gibbons, L. E., Jolley, L., & vanBelle, G. (2006). Differential item functioning with ordinal logistic regression techniques: DIFdetect and difwithpar. *Medical Care*, *44*(Suppl. 3), S115–S123.

Dorans, N. J., & Kulick, E. (2006). Differential item functioning on the Mini-Mental State Examination: An application of the Mantel-Haenszel and standardization procedures. *Medical Care*, *44*(Suppl. 3), S78–S94.

Edelen Orlando, M., Thissen, D., Teresi, J., Kleinman, M., & Ocepek-Welikson, K. (2006). Identification of differential functioning using item response theory and the likelihood-based model comparison approach: Application to the Mini-Mental State Examination. *Medical Care, 44*(Suppl. 3), S134–S142.

Flaherty, J. A., Gaviria, F., Pathak, D., Mitchell, T., Wintrob, R., Richman, J., & Birz, S. (1988). Developing instruments for cross-cultural psychiatric research. *The Journal of Nervous and Mental Disease, 176,* 257–263.

Folstein, M. F., Folstein, S. E., & McHugh, P. R. (1975). The Mini-Mental State: A practical method of grading the cognitive state of patients for the clinician. *Journal of Psychiatric Research, 12,* 189–198.

Folstein, M., Folstein, S., White, T., & Messer, M. (2010). *MMSE-2: Mini-Mental State Examination: User's manual* (2nd ed.). Lutz, FL: Psychological Assessment Resources.

Forrest, C. B., Bevans, K., Tucker, C., Riley, A., Ravens-Sieberer, Gardner, W., & Pajer, K. (2012). The Patient-Reported Outcome Measurement Information System (PROMIS®) for children and youth. *Journal of Pediatric Psychology, 37,* 614–621.

Gregorich, S. (2006). Do self-report instruments allow meaningful comparisons across diverse population groups? Testing measurement invariance using the confirmatory factor analysis framework. *Medical Care, 44*(Suppl. 3), S78–S94.

Hambleton, R. K. (1994). Guidelines for adapting educational and psychological tests: A progress report. *European Journal of Psychological Assessment, 10,* 229–244.

Hambleton, R. K. (2001). The next generation of the ITC test translation and adaptation guidelines. *European Journal of Psychological Assessment, 17,* 164–172.

Hambleton, R. K. (2006). Good practices for identifying differential item functioning. *Medical Care, 44*(Suppl. 3), S182–S188.

Herdman, M., Fox-Rushby, J., & Badia, X. (1997). "Equivalence" and the translation and adaption of health-related quality of life questionnaires. *Quality of Life Research, 6,* 237–247.

Holland, P. W., & Wainer, H. (Eds.). (1993). *Differential item functioning.* Hillsdale, NJ: Lawrence Erlbaum Associates.

Hui, C. H., & Triandis, H. (1985). Measurement in cross-cultural psychology: A review and comparison of strategies. *Journal of Cross-Cultural Psychology, 16,* 131–152.

Johnson, T. P. (2006). Methods and frameworks for cross-cultural measurement. *Medical Care, 44*(Suppl. 3), S17–S20.

Jones, P. S., Lee, J., Phillips, L., Zhang, X., & Jaceldo, K. (2001). An adaptation of Brislin's translation model for cross-cultural research. *Nursing Research, 50,* 300–304.

Jones, R. (2006). Identification of measurement differences between English and Spanish language versions of the Mini-Mental State Examination: Detecting differential item functioning using MIMIC modeling. *Medical Care, 44*(Suppl. 3), S124–S133.

Keller, S. D., Ware, J. E., Gandek, B., Aaronson, N. K., Alonso, J., Apolone, G., . . . Wood-Dauphinee, S. (1998). Testing the equivalence of translations of widely used response choice labels: Results from the IQOLA project. *Journal of Clinical Epidemiology, 51,* 933–944.

Lane, D. A., Jajoo, J., Taylor, R., Lip, G., & Jolly, K. (2007). Cross-cultural adaptation into Punjabi of the English version of the Hospital Anxiety and Depression Scale. *BMC Psychiatry, 7,* 5.

Le Gal, M., Mainguy, Y., LeLay, K., Nadjar, A., Allain, D., & Galissié, M. (2010). Linguistic validation of six patient-reported outcome instruments into 12 languages for patients with fibromyalgia. *Joint Bone Spine, 77,* 165–170.

Lix, L. M., Osman, B. A., Adachu, J., Towheed, T., Hopman, W., Davison, K., & Leslie, W. (2012). Measurement equivalence of the SF-36 in the Canadian multicenter osteoporosis study. *Health and Quality of Life Outcomes, 10,* 29.

Mallinckrodt, B., & Wang, C. (2004). Quantitative methods for verifying semantic equivalence of translated research instruments. *Journal of Counseling Psychology, 51,* 368–379.

Marin, G., & Marin, B. V. (1991). *Research with Hispanic populations.* Newbury Park, CA: Sage.

Meredith, W. (1993). Measurement invariance, factor analysis and factorial invariance. *Psychometrika, 58,* 525–543.

Meredith, W., & Teresi, J. (2006). An essay on measurement and factorial invariance. *Medical Care, 44*(Suppl. 3), S69–S77.

Mokkink, L. B., Terwee, C., Patrick, D., Alonso, J., Stratford, P., Knol, D. L., . . . DeVet, H. C. W. (2010). The COSMIN study reached international consensus on taxonomy, terminology, and definitions of measurement properties for health-related patient-reported outcomes. *Journal of Clinical Epidemiology, 63,* 737–745.

Nápoles-Springer, A. M., Santoyo-Olsson, J., O'Brien, H., & Stewart, A. L. (2006). Using cognitive interviews to develop surveys in diverse populations. *Medical Care, 44*(Suppl. 3), S21–S30.

Nápoles-Springer, A. M., & Stewart, A. L. (2006). Overview of qualitative methods in research with diverse populations: Making research reflect the population. *Medical Care, 44*(Suppl. 3), S5–S9.

Neziraj, M., Sarac Kart, N., & Samuelson, K. (2011). The Intensive Care Delirium Screening Checklist: Translation and reliability testing in a Swedish ICU. *Acta Anaesthesiologica Scandinavica, 55,* 819–826.

Osterlind, S. J., & Everson, H. T. (2009). *Differential item functioning* (2nd ed.). Thousand Oaks, CA: Sage.

Paz, S. H., Spritzer, K., Morales, L., & Hays, R. (2013). Evaluation of the Patient-Reported Outcomes Information System (PROMIS®) Spanish-language physical functioning items. *Quality of Life Research, 22,* 1819–1830.

Ramirez, M., Teresi, J., Holmes, D., Gurland, B., & Lantingua, R. (2006). Differential item functioning (DIF) and the Mini-Mental State Examination (MMSE): Overview, sample, and issues of translation. *Medical Care, 44*(Suppl. 3), S95–S106.

Scorza, P., Stevenson, A., Canino, G., Mushashi, C., Kanyanganzi, F., Munyanah, M., & Betancourt, T. (2013). Validation of the "World Health Organization Disability Assessment Schedule for Children, WHODAS-Child" in Rwanda. *PLoS One, 8*(3), e57725.

Scott, N. W., Fayers, P., Aaronson, N., Bottomley, A., de Graeff, A., Groenvold, M., . . . Sprangers, M. A. (2010). Interpretation of differential item functioning analyses using external review. *Expert Review of Pharmacoeconomics & Outcomes Research, 10*, 253–258.

Sidani, S., Guruge, S., Miranda, J., Ford-Gilboe, M., & Varcoe, C. (2010). Cultural adaptation and translation of measures: An integrated method. *Research in Nursing & Health, 33*, 133–143.

Streiner, D. L., & Norman, G. R. (2008). *Health measurement scales: A practical guide to their development and use* (4th ed.). Oxford: Oxford University Press.

Sudano, J. J., Perzynski, A., Love, T., Lewis, S., Murray, P., Huber, G., . . . Baker, D. (2011). Measuring disparities: Bias in the SF-36 v2 among Spanish-speaking medical patients. *Medical Care, 49*, 480–488.

Teresi, J. (2006). Overview of quantitative measurement methods: Equivalence, invariance, and differential item functioning in health applications. *Medical Care, 44*(Suppl. 3), S39–S49.

Terwee, C. B., Mokkink, L. B., Knol, D. L., Ostelo, R., Bouter, L. M., & DeVet, H. C. W. (2012). Rating the methodological quality in systematic reviews of studies on measurement properties: A scoring system for the COSMIN checklist. *Quality of Life Research, 21,* 651–657.

Torres, C. T., Paiva, S., Vale, M., Pordeus, I., Ramos-Jorge, M., Oliveira, A., & Allison, P. (2009). Psychometric properties of the Brazilian version of the Child Perceptions Questionnaire (CPQ$_{11-14}$)—short forms. *Health and Quality of Life Outcomes, 7*, 43.

Wagner, A. K., Gandek, B., Aaronson, N., Axquadro, C., Alonso, J., Apolone, G, . . . Ware, J. E. (1998). Cross-cultural comparisons of the content of SF-36 translations across 10 countries: Results from the IQOLA project. *Journal of Clinical Epidemiology, 51*, 925–932.

Ware, J. E., & Sherbourne, C. D. (1992). The MOS 36-item Short Form Health Survey (SF-36). *Medical Care, 30*, 473–483.

Wild, D., Grove, A., Martin, M., Eremenco, S., McElroy, S., Verjee-Lorents, A., & Erikson, P. (2005). Principles of good practice for the translation and cultural adaptation process for patient-reported outcome (PRO) measures: Report of the ISPOR task force for translation and cultural adaptation. *Value in Health, 8*, 94–104.

Yu, D. S. F., Lee, D. T. F., & Woo, J. (2004). Issues and challenges of instrument translation. *Western Journal of Nursing Research, 26*, 307–320.

16

Interpretation of Scores

Chapter Outline

When instrument developers gather evidence of their measure's good reliability and validity, and present their evidence in professional papers and reports, the new measure may be ready for adoption by clinicians and researchers. Yet, the utility of the measure may be constrained if its scores cannot be properly interpreted. Although interpretability is not a measurement property per se, it is a measurement characteristic that can limit or enhance the usefulness of an instrument. Interpretation should always be tempered by consideration of the measure's measurement properties (i.e., its reliability, measurement error, and validity).

Some "scores" are so widely used and familiar that clinicians and lay people alike understand what the score values mean. For example, most people in developed countries would recognize that a body temperature of 104°F (or 40°C) indicates a worrisome elevation, even though the numbers 104 and 40 are not inherently meaningful. But what does a score of 40 mean on the Center for Epidemiologic Studies Depression Scale (CES-D) (Radloff, 1977) or on other patient-reported outcomes (PROs)?

The Consensus-based Standards for the selection of health Measurement Instruments (COSMIN) group defined **interpretability** as "the degree to which one can assign qualitative meaning—that is, clinical or commonly understood connotations—to an instrument's qualitative scores or change in scores" (Mokkink et al., 2010, p. 743). This chapter focuses on interpretation of scores generated at a single point in time, and Chapter 19 discusses interpretability in terms of change scores—a topic that has received considerably more attention.

Strategies for interpreting health measurement scores vary by the use to which the scores will be put. Clinicians (and patients) need assistance in interpreting individual scores. For example, what does Alan's score of 22 on the Mini-Mental State Examination (MMSE) mean? Researchers and research consumers, on the other hand, tend to need help in understanding and interpreting scores for a group (e.g., what does a mean MMSE of

22.0 for patients in a nursing home mean?). Whether the interpretation is for individuals or groups, the interpretation must take into consideration the characteristics of the population of interest. We begin with the interpretation of an individual score.

16.1 Interpretation of Individual Scores

Interpretation of a person's score on a health measure is largely a matter of putting a score into context; in other words, providing a mechanism for making an appropriate comparison. The context is usually the scores of other people but can also be the person's scores on other measures. Those who develop a new measure that could be used by clinicians to evaluate individual patients need to consider how best to assist users in interpreting single scores.

16.1.a Reference Ranges

For most measurements that are subjected to laboratory analysis, the lab provides a **reference range** to aid in interpreting values. The reference range is calculated based on thousands of values and is usually defined as the values within which 95% of the cases fall. Values that are higher than the upper limit (greater than approximately two standard deviations [*SD*] above the mean) or below the lower limit (lower than about two *SD*s below the mean) lie outside the reference range.

To establish a reference range, an appropriate population needs to be defined, and this may be a general population (e.g., healthy adults) or a more specific one (e.g., healthy women aged 30 to 45 years). Then, a very large sample from the population is assessed, and the score distribution is examined to establish the reference range.

Because score values outside the reference range are not necessarily "abnormal," additional information is usually needed for a proper interpretation. Clinicians evaluate out-of-range scores within the context of a patient's medical and medication history, lifestyle choices, physical examinations, and values on other tests. For example, a score of 155 for low-density lipoprotein (LDL) "bad" cholesterol (higher than the usual reference range) would likely be interpreted differently for a patient whose high-density lipoprotein (HDL) cholesterol was 70 than for one whose HDL was 30 (i.e., high and low values for "good" cholesterol). This example illustrates how the interpretation of scores is facilitated by various comparisons: external comparisons (with other people) and internal comparisons (for the focal person on other measures).

16.1.b Percentiles

Raw score values can be made more interpretable by converting them into percentiles. A **percentile** indicates the percentage of people who score below a particular score value. Percentiles provide information about how a person performs relative to others and are easily interpreted by most people. Percentiles can range from zero to the 99th percentile, and the 50th percentile corresponds to the median (and the mean, when scores are normally distributed). For scores that are normally distributed, percentiles correspond to a specified area of the normal curve, as shown in Figure 16.1.

Percentiles are widely used to communicate information about scores on standardized tests and also for interpreting children's height and weight relative to other children. When percentile values are presented for a given measure, there may be guidance about percentiles that are considered outside the usual range (e.g., below the 5th percentile for children's height or weight).

Percentiles are not difficult to calculate manually, but there are actually several different formulas that can lead to slightly different results. Calculations become complex when there are many cases and when there are multiple cases with the same score (i.e., scores with tied

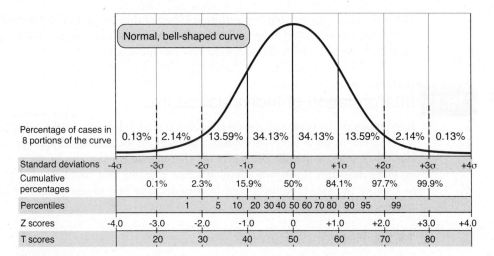

Figure 16.1

Comparison of score interpretation methods for normally distributed scores.

rankings). Many online calculators are available, and statistical software readily converts raw values from a score distribution into percentiles (e.g., in Statistical Package for the Social Sciences [SPSS] in the Frequencies or Explore procedures).

As with reference ranges, percentile values are most useful when they are determined on the basis of a large, representative, and appropriate reference sample. Also similar to reference ranges, the interpretation of percentiles sometimes benefits from internal comparisons. For example, there would be greater concern about a school-aged child's development if his or her percentile for weight was dramatically higher than his or her percentile for height.

Percentiles are often calculated for specific demographic or clinical subgroups. For example, percentiles for age and education subgroups were calculated and published for the MMSE (Crum, Anthony, & Folstein, 1993). When widely used patient-reported outcomes have been subjected to adequate testing and made available commercially, developers usually create a user's manual that provides information about percentiles or about other ways to interpret scores.

One drawback of percentiles is that the units are not at equal intervals at all points on the scale of raw scores, as shown in Figure 16.1. Because more people obtain scores near the middle of the distribution, a percentile difference of, say, 5 points near the middle of the scale (e.g., the 47th vs. 52nd percentile) represents a smaller raw score difference than percentile differences near the extreme (e.g., 92nd vs. 97th percentile).

16.1.c Standard and Transformed Scores

Standard scores transform raw scores into values that have been stripped of the original measurement metric. The transformation makes it possible to compare people on a measure along an easily interpretable scale, without needing to understand the meaning of a raw score value. Standard scores also make it possible to compare a person's performance on multiple measures that have different metrics (e.g., a 10-item fatigue scale and a 5-item pain scale).

Standard scores (or **z-scores**) are expressed in terms of their relative distance from the mean, in standard deviation units. A z-score of 0.0 corresponds to a raw score exactly at the mean on the original scale, regardless of what that mean is. A z-score of 1.0 corresponds to a score 1 *SD* above the mean, and a z-score of −1.0 corresponds to a score 1 *SD* below the mean. Standard scores can be readily calculated from raw scores once the mean and *SD* have been calculated. As a review, the formula is:

$$z = \frac{X - \overline{X}}{SD}$$

For example, if a mean raw score on a quality-of-life scale is 26 and the standard deviation is 4.2, then a person with a score of 20 would have a *z*-score of -1.43, that is, about 1.5 *SD*s below the mean. This *z*-score immediately communicates information about a person's quality of life, relative to others in the population, whereas a raw score of 20 does not.

It is often easier to work with score values that do not have negative values and decimal points. Standard scores can be further transformed to have any desired mean and standard deviation, and certain transformations are particularly common. IQ scores, for example, typically have a mean of 100 and an *SD* of 15. Many standardized tests (e.g., the Scholastic Assessment Test, or SAT) have a mean of 500 and an *SD* of 100. Standard scores with a mean of 50 and an *SD* of 10 are widely used and are often called **T scores**. For example, version 2 of the SF-36 uses a scoring algorithm that creates T scores (Maruish, 2011). The formula for converting raw scores to T scores is as follows:

$$T = \left(\left(\frac{X - \overline{X}}{SD} \right) \times 10 \right) + 50$$

Such T scores are created for all eight subscales on the SF-36. This allows people to be compared to those in the normative sample with respect to, say, physical functioning. It also allows a **profile** to be created for each person, so that internal or *ipsative* comparisons can be made (e.g., performance on the Physical Functioning subscale compared to the Vitality subscale).

In item response theory (IRT) and Rasch model analyses, latent trait scores are more directly interpretable than raw total scores on a scale developed using classical test theory (CTT). Yet, transformations are also used to convert estimates of the latent trait (logits) into "scores" that are easier for people to understand. In some cases, scores are transformed into T scores with a mean of 50 (e.g., Varni et al., 2014), but sometimes, trait estimates are transformed to a scale that ranges from 0 to 100 (e.g., Khan, Chien, & Brauer, 2013).

16.1.d Norms

Score interpretation can be facilitated by establishing **norms**, which indicate the "normal" or standard values on a measure and are thus similar to reference ranges. Norms may be presented as percentiles or as standard scores or, often, both. Norms are typically developed not only for a general population but also for key demographic subgroups. For example, in the user's manual for the revised version of the MMSE (MMSE-2), T-score norms are presented for age and education subgroups (Folstein, Folstein, White, & Messer, 2010). As an illustration, a raw score of 26 (out of a maximum raw score of 30), equates to a T score of 32 for people aged 18 to 39 with a college degree (nearly 2 *SD*s below the mean for that group), but it equates to a T score of 54 for those in the 70- to 74-year-old age bracket who have a 7th or 8th grade education (i.e., slightly above the mean for that group). For measures that are used internationally, norms are typically developed for different countries.

Standard scores used to create norms are sometimes *normalized*. When the original distribution is not normal, normalization can further aid in the interpretation of score values because the standard scores can then be evaluated in terms of percentages within a normal distribution (Fig. 16.1). To convert a score distribution to a normal distribution, the obtained scores are converted to percentiles. Then, a *z*-score is determined for each percentile. These *z*-scores are normally distributed, even when the raw scores were not. If the original distribution was approximately normal, normalization is likely unnecessary.

Sampling is a critical issue in norming an instrument. To establish norms, researchers must administer their measure to a very large sample so that subgroup scores are stable. For example, in the original norming of the MMSE, more than 18,000 people were included in the sample (Crum et al., 1993). Most of the age-based subgroups had over 1,000 people; for example, nearly 2,000 people in the 60- to 64-year-old age range were tested. A rigorous sampling design (preferably probability sampling) is needed to ensure adequate regional, educational, and cultural group representation. Studies that are intended to be representative of a well-defined population often use sampling weights to better represent that population.

Another sampling issue of great importance in creating norms concerns how the population is defined. Sometimes the population is specified as an entire general population, including those who might be "cases" for a condition. For example, the SF-36 is normed for a general population of adults (Ware & Kosinski, 2001). In other cases, the norms are developed in a sample of healthy, functioning people that excludes known "cases." For example, the normative sample for the MMSE-2 included 1,531 healthy adults living independently in the community. Patients who had a hearing or visual impairment, who had dementia, or who had a psychiatric disorder were excluded (Folstein et al., 2010). Sometimes the norms are based on heterogeneous groups that confound key determinants of the target attribute. For example, the growth charts for infants produced by the Centers for Disease Control and Prevention (CDC) in 2000 were for a general population that included both breastfed and formula-fed infants, who have different growth patterns. By contrast, the World Health Organization's (WHO, 2006) infant growth norms are based on the growth of healthy infants in optimal conditions, which include being breastfed.

Clearly, clinicians or researchers who use normed values to interpret scores should be aware of how the population was defined and how rigorous the sampling plan was. Another consideration concerns the possibility of a biased sample. Low response rates in the norming study may signal a problem with the norms. Another issue is the recency of the norming procedure. Norms can become outmoded due to changes in lifestyle and medical progress, so norms for certain traits need to be updated periodically.

16.1.e Cutpoints

Interpretation of scores is facilitated to an even greater degree when the instrument developer (or a subsequent researcher) establishes **cutpoints** for classification purposes. Cutpoints are typically used as the basis for making decisions about needed treatments or further assessments.

In some cases, cutpoints are defined in terms of percentiles. For example, for children's weights, those below the 5th percentile are often interpreted as underweight (or, in infants, "failure to thrive"), whereas those above the 95th percentile are considered overweight. Sometimes, standard scores are used to designate cutpoints. As an example, the WHO (2003) has defined osteoporosis as a standard score on a bone mineral density test at or below -2.5 (i.e., 2.5 SDs below the mean for a general population of women in their 30s). Cutpoints that are linked to the measure's distribution can be considered **norm-referenced**.

Cutpoints can also be based on raw score values. For example, the American Heart Association uses cutpoint values for LDL cholesterol (in milligrams per deciliter [mg/dl]) to define five categories: optimal (<100); near or above optimal (100 to 129); borderline high (130 to 159); high (160 to 189); and very high (≥190) (http://www.heart.org). When cutpoints are based on such raw score values, the measurement can be called **criterion-referenced**. These cutpoints designate a desired standard or criterion, not performance relative to others. Using the American Heart Association cutpoints, for example, it would theoretically be possible for everyone's cholesterol to be classified as optimal.

Cutpoints are sometimes established on the basis of distributional characteristics (as in the height–weight example) and sometimes based on expert clinical opinion (as in the cholesterol example). In some cases, cutpoints are established based on an independent criterion or *anchor*. For example, Tubach and colleagues (2005, 2006) developed a cutpoint threshold for what they called the *patient acceptable symptom state* (PASS). The cutpoint was determined by calculating the mean score on pain and physical function measures for patients who reported that they were satisfied with their treatment. The PASS will be described more fully in Chapter 19.

Ideally, cutpoints are based on rigorous research to determine values that maximize specificity and sensitivity—for example, using receiver operating characteristic (ROC) analysis (Chapter 12). When a reliable "gold standard" is used to establish a cutpoint, clinical decisions can be grounded in evidence of an at-risk status rather than on whether a value falls into a statistically "normal" range.

16.1.f Content-Based Interpretations

Inspection of an instrument's content can also help with the interpretation of scores. However, on most patient-reported outcomes developed using CTT, there are typically numerous ways of achieving the same raw score, so there is no necessary correspondence between a scale score and item-level responses. For example, a score of 12 on the CES-D can be achieved with responses of "some of the time" to 12 items (12 × 1), or "a moderate amount of the time" to 6 items (6 × 2), or "most of the time" to 4 items (4 × 3), with all other items answered as "none of the time" (0). Moreover, a score of 12 provides no clues regarding *which* items were rated as being experienced in the previous week. Inspection of item-level responses may thus be needed to better grasp what a score means in terms of content.

For widely used tests, user's manuals sometimes offer content-based interpretations. For example, in the original version of the SF-36, the user's manual provided interpretive information relating to specific items. Among people in the norming sample whose T score was less than 30, 81% reported a limitation in walking a block, whereas for those with a score of 60, fewer than 1% had such a limitation (Ware & Kosinski, 2001). Even when such norms are not available, researchers can provide content-based guidance by linking their own scale-level data to a meaningful single item on the scale (Guyatt et al., 2002). For example, it could be reported that 54% of the people whose score on the CES-D was 10 or lower said they "felt depressed" at least some of the time the previous week, compared to 100% of the people whose score was between 20 and 30.[1]

Content-based interpretations are also possible when scales have either been developed using IRT techniques, or have been found to have a good IRT or Rasch model fit, because items have different locations on the latent trait continuum. For example, several researchers have performed an IRT analysis on the 10 items in the Physical Functioning (PF) subscale of the SF-36 (e.g., Haley, McHorney, & Ware, 1994; Hays, Liu, Spritzer, & Cella, 2007; Jenkinson, Fitzpatrick, Garratt, Peto, & Stewart-Brown, 2001). A person with the highest possible score has no limitations performing any of the activities, including "vigorous activities such as running, lifting heavy objects, or participating in strenuous sports," which is the item with the highest difficulty. A person with the lowest score on the PF subscale would have a limitation with regard to "bathing or dressing"[2] and with all other (more difficult) activities.

Valderas, Alonso, Prieto, Esparrargues, and Castells (2004) offered a good illustration of how IRT analysis can be used to create "interpretation aids." These researchers

---

[1]These are the percentages that were obtained using the sample of 1,000 low-income women, as described in Chapter 5.
[2]Jenkinson et al. (2001) found a different hierarchy in samples in the United Kingdom. In a normative sample of nearly 9,000 respondents, "walking 100 yards" was slightly less difficult than bathing or dressing oneself.

administered the Visual Function Index (VF-14) to a sample of patients scheduled for cat-aract surgery. Data from the scale, which measures perceived functional capacity related to vision, was analyzed using a Rasch model. The VF-14 has 14 items that form a hierarchy of visual abilities, from "Recognizing people when they are close to you" to "Driving at night." Respondents rate the difficulty of performing each activity. One interpretation aid that Valderas et al. created was a "ruler" that calibrated specific vision abilities against a patient's total score (values that transformed logit values to a scale of 0 to 100) based on item dif-ficulty. For example, as shown in Figure 16.2, a patient with a score of 65 would be expected to have difficulty doing fine handwork, reading small print, and driving during the day or night but little difficulty doing the other 10 activities. Thus, one way to interpret a score is in

Score	Ruler interpretation aid: Specific abilities for different scores	Clinical scenario interpretation aid: Benchmarks
100		
	⬅ Driving at night	Driving at night
95		
90		
85		
80		
	⬅ Driving during the day	
75	⬅ Reading small print	Reading small print
70		
	⬅ Doing fine handwork	Doing fine handwork
65		
	⬅ Reading a newspaper	
60	⬅ Writing checks	
	⬅ Reading traffic signs	
55	⬅ Watching TV/Seeing steps	Watching TV
	⬅ Taking part in sports	
50	⬅ Playing games	
45		
	⬅ Preparing meals	
40	⬅ Reading large print	
35	⬅ Recognizing people	Recognizing people
30		
25		
20		

* Adapted from information provided by Valderas et al., 2004

Figure 16.2

Example of a content-based interpretation aids for the visual function index.

terms of the most difficult activity that the patient would be expected to perform with ease. Valderas and colleagues also identified five "significantly different clusters of visual capacity items within the VF-14" (p. 40). The benchmarks for these "clinical scenarios" are shown in the right panel of Figure 16.2. Such interpretation aids can be extremely useful for clinical users of PROs but are seldom created.

16.1.g Confidence Intervals

Clinicians who understand measurement principles may be able to compute a confidence interval (CI) around an obtained score using the standard error of measurement (Chapter 10). CIs help with interpretation because they provide a better sense of the range of score values within which a true score value probably lies. User's manuals sometimes provide 95% CIs around standard scores.

16.2 Interpretation of Group Scores

Researchers are most often concerned with interpreting scores from a sample of patients rather than an individual. We offer a few comments relating to such interpretations, directed primarily at those who are making sense of their data based on a scale created by others.

16.2.a Descriptive Statistics

Interpretation of scores begins with basics, namely examining a frequency distribution for evidence of skewness, outliers, floor and ceiling effects, and missingness. A frequency distribution also shows whether the scores are distributed over the full range of possible score values. Visual diagrams (e.g., histograms or box plots) can facilitate understanding key aspects of a distribution, such as whether scores tend to cluster in a narrow range. For continuous scores, indexes of central tendency and dispersion should be inspected. In SPSS, the Explore procedure provides many ways of examining data characteristics. If the research specifically concerns an assessment of a new instrument, then understanding variability within the development sample is essential for interpreting evidence of the instrument's reliability and validity.

16.2.b Measurement Properties

Interpretations of scores should also take into consideration the measurement properties of the instrument. When evidence for the reliability or validity of an instrument is unfavorable or slim, caution should be exercised in interpreting its scores. However, the utility of information from an instrument development paper relies on the similarity of a researcher's population with the development population. If the measure is used in research with a very different population, new estimates of the scale's measurement properties for the population would need to be calculated.

16.2.c Normative and Other Comparisons

If normative information is available for an instrument, then researchers using the instrument can readily use it in interpreting average scores for their sample or for groups within their sample. For example, using the SF-36, one can develop a sense of the burden of a research sample's illness by comparing their profile of mean T scores against normed values. Table 16.1 presents hypothetical results for a study showing mean T scores on the eight subscales of the SF-36 for a sample of patients with sleep apnea and percentages of patients below the normative mean of 50. This table provides both internal and external comparisons to facilitate interpretation. It shows that the sample of patients with sleep apnea had lower scores that those in the norming population with respect to all eight domains of the

Table 16.1	Fictitious Table Summarizing Scores on the Eight Subscales of the SF-36 for Patients With Sleep Apnea ($N = 250$) Compared to Population Norms		
SF-36 Subscale	**Mean T Scores**	**Standard Deviation**	**Percentage (%) of Patients Below Normative Mean of 50**
Physical Functioning (PF)	42.5	10.2	70.3
Role Limitations–Physical (RP)	47.9	11.0	56.7
Bodily Pain (BP)	46.1	9.8	61.0
General Health (GH)	42.4	9.4	77.2
Vitality (VT)	41.9	8.9	78.9
Social Functioning (SF)	48.1	9.3	54.4
Role Limitations–Emotional (RE)	46.2	11.8	61.2
Mental Health (MH)	44.0	8.1	67.9

Note: For each SF-36 subscale, the normative mean is 50 with an *SD* of 10.00.

SF-36. The table also shows that the burden of sleep apnea was especially severe with regard to the Vitality domain but modest with regard to Social Functioning.

Even when norms are not available, researchers can put their sample's mean scores in context by examining mean values for the instrument development sample and for other samples if the scale has been used by other researchers. The more an instrument has been used by other researchers, the easier it is to interpret mean scores.

Because comparisons are at the heart of most interpretative efforts, researchers can create their own context by computing descriptive information for subgroups of their sample. This includes key demographic subgroups as well as subgroups based on clinical information, such as illness severity or length of time since diagnosis.

16.2.d Construct-Based Interpretations

One final interpretative approach is to consider available evidence regarding how scores on the scale in question correlate with scores for other constructs. If the measure has several subscales, it is important to consider how the subscales are intercorrelated; such information is usually available in instrument development papers. If a rigorous construct validation was undertaken, information about how scores on the measure relate to measures of other constructs also helps to interpret scores on the measure. Subsequent use of the scale by other researchers should also be reviewed to better understand both the instrument and the construct it represents.

References

Centers for Disease Control and Prevention. (2000). *2000 CDC growth charts for the United States.* Washington, DC: National Center for Health Statistics.

Crum, R. M., Anthony, S. S., & Folstein, M. F. (1993). Population-based norms for the Mini-Mental State Examination. *Journal of the American Medical Association, 269,* 2386–2391.

Folstein, M., Folstein, S., White, T., & Messer, M. (2010). *MMSE-2: Mini-Mental State Examination: User's manual* (2nd ed.) Lutz, FL: Psychological Assessment Resources.

Guyatt, G. H., Osoba, D., Wu, A., Wyrwich, K., & Norman, G. (2002). Methods to explain the clinical significance of health status measures. *Mayo Clinic Proceedings, 77*, 371–383.

Haley, S. M., McHorney, C. A., & Ware, J. E. (1994). Evaluation of the MOS SF-36 Physical Functioning scale (PF-10). Dimensionality and reproducibility of the Rasch item scale. *Journal of Clinical Epidemiology, 47*, 671–684.

Hays, R. D., Liu, H., Spritzer, K., & Cella, D. (2007). Item response theory analysis of physical functioning items in the Medical Outcomes Study. *Medical Care, 45*(Suppl. 1), S32–S38.

Jenkinson, C., Fitzpatrick, R., Garratt, A., Peto, V., & Stewart-Brown, S. (2001). Can item response theory reduce patient burden when measuring health status in neurological disorders? Results from Rasch analysis of the SF-36 physical functioning scale (PF-10). *Journal of Neurology, Neurosurgery, and Psychiatry, 71*, 220–224.

Khan, A., Chien, C., & Brauer, S. (2013). Rasch-based scoring offered more precision in differentiating patient groups in measuring upper limb function. *Journal of Clinical Epidemiology, 66*, 681–687.

Maruish, M. E. (2011). *User's manual for the SF-36v2 Health Survey* (3rd ed.). Lincoln, RI: QualityMetric

Mokkink, L. B., Terwee, C., Patrick, D., Alonso, J., Stratford, P., Knol, D. L., . . . DeVet, H. C. W. (2010). The COSMIN study reached international consensus on taxonomy, terminology, and definitions of measurement properties for health-related patient-reported outcomes. *Journal of Clinical Epidemiology, 63*, 737–745.

Radloff, L. S. (1977). The CES-D scale: A self-report depression scale for research in the general population. *Applied Psychological Measurement, 1*, 385–401.

Tubach, F., Dougados, M., Falissard, B., Baron, G., Logeart, I., & Ravaud, P. (2006). Feeling good rather than feeling better matters more to patients. *Arthritis & Rheumatism, 55*, 526–530.

Tubach, F., Ravaud, P., Baron, G., Falissard, B., Logeart, I., Bellamy, N., . . . Dougados, M. (2005). Evaluation of clinically relevant states in patient reported outcomes in knee and hip osteoarthritis: The patient acceptable symptom state. *Annals of the Rheumatic Diseases, 64*, 34–37.

Valderas, J. M., Alonso, J., Prieto, L., Esparrargues, M., & Castells, X. (2004). Content-based interpretation aids for health-related quality of life measures in clinical practice. An example for the Visual Function Index (VF-14). *Quality of Life Research, 13*, 35–44.

Varni, J. W., Magnus, B., Stucky, B., Liu, Y., Quinn, H., Thissen, D., . . . DeWalt, D. (2014). Psychometric properties of the PROMIS® pediatric scales: Precision, stability, and comparison of different scoring and administration options. *Quality of Life Research, 23*(4):1233–1243.

Ware, J. E., & Kosinski, M. (2001). *SF-36 Physical & Mental Health summary: A manual for users of version 1* (2nd ed.). Lincoln, RI: QualityMetric.

World Health Organization. (2003). *Prevention and management of osteoporosis. WHO Technical Report No. 921.* Geneva, Switzerland: Author.

World Health Organization. (2006). *WHO child growth standards.* Geneva, Switzerland: Author.

CHANGE SCORES AND THE RESPONSIVENESS DOMAIN

chapters

17

Change Scores and
Their Reliability

Chapter Outline

The last three chapters in this book focus on a topic that is fraught with controversy, divergent viewpoints, and new advances: the measurement of change on a construct of interest. Although there are many different opinions regarding terminology, definitions, and approaches to change measurement, much of our presentation is consistent with Consensus-based Standards for the selection of health Measurement Instruments (COSMIN; Mokkink et al., 2010).

In Chapter 3, we noted that six questions are relevant to the use and understanding of health measurements, each corresponding to a measurement property within an overall taxonomy (Fig. 3.1). Three questions relate to changes in scores over time, such as changes that result from either a natural progression of a construct or trait or from a health care intervention. As a review, these three questions are as follows:

1. *Reliability of change:* Does a change in scores truly represent change, or does it merely reflect random fluctuations in measurement?

2. *Responsiveness:* Does a person's change in scores on a measure correspond to a commensurate improvement (or deterioration) in the construct?

3. *Interpretation of a change score:* What does a change score *mean*? Is the change large enough to be considered clinically significant?

This chapter focuses primarily on the first of these questions, and the next two chapters cover the last two. Before discussing the reliability of change scores, however, we offer a brief overview of the broader topic of measuring change.

17.1   Measuring Change

How does one measure whether a change in an attribute has occurred?[1] For some attributes, there is only one option: measuring it on two occasions and comparing the values; in other words, subtracting one value from the other to calculate the amount of change. If we want to learn, for example, whether a patient's blood pressure has decreased, we need to know what it was initially and what it is now and calculate the difference. For patient-reported outcomes (PROs), there are two other alternatives: asking patients directly whether a change has occurred, and asking them to report retrospectively what their status was previously and then comparing it to their current status. Unfortunately, all three methods have potential problems. Figure 17.1 illustrates the three approaches to change measurement for PROs.

17.1.a   Direct Questioning About Change

In clinical settings, patients are often asked about change they have noticed: Has your pain lessened? Are you getting more sleep? Are you better able to perform usual daily activities? Thus, one approach to assessing change is through direct questioning.

There are several reasons for being cautious about self-reported change, particularly in research contexts in which there is little opportunity for clarification or amplification of responses. For one thing, direct measures of change are almost always single items rather than multi-item scales[2]—for example, "Has your pain gotten a lot better, somewhat better, stayed the same, gotten somewhat worse, or gotten a lot worse?" Single items are inherently less reliable than multi-item scales, which is a key reason for constructing scales in the first place. Nevertheless, as we shall see in the next two chapters, such single *health transition ratings* do play a role in assessing responsiveness and in interpreting change scores.

Much has been written about how responses to direct change questions can be subject to **recall biases** (errors or incompleteness of retrieved recollections as a result of various cognitive and emotional forces). One formal explanation of such a bias is called the *implicit theory of change* (Ross, 1989). Ross contended that because people do not truly remember a previous state, their responses to change questions are not likely to be accurate. Ross's theory is that the memory of a prior personal attribute encompasses two steps. People begin by considering their *present* state on the attribute, and this evaluation serves as a benchmark for answering a change question because it is more salient than a previous state. Then, in the second step, "people may invoke an implicit theory of stability or change to guide their construction of the past" (p. 342). Thus, respondents work backward in time to infer what their previous state must have been. To estimate their previous state, people might ask whether there is any reason to think they were different in the past than in their present state, and their evaluation may be biased by strongly held beliefs, memories, and social norms (e.g., "I must have been in better physical condition a year ago because I was younger"). In support of this theory, there is considerable evidence that responses to direct questions about change are more highly correlated with posttest outcome scores than with pretest scores (e.g., Meyer et al., 2013; Schmitt & DiFabio, 2005). Because of such problems with direct questions, important research outcomes are often measured through change scores.

---

[1]Given that this book focuses on *measurement,* we do not describe efforts to model change or growth, topics addressed in (for example) the growth curve literature (e.g., Dudley, McGuire, Peterson, & Wong, 2009; Speer & Greenbaum, 1995). We also omit discussion of *residual change scores* (RCS), which reflect the difference between actual Time 2 scores and Time 2 scores predicted through linear regression based on Time 1 scores. Theoretically, RCSs are more reliable than simple change scores, but they are primarily appropriate for studying the correlates of group change and not for assessing change at the individual level (Kim-Kang & Weiss, 2008).

[2]To our knowledge, scales with multiple questions asking directly about change have been created by only two research teams (Meyer, Richter, & Raspe, 2013; Middel et al, 2002). The Meyer et al. scale was developed as part of a methodologic inquiry into change measurement, not as a proposed instrument for actually measuring change.

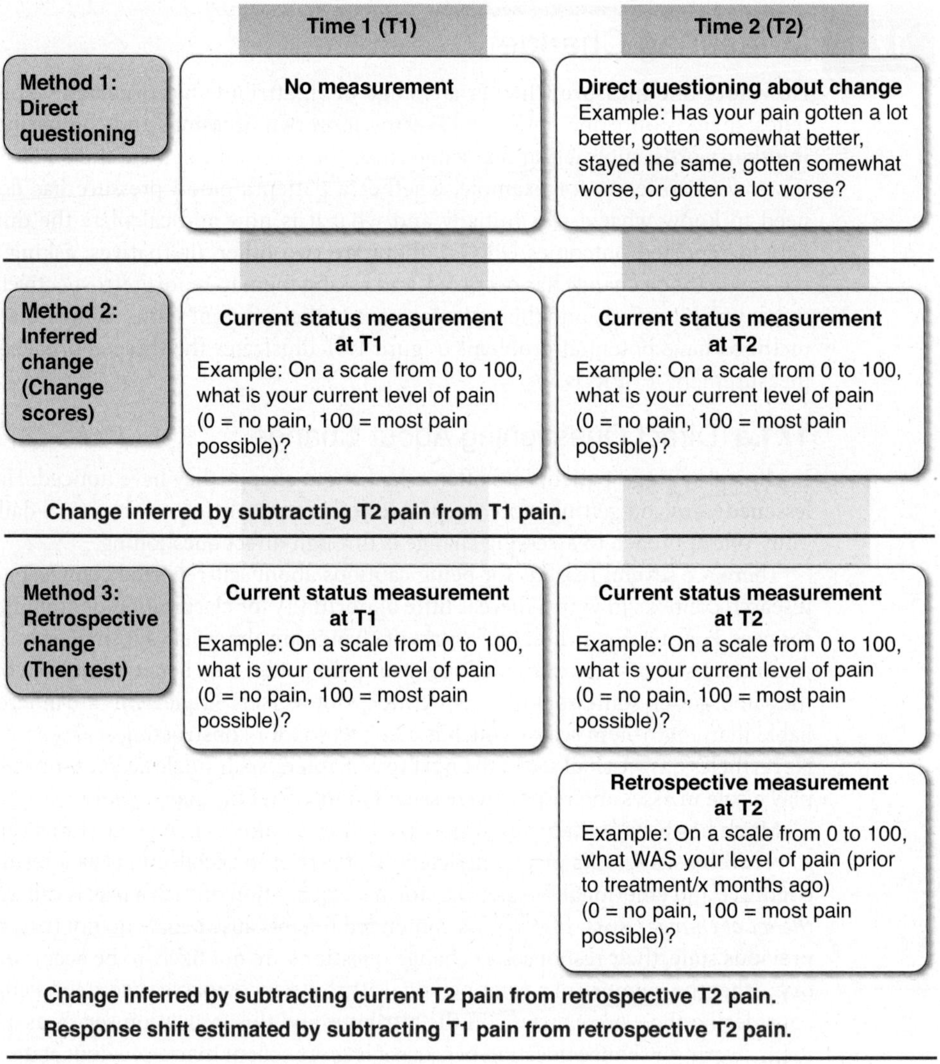

	Time 1 (T1)	**Time 2 (T2)**
Method 1: Direct questioning	No measurement	**Direct questioning about change** Example: Has your pain gotten a lot better, gotten somewhat better, stayed the same, gotten somewhat worse, or gotten a lot worse?
Method 2: Inferred change (Change scores)	**Current status measurement at T1** Example: On a scale from 0 to 100, what is your current level of pain (0 = no pain, 100 = most pain possible)?	**Current status measurement at T2** Example: On a scale from 0 to 100, what is your current level of pain (0 = no pain, 100 = most pain possible)?

Change inferred by subtracting T2 pain from T1 pain.

	Time 1 (T1)	**Time 2 (T2)**
Method 3: Retrospective change (Then test)	**Current status measurement at T1** Example: On a scale from 0 to 100, what is your current level of pain (0 = no pain, 100 = most pain possible)?	**Current status measurement at T2** Example: On a scale from 0 to 100, what is your current level of pain (0 = no pain, 100 = most pain possible)?
		Retrospective measurement at T2 Example: On a scale from 0 to 100, what WAS your level of pain (prior to treatment/x months ago) (0 = no pain, 100 = most pain possible)?

Change inferred by subtracting current T2 pain from retrospective T2 pain.

Response shift estimated by subtracting T1 pain from retrospective T2 pain.

Figure 17.1

Three approaches to measuring change in health outcomes (pain measurement example).

17.1.b Indirect Change: Change Scores

A **change score** is easy to calculate by simply subtracting a score at one point in time from the score at an earlier point in time (Fig. 17.1):

$$X_{\text{Change}} = X_{\text{T1}} - X_{\text{T2}} \tag{17.1}$$

Computing such a change score has intuitive appeal.[3] Yet, such a calculation can be problematic, and the resulting value can be difficult to interpret, a topic to which we devote more attention in Chapter 19.

In clinical trials, statisticians have argued against using change scores as the dependent variables in the analysis of treatment effects (e.g., Senn, 2006; Van Breukelen, 2006; Vickers & Altman, 2001). When patients are randomized to groups, it is recommended that scores at the posttest be used as the outcome variables rather than change scores. Baseline scores, if used in the analysis of group differences, are usually used as covariates to enhance initial

---

[3]The formula could also be $X_{\text{T2}} - X_{\text{T1}}$, depending on whether high scores are considered advantageous or disadvantageous.

group comparability.[4] Effect size estimates for trials are computed as the difference between the treatment and control groups at posttest. Thus, a major emphasis in clinical trials is on *difference scores* (the difference between the randomized groups at posttest) rather than on *change scores*.

Yet, it is of inherent substantive interest to understand how much the patients in a study have changed, including those in different arms of a randomized trial. Moreover, not all health care studies are trials. Some investigations seek to describe outcomes over the course of an illness, for example, which requires a direct examination of how scores have changed. Observational prospective studies sometimes seek to identify factors associated with increases or decreases in patients' symptoms or behaviors. For example, investigators testing hypotheses about factors affecting declines in pulmonary function (e.g., smoking) would likely use change scores in the analysis (Van Breukelen, 2006). And, at the level of an individual patient, assessments of improvement or deterioration (or stability) over time as measured by change scores may be the focus of clinical assessment and decision making. Whenever change scores are computed, it is important to understand their reliability and validity and to rely on mechanisms for interpreting change score values.

Change scores are affected by several factors that can threaten their accuracy and validity. Indeed, some of the issues relating to change scores are similar to ones we described in Chapter 8 with regard to test–retest reliability, except in reverse. In test–retest reliability, the emphasis is on measuring a stable trait, but the worry is that the trait may have changed. In computing change scores, the emphasis is on capturing a change, but the worry is that the measure may suggest change when none exists, or vice versa. Among the factors that can affect a change score are the following:

1. *Measurement error.* A basic problem with change scores is that measurement is never perfectly reliable, as discussed in Chapter 8. Change scores—the difference between an imperfectly reliable score at Time 1 and another imperfectly reliable score at Time 2— potentially can magnify a small change, or mask a large one. The greater the degree of unreliability, the greater the risk that a change score will be misleading. This chapter focuses primarily on this issue: How do we know when a change score is a reliable one and not merely a random fluctuation?

2. *Regression to the mean.* Another problem with change scores concerns **regression to the mean**, which is a statistical phenomenon in which scores that are at the extreme (very high or very low) at an initial measurement tend to be closer to the mean on the same measure on a subsequent measurement. Regression to the mean can result in change scores that make natural variation in repeated measurements look like a change has occurred when it has not. The effects of regression to the mean are especially severe when measurement error is high (Barnett, van der Pols, & Dobson, 2005).

3. *Floor and ceiling effects.* A problem can arise in measuring change if the instrument is incapable of capturing improvements or deteriorations beyond what was measured at baseline. Whenever it is expected that change scores will be computed, it is important to use measures that provide room to register higher or lower scores at a follow-up.

4. *Missing data.* The computation of a change score requires two separate measurements, and sometimes one of the measurements (usually the second one) is missing. Imputation of the missing Time 2 score using standard methods may be ill-advised because such imputations are based on the assumption that data are *missing at random* (MAR). However, in health research, missingness may depend on the unobserved outcome. For example, a person may fail to complete a follow-up quality of life questionnaire because his or her health has dramatically deteriorated, which results in nonignorable missing data.

---

[4]An analysis using analysis of covariance (ANCOVA) generally has greater statistical power to detect a treatment effect than an analysis using change scores as the outcome variable, especially if the correlation between the baseline and posttest scores is not extremely high (e.g., <.80) (Vickers & Altman, 2001).

5. *Response shift*. According to the theory of **response shift** (Rapkin & Schwartz, 2004; Schwartz & Sprangers, 1999), a person's understanding of a health construct—the cognitive appraisal of one's attribute—can shift over time, even when the construct itself has not changed or when it has changed in the opposite direction. In response shift theory, such revised appraisals are triggered by a catalyst, such as a change in health status as a result of disease or injury or a health treatment. Response shift is a phenomenon that is often used to explain seemingly paradoxical results with PROs, such as the observed stability of health-related quality of life among terminally or chronically ill patients with deteriorating health (e.g., Albrecht & Devlieger, 1999; Groenvold, et al., 1999). Response shift can occur for various reasons that can be subsumed under three categories, sometimes referred to as the three Rs: recalibration, reprioritization, and reconceptualization of internal standards used in self-appraisal. *Recalibration* is a change in the person's use of the scale on which the trait is being measured. For example, a patient's internal definition of pain may change following a surgical intervention. Patients might say that their presurgical pain was 85 (out of 100), but immediately after surgery their more severe pain might also be rated at 85 because they are using a different pain yardstick, and if asked to rate their presurgical pain retrospectively, their response might now be 50. *Reconceptualization* is a change in a patient's definition of a construct or a change in his or her interpretation of items that measure the construct. For example, a patient's definition of autonomy might be modified to incorporate different activities after an assistive device has become necessary. *Reprioritization* is a revision of patients' preferences, values, and goals that affect their view of health constructs such as quality of life. For example, a patient might come to view family relationships as a more important component in quality-of-life assessments following a diagnosis of cancer.

Response shift is problematic for change scores in PROs because patients respond to the same questions differently at different points of their health trajectory, such as over the course of a chronic illness or at pretreatment and posttreatment measurements. Response shift can sometimes attenuate or inflate estimates of treatment effects.

The response shift phenomenon has given rise to an entire body of research—particularly in quality-of-life research—in efforts to better detect it, understand it, and control for it in studies of change. One approach to response shift is described next.

17.1.c Retrospective Change: The Then-Test Approach

A widely used approach to dealing with response shift is called the **then test** (Barclay-Goddard, Epstein, & Mayo, 2009; Schwartz & Sprangers, 2010). As shown in Figure 17.1, the then test yields a change measurement by comparing a patient's present appraisal of a construct (T2) with a retrospective appraisal of a construct at an earlier point, for example, at the point of a pretest in a pretest–posttest design. These retrospective ratings are construed as more appropriate for use as a standard for a change assessment than the actual pretest ratings if there is a response shift effect. The assumption is that the patient is using the same "yardstick" or scale calibration for both the current and retrospective ratings because the measurements are made at the same time. In this approach, then, a change score is the difference between the T2 current scores and the T2 retrospective scores:

$$X_{Change} = X_{RetrospectivePretest} - X_{T2} \tag{17.2}$$

A response shift is inferred if there are significant differences between the T1 actual pretest scores and the T2 retrospective pretest scores. If no significant response shift effect is found, researchers can use either the original or the retrospective baseline scores to compute a change score.

Careful attention is needed in designing a then test (Schwartz & Sprangers, 2010). First, the retrospective questions must refer to a previous point in time that is *salient* to patients.

Asking patients about an arbitrary point in time, such as "6 months ago" may yield meaningless data. The retrospective questions ideally are about a well-defined baseline, such as "prior to your chemotherapy" or "3 months ago when you came in for your follow-up appointment."

Questions and instructions for a then test need to be carefully crafted. The instructions should encourage recall and reflection, such as in the following example that might prepare people for completing a retrospective SF-36:

> *Back in April of this year, just prior to your knee replacement surgery, we asked you some questions about your health and your activities. Please take a minute and try to remember how you were doing just before you had the surgery.*

Questions on the measure also have to be modified to reflect the changed time frame. For example, the SF-36 question on the Physical Functioning subscale about climbing a flight of stairs might be worded:

> *Before your knee replacement surgery, did your health limit you in activities you might have done in a typical day—for example, were you limited in climbing one flight of stairs?*

One of the shortcomings of many studies that have used the then-test approach is that the investigators have failed to assess the psychometric adequacy of the then-test scales. Clearly, it is important to use measures that have good reliability and validity, whether they are current status or retrospective status measures. It should not be assumed that the retrospective scale will have similar measurement properties to those for a scale used to assess a current status.

17.1.d How Should Change Be Measured?

Given that all three approaches to measuring change have problems and complexities, there is no straightforward answer to how change should best be measured.[5] It is a thorny issue for which measurement experts, theorists, and statisticians will undoubtedly continue to pursue solutions. At the moment, the most common approach is to compute a T2–T1 change score (method 2 in Fig. 17.1). Yet, such change scores are vulnerable to myriad problems, as previously discussed.

Response shift is a particularly stubborn problem because there are individual differences in susceptibility to response shift, making it more difficult to model. Indeed, one of the challenges in the field of response shift research is that it has proved difficult to predict who will undergo a response shift, how large an effect it will be, and even what direction it will take (Barclay-Goddard et al., 2009). Response shift is an issue that affects the *interpretation* of change scores, and so it is a topic to which we return in Chapter 19. The remainder of this chapter deals with one particular threat to change score measurement: the reliability of such scores.

17.2 The Reliability of a Change Score: Traditional Methods

In this section, we discuss methods of assessing whether a change score is reliable—that is, whether a change in score is not merely a reflection of random variation. This section discusses "traditional" approaches to assessing change score reliability, and a later section discusses change scores for measures derived from item response theory (IRT) models.

---

[5]Many new analytic strategies have been proposed or are under development to sort out "true" change from response shift and other threats to change interpretation. This book focuses primarily on *measurement* and not on statistical analysis, and so it is beyond the scope of this book to review recent advances in modeling change and detecting response shift. For recent reviews, readers are encouraged to consult Swartz et al. (2011) or Barclay-Goddard et al. (2009).

In the COSMIN taxonomy, the approaches described in this chapter are included as an aspect of *interpreting* change scores. We offer a modified version of the COSMIN taxonomy (Fig. 3.1) because we think that both reliability and validity have cross-sectional and longitudinal aspects. Cross-sectional reliability concerns how much faith can be put in a score at a single point in time, and longitudinal reliability concerns how much faith can be put in a change score.

17.2.a Smallest Detectable Change

The usual approach to assessing the reliability of group-level change is to test the statistical significance of a group's change in scores from one point in time to another. One can use a paired t test for interval or ratio-level scores, a Wilcoxon signed-ranks test for ordinal scores, and a McNemar test for nominal-level data, for example.

From a measurement perspective, however, statistical significance may not be an adequate or informative way to understand change, and significance tells us nothing about reliable change for an individual. Statistical significance is a function of not only the magnitude of a change but also of sample size and variability. With a sufficiently large sample, modest change scores can be statistically significant, even when the change for most study participants is not reliable. Several methods of evaluating the reliability of an individual change score have been developed, and this section describes one such approach.

Reliable change for continuous data is often estimated using an index called the **smallest detectable change (SDC)** or the *minimal detectable change* (MDC).[6] An SDC can be defined as a change in scores that is beyond measurement error—a change of sufficient magnitude that the probability of it being the result of random error is low.

Operationally, the SDC has been defined as a change score that falls outside the limits of agreement (LOA) on a Bland–Altman plot (DeVet, Terwee, Mokkink, & Knol, 2011). As noted in Chapter 10, a Bland–Altman plot can be constructed with test–retest data from a stable population, which in turn requires a time interval between testings that maximizes the potential for trait stability while minimizing the risk of carryover effects. The limits of agreement on a Bland–Altman plot indicate how much the test–retest score differences can be expected to vary in a stable population. If a change score falls outside the LOA, there can be greater confidence that the change is "real." High measurement error makes it more difficult to detect true change than when measurement error is small, further underscoring the importance of using measures with high reliability.

As noted in Chapter 10, one does not need to actually create a Bland–Altman plot to calculate the limits of agreement; the elements for the calculation formula can be obtained from paired t-test output. As a review, the basic formula for the LOA with a 95% confidence interval (CI) is:

$$\text{LOA} = \bar{d} \pm 1.96 \times SD_{\text{Difference}} \tag{17.3}$$

where $\bar{d}$ is the mean difference in T1-T2 scores and $SD_{\text{Difference}}$ is the standard deviation of difference scores.

If the standard error of measurement (*SEM*) has been calculated, an alternative formula is:

$$\text{LOA} = \bar{d} \pm 1.96 \times (\sqrt{2} \times SEM) \tag{17.4}$$

When using this second formula, the *SEM* should be one that has been calculated on the basis of a test–retest reliability assessment and not the *SEM* from an internal consistency assessment. The SDC represents an effort to sort out temporal instability in scores (*transient error*) from a true change in scores, so the *SEM* based on coefficient alpha is not considered appropriate (DeVet et al., 2011).

---

[6]The term *minimal detectable change* is often used in the medical and physical therapy literature. We have used "smallest detectable change" to be consistent with the COSMIN group. We also think this acronym reduces the risk of confusion with another index called MIC ("minimal important change"), which is discussed in Chapter 19. The SDC index has also been called the "smallest detectable *difference*" or "minimal detectable *difference*" but, like the COSMIN group, we prefer "smallest detectable *change*" to emphasize the focus on *change* scores.

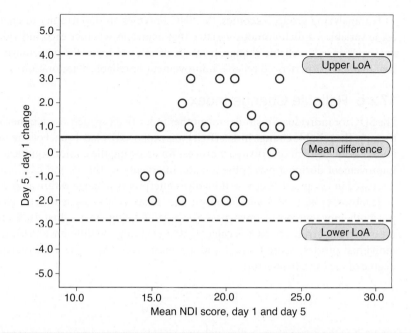

Mean difference = 0.60 (non-significant), $SD_{Difference}$ = 1.76; Upper LOA = 4.05, Lower LOA = 2.85

Smallest detectable change (SDC) for mean difference = 0.0: ± 3.45

Figure 17.2
Bland–Altman plot for 25 Neck Disability Index (NDI) scores, with a 5-day retest interval.

Figure 17.2 presents a fictitious example of a Bland–Altman plot that shows 5-day test–retest difference scores on the Neck Disability Index (NDI) for 25 patients with chronic neck pain. The NDI is a widely used measure of neck pain and dysfunction and consists of 10 items scored on a 5-point scale, with scores ranging from 0 (least disability) to 50 (highest disability) (Vernon & Mior, 1991). Based on a paired t test, we learn that the mean difference between the two administrations was 0.60 (means = 19.4 and 20.0), a nonsignificant difference. The $SD_{Difference}$ was 1.76. Thus, the limits of agreement are:

$$Upper\ LOA = 0.60 + (1.96 \times 1.76) = 4.05$$
$$Lower\ LOA = 0.60 + (-1.96 \times 1.76) = -2.85$$

Because the mean 5-day retest difference was not significant (the 95% CI around the mean of 0.60 includes 0.0), the LOA calculation can be simplified by dropping the term for the average difference score, in which case, the SDC would be ± 3.45. Thus, if a person's change score on the NDI after a 10-week intervention was 4.0 points (e.g., from 24.0 at baseline to 20.0 at follow-up), we could conclude that the change score was reliable on the basis of this SDC. If the person's follow-up score was 21.0, however, we could not rule out the possibility that the drop in score was the result of measurement error, with confidence set at 95%.

It is important to note that for group-level analysis (e.g., for groups of patients in a clinical trial), both measurement error and the SDC are reduced through the effects of averaging. The reliability of a change score for a group is reduced by a factor of $\sqrt{n}$, which in our example of 25 patients would be 3.45 ÷ 5 = .69. This index is sometimes referred to as SDC_{Group} (De Boer et al., 2005).

For analyzing group outcomes, the SDC provides an opportunity to create a new outcome variable—a dichotomous variable that expresses whether each individual has or has not experienced a reliable change. It can be of value to know the percentage of people in a trial that have experienced reliable improvement or reliable deterioration.

17.2.b Reliable Change Index

The SDC for individuals is similar to another index that is widely used in the field of psychotherapy. The **reliable change index (RCI)** was proposed by Jacobson, Follette, and Revenstorf (1984) as an element of a two-part process for assessing the clinical significance of patients' improvement during a psychotherapeutic intervention. The second part of this process is discussed in Chapter 19 because it involves interpreting change within a normative context.

Jacobson et al. (1984) and Jacobson and Truax (1991) argued that a change score on psychotherapy outcomes must pass the test of being "real"—that is, a change beyond measurement error. The RCI is calculated by dividing the difference between an observed individual posttest score (X_{POST}) and a pretest score (X_{PRE}) by a factor representing the degree of measurement error:

$$RCI = \frac{X_{POST} - X_{PRE}}{\sqrt{2 \times SEM^2}} \tag{17.5}$$

where X is the score of an individual and SEM is the standard error of measurement. As a review, the SEM is computed from the following formula, which we presented in Chapter 10 as formula 10.3:

$$SEM = SD \times \sqrt{(1 - R)} \tag{17.6}$$

where R is the reliability of the instrument, and SD (in the context of the RCI formula) is the standard deviation of a "control group, normal population, or pretreatment experimental group" (Jacobson & Truax, 1991, p. 14).

Table 17.1 presents some fictitious data to illustrate calculation of the RCI. The table shows scores on the 20-item Center for Epidemiologic Studies Depression Scale (CES-D) (Radloff, 1977) for 10 patients at three points in time. T1 and T2 scores are scores prior to an intervention administered 1 week apart. The third set of scores (T3) are measurements following a 12-week intervention.[7] All of the information needed to compute the RCI is shown in the panel beneath the score values. The test–retest reliability, based on T1 and T2 scores, is .824 ($ICC_{Consistency}$). The SD is 3.592—the standard deviation of the 10 scores at T2, which is considered the pretest. Therefore:

$$SEM = 3.592 \times \sqrt{(1 - .824)} = 1.507$$

This denominator of the RCI formula is thus:

$$\sqrt{2 \times 1.507^2} = 2.131$$

We can use this value to assess whether any particular patient had a reliable improvement in CES-D scores following the intervention. For example, for the first two patients:

Patient 1: $(14 - 17) \div 2.131 = -1.408$

Patient 2: $(13 - 19) \div 2.131 = -2.816$

These RCI values are compared to the z value for the desired criterion, which is usually ± 1.96. In this example, the reduced score on the CES-D for Patient 1 is not reliable, but the change for Patient 2 is reliable, according to this RCI.

---

[7]As a measure intended to assess depression in a general population, the CES-D would not be used as an outcome for a clinical intervention. We use the scale in our example for illustrative purposes because the CES-D has been well described in this book.

Table 17.1	**Fictitious Scores for 10 Patients on the CES-D, Illustrating the Reliable Change Index**			
		Pretest		Posttest
Patient	T1 Week 1	T2 Week 2	12-Week Intervention	T3 Week 14[a]
1	18	17		14
2	16	19		**13**
3	27	24		20
4	20	21		**15**
5	19	22		**14**
6	19	19		16
7	17	18		**11**
8	26	29		**13**
9	22	20		16
10	26	24		**17**
Mean	21.0	21.3		14.9
SD	4.03	3.59		2.51

$\longleftarrow$ Test–Retest $\longrightarrow$ $\longleftarrow$ Assessment of Reliable Change $\longrightarrow$

Mean (SD) change for retest (T1–T2) $=$ $-.30$ (2.263), $t = 0.42, p = .69$

Mean (SD) change for trial (T2–T3) $=$ 6.4 (3.806), $t = 5.32, p < .001$

Test–retest reliability (T1–T2) $=$ .824 ($ICC_{Consistency}$)

$SEM = 3.592 \times \sqrt{(1 - .824)}$ $=$ 1.507

Denominator for RCI $=$ $\sqrt{2 \times 1.507^2} = 2.131$

RCI score to exceed at 95% CI $=$ $1.96 \times 2.131 = 4.18$

[a]Bolded values indicate that the pretest–posttest change was reliable (60% of the sample).

A more convenient way to draw conclusions about a reliable change for an entire sample is to calculate the change score value that must be exceeded. In this example, the cutoff value for 95% confidence is $\pm 1.96 \times 2.131 = \pm 4.18$. In Table 17.1, we can be 95% confident that 6 out of 10 patients had reliable improvements in CES-D scores between T2 and T3, as shown by the bolded values in the far right column.

The RCI has been reported as the most widely used index of reliable change in psychotherapy (Ogles, Lunnen, & Bonesteel, 2001), but it is not without controversy. The Jacobson–Truax (J–T) formula for calculating the RCI has been criticized by statisticians on several grounds, most notably that it fails to take regression toward the mean into account. At least five other RCI formula have been proposed (e.g., Hsu, 1989; Speer

& Greenbaum, 1995), but these have also been found to be problematic. Several studies have found, using either real data sets or simulations, that classifications of people in terms of reliable change are similar for different RCI formulas (e.g., Atkins, Bedics, McGlinchey& Beauchaine, 2005; Bauer, Lambert, & Nielsen, 2004). These findings have, in turn, led several writers to recommend the J–T approach because of its ease of calculation and history of use (e.g., Atkins et al., 2005; Lambert & Ogles, 2009).

Another controversy concerns the reliability parameter that should be used in estimating the *SEM*. In their paper, Jacobson and Truax (1991) used a test–retest reliability coefficient as the value of *R* in the formula for the *SEM* formula (formula 17.3). However, psychologists have long worried that the possibility of true change in the trait over a retest interval makes it risky to trust retest reliability coefficients, as discussed in Chapter 8. Consequently, several writers have asserted that the appropriate coefficient to use in the *SEM* formula for the RCI is Cronbach's alpha (e.g., Lambert & Ogles, 2009; Martinovich, Saunders, & Howard, 1996; Tingey, Lambert, Burlingame, & Hansen, 1996). Given that the RCI concerns the reliability of *change,* however, we agree with others in the medical field (e.g., DeVet et al., 2011; McHorney & Tarlov, 1995) in preferring a retest reliability coefficient in calculating the RCI because it is an index of how much random fluctuation over a short time period can be expected in a presumably stable trait. The importance of doing a retest study with rigor, including making evidence-based decisions about the retest interval, cannot be overemphasized (Polit, 2014).

17.2.c The Smallest Detectable Change Versus the Reliable Change Index

Cutoff values for a reliable change according to the SDC and RCI, when they are computed as described in the previous two sections, are similar but not identical. For example, for the data in Table 17.1, the RCI value that had to be exceeded for a change score to be deemed reliable was ±4.18. For the same data, the SDC cutoff is ±4.44. The disparity is the result of differences in what is used to capture variability in the *SEM* formula. For the SDC, the $SD_{\text{Difference}}$ is used—that is, the *SD* from two administrations of a measure. For the RCI, the *SD* recommended by Jacobson and Truax (1991) is from a single set of scores, such as baseline scores in a trial. In Chapter 10, we noted that in the context of a test–retest reliability assessment, it is better to use a *pooled SD*, rather than the *SD* from one administration or the other, in estimating *SEM*. With the data in Table 17.1, the *SEM* was calculated as 1.507 when the T2 *SD* was used because this administration was designated as the pretest. Had the *SD* from Time 1 been used, the *SEM* would have been calculated as 1.69. Using the pooled T1-T2 *SD*, the *SEM* would have been 1.60, which is exactly the same as the *SEM* based on the $SD_{\text{Difference}}$ ($2.263/\sqrt{2} = 1.60$).

When researchers calculate the value for the SDC for a measure, they typically rely on information from a sample of people other than their own. For example, in a clinical trial, the investigators depend on information provided by the instrument developers regarding retest reliability, the *SEM*, and the SDC because retest reliability is seldom recomputed in a trial. By contrast, the RCI is often computed using data from the research sample itself. If Cronbach's alpha is used as the reliability estimate, as is often the case among psychotherapists, then the *SEM* can be computed from the baseline administration of the measure, using alpha for R and SD_{Pretest} as the *SD* in formula 17.6. As noted earlier, we think it is more appropriate to estimate reliable change in relation to an assessment of measurement error from a retest study. However, unless retest reliability is reassessed, reliance on existing retest data for the SDC or the RCI means that it is essential to ensure the comparability of a research sample and the sample used to estimate the psychometric properties of the instrument.

17.2.d Alternative Confidence Intervals for Smallest Detectable Changes and Reliable Change Indexes

At the individual level, the detection of reliable change based on the standard SDC or RCI relies on a strict criterion for a change as "probably real": a 95% CI. In Table 17.1, for example, two patients improved their level of depression by 4 points on the CES-D following an intervention (Patients 3 and 9), but they were classified as not having reliably changed on the basis of the 95% CI for the RCI.

Several writers in the field of measurement have noted that the 95% CI sets a very stringent standard. For example, Cella, Bullinger, Scott, and Barofsky (2002), participating in a clinical significance meeting group, commented that "a reliable change index is conservative, only allowing classification as changed if the change exceeds a degree that would *only rarely* [emphasis added] be due to chance" (p. 386).

A study by Jordan, Dunn, Lewis, and Croft (2006) illustrates how such a stringent standard can result in seemingly anomalous results. These researchers studied change on the Roland Morris Disability Questionnaire (RMDQ) among patients with low back pain at baseline and 6 months after they began a treatment regimen. The researchers found that nearly two-thirds of the patients who described themselves as "completely recovered" on a global rating scale for back pain at the 6-month point did *not* meet 95% RCI criterion for reliable change on the RMDQ.

Because some researchers may be willing to infer a change as real with a lower degree of certainty, several researchers have used other standards for the SDC or RCI. In particular, several have adopted a 90% CI for calculating the SDC or RCI, which translates to a z-score of 1.65 rather than 1.96 (e.g., Hageman & Arrindell, 1999; Jordan et al., 2006; Stratford et al., 1996). In our example in Table 17.1, an RCI with a 90% CI would be: $1.65 \times 2.131 = 3.52$. With this level of confidence, Patients 3 and 9 would be classified as having improved reliably, meaning that 80% of the sample would now be classified as having experienced a true improvement following the intervention.

As we will see in Chapter 19, some researchers have proposed that a more liberal standard—1 standard error of measurement—be used in interpreting change scores.

17.3 Change Scores and Item Response Theory Models

Traditional approaches to assessing the reliability of change scores, such as those described in the previous section, suffer from a problem that we noted in Chapter 10 on measurement error. In classical test theory (CTT), the *SEM* is assumed to be the same for everyone, which is rarely the case. Measurement error tends to be lower for those in the middle of a score distribution than for those at the extremes. In our CES-D example in this chapter, we estimated that a change score of more than 4 points (using either the SDC or RCI) was needed to conclude that the depression scores were reliably changed with 95% CI, regardless of whether the baseline score was 40 or 20.

In IRT-derived measures, by contrast, the standard errors for different values of the latent trait theta (θ) can vary, and usually do. Because IRT offers greater measurement precision at the individual level, proponents argue that it is better suited than traditional methods to examining reliable change at the individual level.[8]

IRT methods are also considered preferable for measuring trait change in multi-item scales because of another characteristic mentioned in Chapter 6, namely that scales created using classical test theory approaches yield total scores that are not on a true interval scale. Figure 17.3 presents a *scale response curve* (SRC) that displays the relationship between latent trait levels (X axis) and expected raw scores (true scores) on a measure (Y axis). This SRC illustrates several things. First, the relationship between raw scores and theta levels is not linear. A 10-point change in raw scores from 40 to 50 is equal to only 0.5 logits on the trait continuum, but a 10-point change from 80 to 90 corresponds to a change of 1.5 logits on theta. This, in turn, shows that traditional sum-score scales are not especially well suited

---

[8]We note that these advantages of IRT apply only to unidimensional, multi-item, reflective scales. "Traditional" methods apply not only to CTT-derived scales but also apply to formative indexes and non-scaled measurements such as performance tests (e.g., the 6-minute walk test) and biophysiologic measures.

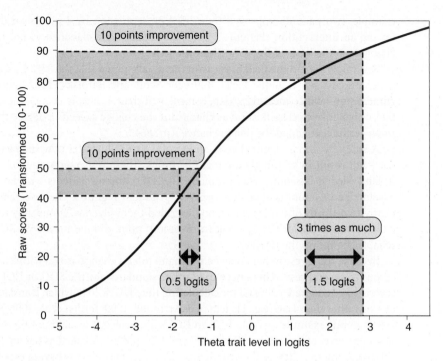

Figure 17.3

Example of a scale response curve showing relationship between theta and raw scores. (Adapted from Figure 2 in Cella and Chang [2000].)

to representing the *amount* of change present on the construct of interest. Second, the relationship between theta and raw scores is nearly linear in the midrange of theta, which corresponds to the range in which total test information is high. Raw scores at the extreme tend to be biased and may underestimate the magnitude of a change score. This is especially unfortunate because for many health measures, the goal is to move patients from an extreme score to a more moderate one (e.g., pain, physical dysfunction, depression).

Several different approaches for detecting reliable individual-level changes within an IRT framework have been developed (e.g., Embretson, 1991; Weiss & Kingsbury, 1984).[9] The one we describe here (the **Z-test**) has been found in simulations to perform well in terms of Type I error rates and power to detect change, compared to an alternative likelihood ratio test (Finkelman, Weiss, & Kim-Kang, 2010; Guo and Drasgow, 2010). The Z-test is used to test the null hypothesis that the value of the latent trait has not changed, against the alternative that it has:

$$H_0: \theta_1 = \theta_2 \qquad H_A: \theta_1 \neq \theta_2 \tag{17.7}$$

where θ_1 is the baseline or Time 1 score on the latent trait scale and θ_2 is the posttest or Time 2 score on the latent trait scale. The test statistic for testing the hypothesis is (Guo & Drasgow, 2010):

$$Z = \frac{\hat{\theta}_2 - \hat{\theta}_1}{\sqrt{SE_2{}^2 + SE_1{}^2}} \tag{17.8}$$

where $\hat{\theta}_i$ is the maximum likelihood estimator of θ_i (for i = T1 or T2), and SE_i is the standard error for a given value of θ_i. The null hypothesis is rejected for a specified level of

---

[9]This section does not describe the efforts that have been made to measure change in IRT models for groups. For a summary, see Kim-Kang and Weiss (2008).

confidence if the absolute value of Z is greater than the relevant z value (i.e., 1.96 for 95% confidence).

A few studies have directly compared change score reliability results for multi-item scales using this IRT approach compared to a traditional approach. For example, Brouwer, Meijer, and Zevalkink (2013) compared reliable change classification outcomes for the Beck Depression Inventory for standard summed total scores, using the RCI, and for IRT-based trait estimates, using the Z-test. Based on both the RCI and Z-test results, the researchers classified patients as reliably improved, reliably deteriorated, or not reliably changed. They found that 92% of the patients were classified in the same manner using the two approaches, but 8% were classified differently. For the RCI, any score change of 9 points or more was deemed reliable; with the Z-test, smaller changes (equivalent to raw score changes of six to eight points) could also be deemed reliable, which is consistent with the view that IRT methods are more sensitive to change.

As we saw in Chapter 6, IRT can place different people (or the same person at different points in time) on the same scale even when different items are used. This is the basis for computerized adaptive testing (CAT). When measuring change is a goal, CAT programs can be instructed to specifically select items to differentiate between θ_1 and θ_2 in what is called *adaptive measurement of change* (AMC). For example, Finkelman and colleagues (2010) used Z-tests to compare alternative item selection criteria at Time 2 measurements and found that using Time 1 responses to select Time 2 items improved the power to detect relatively small (true) changes in their simulations. Kim-Kang and Weiss (2008), in their simulations, compared AMC to various conventional testing methods. Conventional methods estimated individual change fairly well when the individual's trait level matched the difficulty of the test. AMC, however, was found to measure individual change at comparably high levels across the entire range of theta.

Thus, it may be expected that as more people become familiar and comfortable with IRT models, improvements in measuring and detecting change may be realized.

17.4   Reporting Reliability of Change Information

In Chapter 10, we urged researchers who develop a new instrument to report information about measurement error. We also think it is useful to provide potential users of a CTT-based instrument with information about the SDC (or the RCI), which is easy to calculate once the *SEM* is estimated.

Reporting the SDC is fairly common in measurement papers in the fields of sports and rehabilitation medicine and physical therapy. For example, Reurink and colleagues (2013) evaluated the psychometric properties of the Active Knee Extension Test (AKET) and Passive Knee Extension Test (PKET) for monitoring recovery after a hamstring injury. They reported that the SDC was 15 degrees for the AKET and 21 degrees for the PKET. Reporting the SDC appears to be less common in psychometric papers for PROs, but such information may prove useful to potential users of an instrument. For IRT-derived measures, there is no single number that summarizes the amount of change needed to be considered real, but scale developers should consider presenting some examples. For instance, reports on a new IRT-derived scale could report the value of Z (for a specified confidence level) at key theta levels, such as -1.0, 0.0, and 1.0, or at theta levels considered to be critical cutpoints for decision makers.

References

Albrecht, G. L., & Devlieger, P. J. (1999). The disability paradox: High quality of life against all odds. *Social Science and Medicine, 48,* 977–988.

Atkins, D. C., Bedics, J., McGlinchey, J., & Beauchaine, T. (2005). Assessing clinical significance: Does it matter which method we use? *Journal of Consulting and Clinical Psychology, 73,* 982–989.

Barclay-Goddard, R., Epstein, J., & Mayo, N. (2009). Response shift: A brief overview and proposed research priorities. *Quality of Life Research*, *18*, 335–346.

Barnett, A. G., van der Pols, J., & Dobson, A. (2005). Regression to the mean: What it is and how to deal with it. *International Journal of Epidemiology*, *34*, 215–220.

Bauer, S., Lambert, M., & Nielsen, S. (2004). Clinical significance methods: A comparison of statistical techniques. *Journal of Personality Assessment*, *82*, 60–70.

Brouwer, D., Meijer, R., & Zevalkink, J. (2013). Measuring individual significant change on the Beck Depression Inventory-II through IRT-based statistics. *Psychotherapy Research*, *23*, 489–501.

Cella, D., Bullinger, M., Scott, C., & Barofsky, I. (2002). Group vs. individual approaches to understanding the clinical significance of differences or changes in quality of life. *Mayo Clinic Proceedings*, *77*, 384–392.

Cella, D., & Chang, C. (2000). A discussion of item response theory and its applications in health assessment. *Medical Care*, *38*(9, Suppl.), II66–II72.

De Boer, M., DeVet, H. C. W., Terwee, C., Moll, A., Völker-Dieben, H., & van Rens, G. (2005). Changes to the subscales of two vision-related quality of life questionnaires are proposed. *Journal of Clinical Epidemiology*, *58*, 1260–1268.

DeVet, H. C. W., Terwee, C., Mokkink, L. B., & Knol, D. L. (2011). *Measurement in medicine: A practical guide*. Cambridge, MA: Cambridge University Press.

Dudley, W. N., McGuire, D., Peterson, D., & Wong, B. (2009). Application of multilevel growth curve analysis in cancer treatment toxicities: The exemplar of oral mucositis and pain. *Oncology Nursing Forum*, *36*, E11–E19.

Embretson, S. E. (1991). A multidimensional latent trait model for measuring learning and change. *Psychometrika*, *56*, 495–515.

Finkelman, M. D., Weiss, D., & Kim-Kang, G. (2010). Item selection and hypothesis testing for the adaptive measurement of change. *Applied Psychological Measurement*, *34*, 238–254.

Groenvold, M., Fayers, P. M., Sprangers, M., Bjorner, J., Klee, M., Aaronson, N., . . . Mouridsen, H. (1999). Anxiety and depression in breast cancer patients at low risk of recurrence compared with the general population. *Journal of Clinical Epidemiology*, *52*, 523–530.

Guo, J., & Drasgow, F. (2010). Identifying cheating on unproctored Internet tests: The Z-test and the likelihood ratio test. *International Journal of Selection and Assessment, 18*, 351–364

Hageman, W. J., & Arrindell, W. (1999). Establishing clinically significant change: increment of precision and the distinction between individual and group level of analysis. *Behaviour Research and Therapy*, *37*, 1169–1193.

Hsu, L. M. (1989). Reliable changes in psychotherapy: Taking into account regression toward the mean. *Behavioral Assessment*, *11*, 459–467.

Jacobson, N. S., Follette, W. C., & Revenstorf, D. (1984). Psychotherapy outcome research: Methods for reporting variability and evaluating clinical significance. *Behavior Therapy*, *15*, 336–352.

Jacobson, N. S., & Truax, P. (1991). Clinical significance: A statistical approach to defining meaningful change in psychotherapy research. *Journal of Consulting and Clinical Psychology*, *59*, 12–19.

Jordan, K., Dunn, K., Lewis, M., & Croft, P. (2006). A minimal clinically important difference was derived for the Roland Morris Disability Questionnaire for low back pain. *Journal of Clinical Epidemiology*, *59*, 45–52.

Kim-Kang, G., & Weiss, D. J. (2008). Adaptive measurement of individual change. *Zeitschripft für Psychologie/ Journal of Psychology*, *216*, 49–58.

Lambert, M. L., & Ogles, B. (2009). Using clinical significance in psychotherapy outcome research: The need for a common procedure and validity data. *Psychotherapy Research*, *19*, 493–501.

Martinovich, Z., Saunders, S., & Howard, K. (1996). Some comments on "assessing clinical significance." *Psychotherapy Research*, *6*, 124–132.

McHorney, C. A., & Tarlov, A. R. (1995). Individual-patient monitoring in clinical practice: Are available health status surveys adequate? *Quality of Life Research*, *4*, 293–307.

Meyer, T., Richter, S., & Raspe, H. (2013). Agreement between pre-post measures of change and transition ratings as well as then-tests. *BMC Medical Research Methodology*, *13*, 52.

Middel, B., de Greef, M., de Jongste, M., Crijns, H., Stewart, R., & van den Heuvel, W. (2002). Why don't we ask patients with coronary heart disease directly how much they have changed after treatment? *Journal of Cardiopulmonary Rehabilitation*, *22*, 47–52.

Mokkink, L. B., Terwee, C., Patrick, D., Alonso, J., Stratford, P., Knol, D. L., . . . DeVet, H. C. W. (2010). The COSMIN study reached international consensus on taxonomy, terminology, and definitions of measurement properties for health-related patient-reported outcomes. *Journal of Clinical Epidemiology*, *63*, 737–745.

Ogles, B. M., Lunnen, K. M., & Bonesteel, K. (2001). Clinical significance: History, application, and current practice. *Clinical Psychology Review*, *21*, 421–446.

Polit, D. F. (2014). Getting serious about test–retest reliability: A critique of retest research and some recommendations. *Quality of Life Research*, *23*(6), 1713–1720.

Radloff, L. S. (1977). The CES-D scale: A self-report depression scale for research in the general population. *Applied Psychological Measurement*, *1*, 385–401.

Rapkin, B. D., & Schwartz, C. E. (2004). Toward a theoretical model of quality-of-life assessment in light of response shift and appraisal. *Health and Quality of Life Outcomes*, *2*, 14.

Reurink, G., Goudswaard, G., Oomen, H., Moen, M., Tol, J., Verhaar, J., & Weir, A. (2013). Reliability of the active and passive knee extension test in acute hamstring injuries. *American Journal of Sports Medicine, 41*, 1757–1761.

Ross, M. (1989). Relation of implicit theories to the construction of personal histories. *Psychological Review, 96*, 341–347.

Schmitt, J., & DiFabio, R. P. (2005). The validity of prospective and retrospective global change criterion measures. *Archives of Physical Medicine and Rehabilitation, 86*, 2270–2276.

Schwartz, C. E., & Sprangers, M. A. G. (1999). Methodological approaches for assessing response shift in longitudinal health related quality of life research. *Social Science and Medicine, 48*, 1531–1548.

Schwartz, C. E., & Sprangers, M. A. G. (2010). Guidelines for improving the stringency of response shift research using the then test. *Quality of Life Research, 19*, 455–464.

Senn, S. (2006). Change from baseline and analysis of covariance revisited. *Statistics in Medicine, 25*, 4334–4344.

Speer, D. C. (1992). Clinically significant change: Jacobson & Truax (1991) revisited. *Journal of Consulting and Clinical Psychology, 60*, 1044–1048.

Speer, D. C., & Greenbaum, P. E. (1995). Five methods for computing significant individual client change and improvement rates: Support for an individual growth curve approach. *Journal of Consulting and Clinical Psychology, 63*, 1044–1048.

Stratford, P. W., Binkley, J., Solomon, P., Finch, E., Gill, C., & Moreland, J. (1996). Defining the minimum level of detectable change for the Roland Morris Questionnaire. *Physical Therapy, 76*, 359–365.

Swartz, R., Schwartz, C., Basch, E., Cai, L., Fairclough, D., McLeod, L., . . . Rapkin, B. (2011). The king's foot of patient-reported outcomes: Current practices and new developments for the measurement of change. *Quality of Life Research, 20*, 1159–1167.

Tingey, R. C., Lambert, M. J., Burlingame, G., & Hansen, N. (1996). Assessing clinical significance: Proposed extensions to the method. *Psychotherapy Research, 6*, 109–123.

Van Breukelen, G. J. (2006). ANCOVA versus change from baseline: More power in randomized studies, more bias in nonrandomized studies. *Journal of Clinical Epidemiology, 59*, 920–925.

Vernon, H., & Mior, S. (1991). The Neck Disability Index: A study of reliability and validity. *Journal of Manipulative and Physiological Therapeutics, 14*, 409–415.

Vickers, A. J., & Altman, D. G. (2001). Analysing controlled trials with baseline and follow-up measurements. *BMJ, 323*, 1123–1124.

Weiss, D. J., & Kingsbury, G. (1984). Application of computerized adaptive testing to educational problems. *Journal of Educational Measurement, 21*, 361–375.

18 Responsiveness

Chapter Outline

In this chapter, we discuss the measurement property called *responsiveness*—a property that has given rise to extensive debate, controversy, and confusion. Responsiveness is defined and operationalized in many different ways in the medical and psychometric literature. Indeed, Terwee, Dekker, Wiersinga, Prummel, and Bossuyt (2003) did a systematic review of the quality-of-life literature more than a decade ago and found 25 definitions of responsiveness and 31 ways to assess it. We follow Consensus-based Standards for the selection of health Measurement Instruments' (COSMIN) definition in the hope that momentum will build for greater definitional uniformity in the measurement literature.

18.1 Basics of Responsiveness

Similar to COSMIN (Mokkink et al., 2010), we define the measurement property of **responsiveness** as the ability of a measure to detect change over time in a construct that has changed, commensurate with the amount of change that has occurred. Just as the measurement property of reliability can be extended to apply to change scores (Chapter 17), the measurement property of responsiveness represents the extension of validity over time. Validity concerns whether a measure is truly capturing the intended construct, and responsiveness concerns whether a change score is truly capturing a change in the construct.

Our definition of responsiveness differs from that of COSMIN in only one small respect. COSMIN's definition specifies that a responsive measure is capable of detecting change in a construct that has changed. We add the notion of *commensurate* change. If there is a large change over time in the amount of the construct, then the scores on a measure of the construct should not just change, they should change to a corresponding degree.

18.1.a The History of Responsiveness as a Measurement Property

Psychometricians have resisted adding a third measurement property to the well-established properties of reliability and validity. The term *responsiveness*—and other related terms, such as *sensitivity*—do not appear in any of the classic or even more recent psychometric textbooks (e.g., DeVellis, 2012; Furr & Bacharach, 2014; Nunnally & Bernstein, 1994; Rust & Golombok, 2009). The authors of a widely used book on constructing health scales (Streiner & Norman, 2008) specifically rejected the need for a separate property, preferring to consider responsiveness as an aspect of construct validity, namely longitudinal construct validity.

Clinimetricians, however, have long taken a broader view than psychometricians regarding criteria for evaluating clinical measures, especially patient reported outcomes, or PROs (Chapter 7). Feinstein (1987) proposed the overarching concept of *sensibility* for evaluating scales and indexes, and he argued that one important aspect of sensibility is a measure's *sensitivity to change*. Early clinimetric writers were critical of the standard psychometric approach to scale construction for several reasons. One of these reasons was the absence of attention to the desirability of being *sensitive* to change during item development and scale construction (e.g., Wright & Feinstein, 1992).

Gordon Guyatt and his colleagues appear to have been the first to suggest using the term *responsiveness* (Guyatt, Bombardier, & Tugwell, 1986; Guyatt, Walter, & Norman, 1987; Kirshner & Guyatt, 1985). These researchers specifically noted a preference for *responsiveness* in lieu of *sensitivity* as a way to avoid confusion because the latter term has another meaning (i.e., sensitivity vs. specificity in diagnostic accuracy).[1] Guyatt, however, defined responsiveness differently than the COSMIN group. Specifically, Guyatt and his colleagues (1987) identified responsiveness as "the ability to detect minimal clinically important differences" (p. 171). Several important measurement papers (e.g., Liang, 2000) have adopted this definition.

In the years following Guyatt's use of the term, responsiveness gained considerable popularity as a measurement property, especially among quality-of-life researchers. Yet, there has been little agreement about what it is or how to know when it has been achieved. The proliferation of definitions and assessment methods led several writers to suggest ways to organize the burgeoning literature. For example, Beaton, Bombardier, Katz, and Wright (2001) proposed a taxonomy that classified responsiveness approaches on three dimensions: What (definition of responsiveness), Who (individuals or groups), and Which (between- vs. within-subjects approaches). Terwee and colleagues (2003), in their review of responsiveness in the quality of life literature, organized the myriad definitions of responsiveness into three major groupings: as a measure's ability to detect (1) a change, in general; (2) clinically important change; or (3) a true change in the construct being measured.[2] Testa and Simonson (1996) appear to be among the earliest to have espoused this third way of describing responsiveness.

---

[1] The term *responsiveness* is also potentially problematic because it suggests a change in *response* to an intervention when, in fact, a true change on a health construct could be the result of progressive deterioration, aging, or development.
[2] Liang (2000) and Liang, Lew, Stucki, Fortin, and Daltroy (2002) called the ability to detect change *sensitivity* and the ability to detect clinically important change *responsiveness*, adding yet another twist to the definitional turmoil that has characterized this literature.

The COSMIN panel achieved consensus in defining responsiveness in this third manner (i.e., as the *validity* of change scores). Like the COSMIN group, we think it is essential to distinguish whether a change score is a valid reflection of a construct that has changed over time from whether a change simply has occurred or whether it can be interpreted as clinically meaningful, which relates to interpretation and not to a measurement property. Of course, responsiveness—and change score reliability (Chapter 17)—are preconditions for a change to be considered clinically important. Interpretive aspects of change scores are discussed in Chapter 19.

18.1.b Responsiveness and Validity

In several respects, there is some merit to the argument made by Streiner and Norman (2008) and others (e.g., Hays & Hadorn, 1992) that a separately named measurement property to denote longitudinal construct validity is unnecessary. Construct validity and responsiveness share many features in common, the main difference being the time frame. As we shall see later in this chapter, the methods used to assess responsiveness (as we define it) overlap considerably with methods used to assess validity, particularly with regard to the methods discussed in Chapters 12 (criterion validity) and 13 (hypothesis-testing construct validity).

Validity and responsiveness are similar in another way: They are both challenging to assess. Assessments require creativity, firm knowledge of the construct, and technical and substantive skills. Furthermore, both responsiveness and validity rely on ongoing evidence building. The more evidence that can be brought to bear on a measure's responsiveness, the greater the confidence one has in the measure's capacity to capture true change in a construct. Evidence for responsiveness—as with construct validity—can be generated not only by the researchers who developed the measure but also by subsequent users.

This evidence-building feature of both cross-sectional and longitudinal validity (responsiveness) means that there is no single number to quantify its value. With reliability, new instrument developers (in the classical test theory [CTT] tradition) strive for an intraclass correlation coefficient (ICC) of a given magnitude (e.g., greater than .70) as evidence that the measure is reliable and scores are reproducible in stable subjects from a specified population (Chapter 8). If an instrument's retest reliability is reevaluated with representative samples from the same population and for the same retest interval, it would be expected that the ICC value would be similar. In a systematic review of an instrument's measurement properties, one can compute a pooled ICC for a defined population. By contrast, there is no single validity coefficient for an instrument. Evidence for a measure's validity typically comes from a variety of different statistical methods, which often cannot be compared and are not viewed as indicating a *magnitude* of validity (e.g., *t* tests and area under the curve for known-groups validity). Even within a given statistical method, such as correlations coefficients, the values usually vary in magnitude and direction because the focal measure's relationship with measures of different constructs would not be expected to be comparable.

For those who follow COSMIN's path of defining responsiveness as longitudinal validity, it follows that there is no single responsiveness coefficient that can summarize the extent to which a measure is responsive. Yet, much effort has been put into developing "responsiveness coefficients." Debates have raged about the merits of various coefficients and about the design of studies in which they are computed (e.g., Husted, Cook, Farewell, & Gladman, 2000; Norman, Wyrwich, & Patrick, 2007; Terwee et al., 2003; Zou, 2005). We discuss these so-called responsiveness coefficients later in this chapter, but we see them more as providing supportive evidence of responsiveness in the context of hypothesis tests, rather than as indexes whose values encapsulate the degree of responsiveness a measure has.

Despite the similarities and overlap between responsiveness and validity, we support the use of the term responsiveness as a separate measurement property because having a designated property encourages instrument developers to pay attention to it. Although psychometricians may argue against a separate label, the truth is that relatively few psychological or educational measures undergo an assessment for longitudinal validity. This may reflect the fact that many psychological traits are fairly stable attributes (e.g., intelligence, personality). Yet, many psychological constructs, such as depression or anxiety, are amenable to change and indeed are often targeted for improvement in health interventions. Thus, it seems useful to designate responsiveness as a separate measurement property of importance to health care practitioners because it reminds instrument developers and instrument users to worry about it and seek evidence that it is adequate when drawing conclusions about an instrument's quality.

18.1.c Methods of Assessing Responsiveness

Because of differences in the way responsiveness has been defined, researchers have adopted greatly diverse methods to assess responsiveness. For example, those who have defined responsiveness as the ability of a measure to detect change (in general) often use tests of statistical significance as evidence of responsiveness (e.g., paired t tests) as well as various effect size indexes.

Terwee and colleagues (2003) identified more than a dozen approaches to assessing responsiveness by those who defined it as the ability to detect a *clinically important* change. Some of these methods will be discussed in the next chapter because—like the COSMIN group—we think the concept of "clinically important change" involves the interpretation of a change score, not its validity.

Using the COSMIN definition of responsiveness, assessment options are more clearly circumscribed. The two main approaches, as articulated by the COSMIN group (DeVet, Terwee, Mokkink, & Knol, 2011), are the criterion-related approach when there is a gold standard for the measure and the construct-related approach when there is not. The next two sections describe these approaches and provide examples of their use.

Instrument developers would likely benefit from thinking about responsiveness early in the development process, not simply at the stage of formal instrument assessment. If it is anticipated that an instrument will be used to monitor or evaluate change, then thought ought to be given to responsiveness when items are being created and refined. Change scores on a multi-item scale cannot be expected to correspond to a true change on the focal construct if the scale items are not amenable to change. Guyatt, Deyo, Charlson, Levine, and Mitchell (1989) noted the importance of thinking about responsiveness while the item pool is being created. They gave as an example an item such as "I have attempted suicide" on a scale to measure emotional function. Such an item may work well on scales that will be used only for cross-sectional measurement, but it is an item that inherently will constrain responsiveness: If a person answers that he or she has attempted suicide prior to treatment, then he or she would logically have to report that he or she had attempted suicide at the posttest, regardless of the efficacy of the treatment or the amount of improvement in emotional function.

This is partly a content-related responsiveness issue, and so strategies that we described relating to content validity (Chapter 11) could also be adopted to enhance responsiveness. For example, the conceptualization of the construct should encompass ways in which the construct might evolve or be altered over time, and a conceptual map could delineate factors presumed to bring about changes in the construct, which in turn could have implications for item creation.

Another strategy involves getting feedback from clinical experts. For example, a panel of experts could be asked to rate each item on a scale for the degree to which it might be responsive to health trajectories or health interventions, analogous to a formal content validity assessment. Although we could find no examples of studies in which expert feedback regarding the responsiveness of individual *items* was sought, there are examples of expert opinion regarding the responsiveness of entire measures. For example, Goreshi and colleagues (2012) compared two scales to measure skin severity for cutaneous dermatomyositis, both of which required observational ratings by dermatologists. At the end of the study, the 10 physicians who completed ratings were asked to assess the two scales, including which of the two might be more effective in terms of responsiveness to treatment.

18.2   The Criterion Approach to Responsiveness Assessment

Like criterion validation (Chapter 12), the criterion approach to responsiveness requires a gold standard—a well-established and reliable criterion that indicates that a change in the target construct has occurred. Husted and colleagues (2000) refer to this approach as *external responsiveness* because there is an external criterion, and it has also been called an anchor-based approach, with the criterion serving as the anchor.

18.2.a   Responsiveness Assessed by Changes in a Criterion

A criterion-based assessment of responsiveness can involve an examination of the relationship between changes on the target measure and changes on the criterion, which corresponds directly to a longitudinal assessment of criterion validity. As discussed in Chapter 12, it can be challenging to identify gold standard criteria for PRO measures. PROs (self-reports) have been developed to measure constructs that vary along a continuum from highly subjective (e.g., how patients *feel*) to more objective (e.g., what patients *do*).[3] PROs that are toward the objective end of this continuum can often be validated against a reliable gold standard, including laboratory or physiologic measures, clinician ratings, or other PROs. It follows that *changes* in the focal measure can be assessed against *changes* in the gold standard. The implicit hypothesis in such a responsiveness assessment is that change scores on the focal measure are consistent with or correlated with change scores on the criterion. When formal testing supports such a hypothesis, then evidence of the focal measure's responsiveness (longitudinal validity) is obtained.

We offer a hypothetical example based on an elaboration of one of the criterion validity studies listed in Table 12.1 (p. 184). De Vriendt and colleagues (2011) tested the criterion validity of the Adolescent Stress Questionnaire (ASQ) by testing its relationship to a criterion, wake-up salivary cortisol levels. To test the responsiveness of the ASQ using the criterion approach, one could examine the relationship between *changes* in scores on the ASQ following a therapeutic intervention (for example) against *changes* in cortisol levels from baseline to posttest. In this example, it is not the intervention that is being tested; the treatment could be modestly or highly effective. What is at issue is the degree to which changes on the focal measure are mirrored by changes on the criterion.

In this approach to responsiveness assessment, as with validity assessments, the proper statistical approach for analyzing relationships depends on the measurement level of change scores on the focal measure and the criterion (see Table 18.1). In the ASQ-cortisol example, correlation analysis (or regression analysis) would be appropriate because the scores and change scores for both variables are continuous.

In other situations, receiver operating characteristic (ROC) curve analysis or other statistical approaches are suitable. As a hypothetical example of a criterion-based responsiveness assessment using ROC curve analysis, Cornelius, Groothoff, van der Klink, and Brouwer (2013) assessed the criterion validity of the Kessler Psychological Distress Scale against a *Diagnostic and Statistical Manual of Mental Disorders* 4th edition (*DSM-IV*) disorder using the Composite International Diagnostic Interview (CIDI) as the gold standard. To assess responsiveness, one could plot change scores on the Kessler scale against the sensitivity and specificity for a changed mental disorder diagnosis (unchanged versus improved) on the CIDI following therapy.

Schatz, Zeriger, Yang, Chen, and Kosinski (2011) provided an example of a criterion-based responsiveness assessment in a study that focused on the Asthma Impact Survey (AIS-6), a brief disease-specific quality of life instrument. The researchers tested the scale's criterion validity by examining correlations between the AIS-6 with the longer "gold standard" scale,

---

[3]Experts in response shift have called attention to these differences in PROs and have noted that highly subjective PROs are especially susceptible to response shift (e.g., Schwartz & Rapkin, 2004; Schwartz & Sprangers, 2010).

| Table 18.1 | Parameters for Responsiveness by Measurement Levels for Focal Measure Change Score and (Change) Score on a Gold Standard or Measure of a Relevant Construct |

Measurement Level: Focal Measure Change Score[a]			Measurement Level: Gold Standard or Construct Change Score[b]			
Nominal	Ordinal	Continuous	Nominal	Ordinal	Continuous	Responsiveness Parameter
X			X			Sensitivity/specificity; predictive values; phi coefficient; kappa
	X		X			Area under the curve (AUC)—ROC analysis; Mann–Whitney U test
		X	X			*Between groups:* Area under the curve (AUC)—ROC analysis; independent groups t test/ANOVA/ANCOVA; logistic regression; effect size indexes (e.g., $ES_{Between}$, $SRM_{Between}$)[c]
		X	X			*Within groups:* Paired t test; repeated measures ANOVA; effect size indexes (e.g., ES_{Within}, SRM_{Within}, GRI)[c]
	X			X		Spearman's rho
		X			X	Pearson's r; multiple regression

[a]Or, for within-group designs, the measurement level of the Time 1 and Time 2 scores.
[b]The change score for the gold standard (criterion-related responsiveness) or for a measure of a relevant construct (construct-related responsiveness) is usually the difference between measurements made at two points in time but can also be change measured directly using a health transition question (global rating scale).
[c]ES, effect size index (Cohen's d); SRM, standardized response mean; GRI, Guyatt Responsiveness Index.

the mini-Asthma Quality of Life Questionnaire (mAQLQ), and found correlations of the expected magnitude and direction ($-.85$). They reported that responsiveness was demonstrated by significant correlations between changes in AIS-6 scores and changes in mAQLQ scores ($-.58$) 5 months after baseline. The researchers also assessed responsiveness by comparing the mean change scores on the AIS-6 for three groups of patients: those whose change scores on the criterion (the mAQLQ) had improved, stayed the same, or worsened. The mean AIS-6 change scores for the three subgroups were -7.0, -0.5, and $+5.6$, respectively, and the analysis of variance (ANOVA) was significant ($F = 280.5, p < .0001$).

Revicki et al. (2006) and Revicki, Hays, Cella, and Sloan (2008) have urged measurement researchers to use multiple criteria in their assessments of responsiveness, if possible. The triangulation of evidence, both within a study and over multiple studies, is a key aspect of establishing a "portfolio" to support an inference of a measure's responsiveness. In some cases, however, only one "gold standard" criterion might be available.

Please rate the changes you have experienced in the past three months with regard to *your ability to perform regular activities of daily living*, such as standing up from a sitting position or taking a bath or shower:

1. Very much better
2. Much better
3. A little better
4. No change
5. A little worse
6. Much worse
7. Very much worse

Shaded response options show one possible cutpoint on the criterion: Responses 1-3 (any improvement) versus 4-7 (no improvement)

Figure 18.1

Example of a global rating scale for a criterion-related approach to assessing responsiveness.

18.2.b Global Rating Scales as the Criterion

DeVet and others from the COSMIN group (2011) proposed a different strategy for criterion-based responsiveness testing. Arguing that PROs seldom have gold standards, they suggested that an acceptable gold standard might be a single-item **global rating scale** or **GRS** (also known as a **health transition rating** or a *global rating of change* [GRC]). As discussed in Chapter 17, a health transition question or GRS involves asking patients[4] to rate directly the degree to which their status on the focal construct has been altered over a time interval in which change is presumed to have occurred for at least some people. The adjective "global" is somewhat misleading in this context: As a criterion, the GRS should involve ratings of the same *specific* health construct as the measure being assessed for responsiveness. (If a *general* transition rating regarding overall health is used to assess responsiveness, this might better be classified as a construct approach, which we discuss in the next section).

Figure 18.1 provides an example of such a GRS, which asks patients to rate changes in their ability to perform activities of daily living. For example, such a transition question could be asked of patients several months after hip replacement surgery. Note that this GRS does not ask about changes to the patient's general health but rather about changes on a specific construct that is relevant for assessing the responsiveness of a physical function or Activities of Daily Living (ADL) scale.

Response options to such global rating scales are often on a 5- or 7-point scale, but there are examples in the literature of GRSs with as few as 3 response options and as many as 15 (e.g., Eurich, Johnson, Reid, & Spertus, 2006). In the example shown in Figure 18.1, we used a 7-point scale that asks patients to rate changes in the ability to perform ADL, from *very much better* (1) through *no change* (4) to *very much worse* (7) over a 3-month period.

Let us suppose we were assessing the responsiveness of a physical function scale, such as the Western Ontario and McMaster Universities Osteoarthritis Index or WOMAC (Bellamy, 2012). We might administer the WOMAC just prior to hip replacement surgery and then 3 months later. At the 3-month point, patients would also be asked to complete the GRS as shown in Figure 18.1. Several statistical approaches could then be used to test the responsiveness of the WOMAC. For example, the mean WOMAC change scores could be compared for patients who said they had any improvement on the GRS (response options 1, 2, or 3) and patients who did not report improvements (response options 4 to 7), using an

---

[4]Ratings of perceived change by patients have usually been preferred to ratings by clinicians, especially for constructs on which the patient is considered the "expert," such as quality of life. However, for constructs for which there are objective indicators of improvement or deterioration, clinician's ratings may be appropriate. In an early study of responsiveness involving the Sickness Impact Profile, Deyo and Inui (1984) classified patients as improved, unchanged, or deteriorated if *both* patients and clinicians independently gave the same ratings.

independent groups *t* test. Alternatively, change scores could be plotted on an ROC curve against the sensitivity and specificity for predicting the GRS criterion: improved versus did not improve. The analysis is not focused on establishing a cutpoint but rather on evaluating the ability of the change scores to distinguish those who have improved from those who have not, and hence the area under the curve (AUC) is the measure of responsiveness. With such an ROC analysis, the hypothesis being tested is that the AUC is equal to or greater than a designated amount, such as .70.

Several research teams have used a GRS as a criterion for responsiveness. For example, Freeman and colleagues (2013) evaluated the comparative responsiveness of four measures of mobility in people with multiple sclerosis. The measures included two performance-based measures (the 6-minute walk test [6MWT] and walking velocity) and two PROs (the Rivermead Mobility Index and the MS Walking Scale). Patients were tested at baseline and then at two subsequent annual visits. At the follow-up points, patients also completed eight transition questions that asked for ratings of change on specific aspects of mobility (e.g., general mobility, sitting balance, standing balance) on a 7-point scale from *much better* to *much worse*. Responsiveness was assessed by correlating change scores on the four focal measures with the GRS rating on the relevant transition question. The researchers set their standard of responsiveness as an $r \geq .35$. The only measure that met this criterion was the 6MWT. For example, the correlation between change scores on the 6MWT and the GRS ratings for general mobility was .50.

This GRS approach can lend supporting evidence of responsiveness, but it is not an ideal approach. Although a GRS has face validity and clinimetric appeal, it is problematic as a gold standard. Indeed, if a GRS *were* a gold standard, there would be little apparent reason for developing the focal scale because nothing could be more economical, efficient, or undemanding of patients than a single change question. However, a single item is seldom sufficiently reliable. A person who responded *much better* one day might respond *very much better* the next day, even when the degree of improvement had not changed. Multi-item scales are useful precisely because they are more reliable than one question. The reliability and validity of global rating scales are seldom evaluated (Norman et al., 1997).

Another problem with the GRS is that such direct change items suffer from recall bias. As discussed in Chapter 17, people appear to be more affected by their present state than their prior state in responding to direct questions about change. Thus, a GRS appears to be susceptible to various types of measurement error.

To our knowledge, no one has suggested using a single-item GRS as a "gold standard" for cross-sectional criterion validity. For example, consider a researcher developing a depression scale. If the researcher did a criterion validation of the scale using as the criterion a single GRS item that asked people to rate their current level of depression on a 7-point scale from *highly depressed* to *not at all depressed*, few people would consider the resulting analysis as sufficient evidence of the scale's validity. Similarly, a GRS transition item is a weak criterion for assessing the longitudinal validity of a measure.

Thus, we would argue that if the GRS approach is used to assess responsiveness, it should be supplemented with other strategies, including ones discussed in Section 18.2.a or in the next section on construct-based methods. For example, in Freeman et al.'s (2013) study of comparative responsiveness in four mobility measures, they used the criterion approach using eight transition items, but they also used methods we describe as construct-based. They concluded that their results were more sensible using the latter methods and noted various deficiencies in their GRS anchor.

18.3   The Construct Approach to Responsiveness Assessment

When there is no gold standard criterion, researchers must use other methods to assess responsiveness, just as is the case for validity assessment.

18.3.a Different "Types" of Construct-Based Responsiveness

The construct approach to evaluating a measure's longitudinal validity (responsiveness) is analogous to the hypothesis-testing construct validation approach described in Chapter 13. In brief, the researcher must develop and test hypotheses about changes on the focal measure in relation to other phenomena. Sometimes, the hypotheses concern a change on the construct that is expected to occur, such as a change resulting from a treatment of well-established efficacy. Alternatively, the hypotheses concern the nature and magnitude of the relationship between changes on the focal measure on the one hand and changes on measures of constructs that are theoretically linked to the construct of interest on the other.

Using the COSMIN (and our) definition of responsiveness, a construct-based assessment can be a simple extension of construct validation. An example comes from the development of the Food Allergy Quality of Life Questionnaire-Parent Form (FAQLQ-PF), which is a parent-reported measure of the quality of life in children ages 0 to 12 years with food allergies. Construct validity was assessed, in part, by correlating scores on the FAQLQ-PF with scores on a measure of parent's expectations of outcome for a child with a food allergy, the Food Allergy Independent Measure or FAIM (DunnGalvin, Flokstra-de Blok, Burks, Dubois, & Hourihane, 2008). In the assessment of responsiveness, DunnGalvin and colleagues (2010) examined the correlation between *changes* on the FAQLQ-PF and *changes* on the FAIM following a food challenge for diagnosing a food allergy. The correlation of the two change scores from baseline (prechallenge) to a 2-month postdiagnosis follow-up was .70, and the correlation between baselines to 6-month follow-up change scores was .65.

When hypotheses are developed about how changes in a focal measure are related to other measures, a full array of strategies and analytic methods can be used, analogous to those described in Chapter 13. For example, some hypotheses are designed to support what might be called *convergent responsiveness*, the degree to which change scores on the focal measure are correlated with change scores on a measure of a construct with which a relationship is hypothesized, as in the DunnGalvin et al. (2010) example. Similarly, it would be possible to hypothesize that changes on the focal construct, as assessed through change scores on the focal measure, are *not* associated (or only weakly associated) with changes on another, unrelated measure (*divergent responsiveness*). Another option is *known-groups responsiveness*, the longitudinal extension of known-groups (discriminative) validity. In this approach, researchers test the hypothesis that changes on the focal measure are different for two or more groups known (or hypothesized) to have different amounts of change.

As an example of a "known-groups" analysis, McCaskey, Ettlin, and Shuster (2013) assessed the responsiveness of change scores on the German version of the Whiplash Disability Questionnaire (WDQ). Measurements on the WDQ were obtained upon entry into an inpatient rehabilitation program and then at discharge 3 to 4 weeks later. At discharge, patients were also asked to rate on a 5-point scale the degree to which their health in general had changed "compared to before your rehabilitation therapy" (p. 3). Two groups were created based on responses to the GRS: those who had improved and those who had not. Then, change scores on the WDQ were plotted against sensitivity and specificity for accurately classifying patients as improved or not improved. An AUC greater than .70 was obtained, which the researchers interpreted as evidence of responsiveness. Commendably, further support for the WDQ's responsiveness was obtained by convergent evidence. Change scores on the WDQ correlated significantly with change scores for measures of other relevant constructs, such as the bodily pain subscale of the SF-36 ($r = .50$), a visual analog scale for pain ($r = .74$), and the North American Spine Societies Questionnaire ($r = .69$).

18.3.b Responsiveness and Statistical Analysis

As noted earlier, Terwee and colleagues (2003) identified numerous statistical methods that have been used to evaluate a measure's responsiveness. The appropriate method depends on the nature of the hypothesis being tested and the measurement level of the variables in the analysis. Using our definition of responsiveness as longitudinal validity, the methods can include simple inferential tests (such as t tests or ANOVA), correlation coefficients, regression models (an approach advocated by Husted et al., 2000), ROC analysis, and so on. The statistical options outlined in Table 18.1 are appropriate for assessing responsiveness for change scores at different levels of measurement.

Beaton and colleagues (2001) pointed out that another factor affecting the analysis concerns whether the hypotheses predict within-subject change or between-subject *differences* in change. The majority of studies on responsiveness in the literature are based on within-subject analyses, but this may reflect the fact that most studies have not defined responsiveness as longitudinal validity. If responsiveness were defined as change of any kind or as change that is clinically significant, then a within-groups approach would be needed. Using the definition of responsiveness as longitudinal validity, however, both within- and between-groups designs can be used to test relevant hypotheses. Triangulation of evidence is an important option: both types can be combined in a single study. There should not be an expectation that within- and between-group analyses will yield the *same* results, any more than one would expect identical results for diverse tests of construct validity. The hope would be that different tests would yield consistent and confirmatory results about whether an instrument is good at capturing a change in the underlying construct.

Certain statistical approaches to responsiveness have been used with great regularity in the health literature (Terwee et al., 2003). Many of them involve the calculation of an effect size index. These are often called **distribution-based methods** because they are developed on the basis of change score distributions.[5] Most of these indexes are a ratio of the mean score change to a measure of variability of scores. The indexes differ most with regard to the variability statistic in the denominator. DeVet and colleagues (2011) described such methods as "inappropriate measures of responsiveness" (p. 215), except under certain circumstances (p. 218). We think it makes more sense to say that these methods *are* suitable for providing *evidence* of responsiveness when they are used in the context of theoretically or clinically defensible hypothesis tests that predict how changes in the construct will be manifested. The responsiveness of a measure should not, for example, be assessed as part of a clinical trial in which a new intervention is being tested because in a trial, it is not *known* that the groups will be different or that a change will occur. The central hypothesis in trials concerns the efficacy of the intervention, not the measurement properties of the outcome measures. In a clinical trial, if the results are negative, a lack of significant group differences could reflect an unresponsive measure, an ineffective treatment, or inadequate statistical power. Moreover, clinical trials ideally use outcome measures that have previously been demonstrated to have adequate responsiveness.

When there are legitimate hypotheses regarding a measure's change scores, several methods can be used. Four frequently used methods will be described in the sections that follow.

18.3.c *T* tests and Responsiveness

T tests can be used to test both within-group and between-group hypotheses about change scores. If the hypothesis being tested is that two groups are predicted, on the basis of prior evidence or theory, to have different change scores, an independent groups t test (or a nonparametric equivalent such as the Mann–Whitney U test) can be used. As an example, in the previously described study by DunnGalvin and colleagues (2010), the researchers used an independent groups t test to compare change scores on the Food Allergy Quality of Life Questionnaire (FAQLQ-PF) for two groups of children who were tested for a food allergy: those who, on the basis of the food challenge, tested negative for a food allergy, and those who tested positive. The researchers found that, as hypothesized, the children with a negative test (no diagnosis of a food allergy) had significantly greater improvement in their

---

[5]Husted et al. (2000) referred to these approaches as assessing *internal responsiveness*.

6-month FAQLQ-PF scores than children with a positive test, especially for the subscale measuring food anxiety.

Often, a paired *t* test is used to test score changes over time for a single group predicted to improve (or deteriorate). When a change is hypothesized to occur as a result of a patient's exposure to a well-established procedure or regimen (e.g., scores on a physical function test following hip replacement), then such a test can yield evidence regarding the longitudinal validity of the measure. For example, Tseng, Gajewski, and Kluding (2010) tested the responsiveness of the Visual Analog Fatigue Scale (VAFS), which measures exertion fatigue in patients with chronic stroke. To assess responsiveness, they used a paired *t* test to test the hypothesis that the patients' mean VAFS scores would increase following a 15-minute standardized protocol known to induce fatigue. The mean fatigue scores increased from 7.2 (±4.3) at baseline to 69.4 (±30.5) after exercising ($p < .001$), supporting an inference of responsiveness.

T tests have been criticized as a "not particularly appealing method for assessing responsiveness" (Husted, 2000, p. 460). Husted and others (e.g., DeVet et al., 2011) argue that *t* tests are designed to provide information about *statistical significance*, which is partly a function of sample size, not about validity. However, *t* tests enjoy a long history of being used to test hypotheses about group differences or group changes, including construct validity hypotheses. By extension, criticism of the use of *t* tests for responsiveness assessment implies that *t* tests should not be used to test known-groups hypotheses for construct validity assessment. We think that *t* tests are one of many strategies that can yield supportive evidence for longitudinal construct validity.

Researchers who have used *t* tests in their studies of responsiveness almost always go beyond a consideration of *p* values and supplement *t* tests with the calculation of an index to summarize the magnitude of the effect.

18.3.d Effect Size and Responsiveness

The standard **effect size** index **(ES)**, which is also referred to as *Cohen's d* or the *standardized mean difference*, is often used to evaluate the degree of a measure's responsiveness. One reason for the appeal of the ES index is that there are well-known criteria for interpreting effect size estimates. According to Cohen (1988), an ES of .20 is considered small, .50 is moderate, and .80 is large.[6] Although these standards are widely cited in the responsiveness literature, we caution against thinking of an ES or other related indexes as a coefficient that summarizes the amount of responsiveness of a measure. A large ES can offer strong support for an inference of responsiveness on a measure, but it does not denote a specific quantity of responsiveness.

An ES coefficient can be computed from *t* test output, and many statistical software programs calculate it directly. In responsiveness studies, ES has most often been calculated for within-group analyses, quantifying the magnitude of change over time for patients measured twice over an interval in which a change is expected to occur. The formula is:

$$ES_{Within} = \frac{M_{Time2} - M_{Time1}}{SD_{Time1}} \qquad (18.1)$$

where the mean change score from T1 to T2 is in the numerator and the baseline (T1) standard deviation is in the denominator. At the time of the Terwee et al. (2003) review, this ES index was the most widely reported measure of responsiveness in quality-of-life research.

---

[6]Cohen's criteria have sometimes been accused of being arbitrary (e.g., Guyatt, Osoba, Wu, Wyrwich, & Norman, 2002). However, unlike many psychometric criteria, which is based primarily on expert opinion (e.g., standards of acceptability for coefficient alpha), Cohen's benchmarking standards were based on comparisons with external "anchors," such as adolescent height, IQ score differences in difference groups, and so on. The work of Samsa et al. (1999) suggested a reasonable correspondence between Cohen's benchmarks and quality-of-life anchors.

As an example, Paradowski, Witonski, and Roos (2013) used the within-group ES formula to test responsiveness hypotheses in their psychometric evaluation of the Polish translation of the Knee Injury and Osteoarthritis Outcome Score (KOOS), a measure of functional status and quality of life in patients with joint injury or osteoarthritis. Patients undergoing anterior cruciate ligament reconstruction (ACLR) completed the KOOS before and 1 year after surgery. The researchers tested a series of hypotheses regarding the relative magnitude of the ES index across different subscales of the KOOS. They hypothesized that ES would be largest for the Quality of Life (QOL) subscale (hypothesized as an ES >1.0), followed by the ES for the Sports and Recreation Function subscale, and then the subscales for Pain, Symptoms, and ADL. Their data supported the hypothesized pattern of effects following ACLR. For example, the ES_{Within} for the QOL subscale was 1.38, that for Sports and Recreation was .88, and that for Pain was .41.

An ES can also be computed for between-groups analyses in which the goal is to estimate the magnitude of group *differences* in change for two groups whose change is hypothesized to differ. The formula is:

$$ES_{Between} = \frac{\bar{D}_{Group1} - \bar{D}_{Group2}}{SD_{PooledT1}} \tag{18.2}$$

where the *D*s in the numerator are the mean change scores for the groups being compared, and the *SD* is the pooled standard deviation for the two groups from the T1 measurement. Terwee et al. (2003) reported in their review of responsiveness measures that two studies had used this ES formula, but in fact the formula used in the two cited studies fall into the category we describe in the next section (Formula 18.4).

Researchers interested in between-group comparisons more often compute the ES_{Within} index separately for each group being compared and then contrast the ES values qualitatively. As an example, Dauden and colleagues (2012) developed a scale to measure health-related quality of life in psoriasis (PSO-LIFE) for use in Spain. The researchers computed 3-month within-group ES estimates for a sample of patients with active and inactive psoriasis and then compared the groups' ES_{Within} values to assess implied hypotheses about responsiveness. The ES_{Within} on the PSO-LIFE was substantially higher for patients with active psoriasis at baseline (.73) than for those with inactive psoriasis (.29). Patients were also classified into groups based on a GRS for overall health administered at the 3-month point. The ES_{Within} on the PSO-LIFE was 1.01 for those who reported that their health had greatly improved but was negative for groups who said their health was worse (e.g., −.44 for those who rated their health as "much worse."). The pattern of ES magnitudes and directionality were consistent with the expectations for a responsive instrument.

18.3.e The Standardized Response Mean

Another index to express the magnitude of a change on a measure is the **standardized response mean** or **SRM**. The SRM, most often used in within-group situations, uses information from a paired *t* test, using the following formula:

$$SRM_{Within} = \frac{M_{Time2} - M_{Time1}}{SD_{Change}} \tag{18.3}$$

where the numerator is the mean change score of a group of people measured at two points in time, and the denominator is the standard deviation for change. This formula is identical to that for the ES_{Within} index (18.1), except for the *SD* used in the denominator. Different approaches have been proposed for building confidence intervals (CIs) around SRM values (e.g., Beaton, Hogg-Johnson, & Bombardier, 1997; Liang, Larson, Cullen, & Schwartz, 1990), but CIs are seldom reported.

Cohen's (1988) criteria for the ES are often applied to the SRM, even though SRM and ES values are not equivalent. Benchmarks for small, moderate, and large values for the SRM

(.20, .50, and .80, respectively) are used by many, but their use has also been criticized as inappropriate because of both conceptual and statistical differences between the ES and the SRM (Zou, 2005). When the correlation between the baseline and follow-up scores is .50, the ES and SRM have the same value. With higher correlations, the SRM value is greater than the ES value, and with lower correlations, the reverse is true.

Examples of measurement studies using the SRM as an index of responsiveness abound. In fact, many researchers compute and report both the SRM and the ES$_{Within}$, and results are usually consistent, even though the values are different. For example, in the previously described study of the Polish adaptation of the KOOS (Paradowski et al., 2013), the researchers hypothesized the same pattern of subscale differences for the SRM as for the ES following ACLR surgery, and their hypotheses were supported. For instance, the ES for the QOL subscale was 1.38 and the SRM was 1.08. The values for the Pain subscale were .41 and .39, respectively. Given the fact that ACLR is a therapy with well-established benefits, the researchers' use of paired t tests, ESs, and SRMs provided useful evidence of the responsiveness of the KOOS.

Because the *SD* in the denominator of the SRM is the *SD* for change scores, it might appear as though this index is relevant only for within-groups analyses. However, the SRM has been used in many between-groups studies. One application involves qualitative comparisons of the SRMs for groups expected to have different mean change scores, similar to what we described for the ES. For example, in the study by DunnGalvin et al. (2010), children who tested negative for food allergies on the basis of a food challenge were compared to those who tested positive, as previously described. The researchers computed an SRM for both groups of children to capture the magnitude of change over a 6-month period on the Food Allergy Quality of Life Questionnaire. Scores for both groups of children improved over time but, as predicted, those who tested negative had a substantially higher SRM (.87) than those who tested positive (.45).

The SRM formula shown in 18.3 can also be modified for use in between-groups designs:

$$\text{SRM}_{Between} = \frac{\bar{D}_{Group1} - \bar{D}_{Group2}}{SD_{ChangePooled}} \qquad (18.4)$$

where the *D*s in the numerator are the mean change scores for the groups being compared, and *SD* is the standard deviation of the change scores for both groups combined. This formula is identical to the ES$_{Between}$ formula (18.2), except, once again, for the *SD* value in the denominator.

Guyatt, King, Feeny, Stubbing, and Goldstein (1999) used this between-groups SRM in a study designed to compare the responsiveness of several measures of health-related quality of life, including both generic and disease-specific measures. The study was conducted using data from a clinical trial of respiratory rehabilitation versus conventional community care for patients with chronic airflow limitations. After the trial results indicated the efficacy of the intervention, the various outcome measures were assessed for responsiveness, comparing mean changes for the intervention group to those for the control group. The results indicated that the SRM$_{Between}$ was greatest for the disease-specific Chronic Respiratory Questionnaire (CRQ) Mastery subscale (0.90) and substantially lower for generic scales such as the Sickness Impact Profile (SIP) Physical Function subscale (0.30) and the SIP Psychosocial Function subscale (.00). As mentioned previously, responsiveness usually should not be assessed in the context of a clinical trial, but the between-groups formula for the SRM (18.4) could readily be used to test differences in change scores for known-groups hypotheses.

18.3.f Guyatt's Responsiveness Index

In their review of the responsiveness literature, Terwee et al. (2003) found that researchers who defined responsiveness as the ability to detect change (in general) used the ES and SRM as responsiveness measures. Those who defined responsiveness as the ability to detect clinically important change were more likely to use one of several variants of an index that has been called **Guyatt's responsiveness index** or **GRI** (or sometimes called the *responsiveness statistic* or *responsiveness ratio*). Guyatt and colleagues (1987) proposed an index that puts the minimum important change of a measure in the numerator and the SD_{Change} in stable subjects (e.g., control group subjects) in the denominator. Such a formula requires information about the value of a clinically important change. In COSMIN's taxonomy and in ours, *minimum important change* is considered to be *interpretive* (i.e., an index used to make sense of a change score) rather than a *property* of a measure (responsiveness). Chapter 19 addresses interpretation and change scores.

Guyatt and colleagues (1987) recognized that for many instruments, especially newly developed ones, information about the minimum important change is lacking. They therefore suggested using the mean change score for a group exposed to "an intervention of known efficacy" (p. 176) in the numerator of the formula, as in the following:

$$\text{GRI} = \frac{M_{\text{Time2(IGroup)}} - M_{\text{Time1(IGroup)}}}{SD_{\text{Change(SGroup)}}} \qquad (18.5)$$

where the means are for T1 and T2 measurements for a group expected to improve (the improved or I group), and the SD_{Change} is the variability in change scores for a group expected *not* to change (the stable or S group).

The GRI is used less often than ES or SRM as the index of responsiveness, perhaps because the formula suggests the need for two separate samples. Researchers have interpreted the "improved" and "stable" requirements of this formula in various ways, however. Some researchers simply divide their sample into two subgroups: one that has improved on some measure and another that has not. Then, they use the improved subgroup's means in the numerator and the "not improved" subgroup's variability in the denominator. As an example, Macedo and colleagues (2011) compared the responsiveness of four different versions of the Roland Morris Disability Questionnaire (RMDQ) with a large sample of patients with lower back pain before and after treatment. At the end of treatment, patients were also asked to complete an 11-point GRS, with ratings from -5 (vastly worse) to $+5$ (completely recovered/much better). In computing the responsiveness index, the researchers used in the numerator the mean change scores for those who had a score of at least $+3$ on the GRS. Those with lower transition scores were deemed not to have improved, and the variability of their change scores on the RMDQ was used in the denominator. The value of the GRI ranged from 1.30 (for the 11-item RMDQ) to 1.55 (for the full 24-item RMDQ). When this approach to responsiveness assessment is used, it essentially combines a criterion (anchor) approach with a distribution approach.

Like the ES and SRM, the GRI quantifies the magnitude of changes on a measure, and larger values are considered greater evidence of a measure's responsiveness. Liang (2000) noted that variation in stable patients (in the denominator) provides "an intuitive estimate of background noise" (p. 86) but criticized the GRI because its numerator and denominator are based on different samples. His concern is that this approach is prone to bias because it assumes that the variance for subjects who do not change is approximately equal to that for subjects who do change. It does not appear that standards for interpreting GRI values as *small*, *medium*, or *large* have been proposed.[7]

18.4   The Design of Responsiveness Studies

This section describes some issues to consider in designing and reporting assessments of a measure's responsiveness.

---

[7]Crosby, Kolotkin, and Williams (2003) have stated with regard to the GRI that "values of 0.20, 0.50, and 0.80 have been used to represent *small*, *moderate*, and *large* responsiveness" (p. 402), but we did not find examples of studies using these standards.

18.4.a Explicit Hypotheses and Criteria

Using our definition of responsiveness as longitudinal validity, it follows that much of the advice we offered with regard to construct validation in Chapter 13 is relevant here. In validating new measures, it is customary to test multiple hypotheses. For example, researchers often test hypotheses about the dimensionality of a new scale (structural validity) as well as hypotheses relating to its criterion-related and/or construct validity. Furthermore, efforts to assess construct validity may involve multiple tests of convergent validity using measures of several related constructs. Tests for known-groups validity may also entail hypotheses regarding differential outcomes for several groups expected to differ on the underlying construct. In other words, the triangulation of multiple types of evidence is considered valuable in validating a measure.

Multiple hypothesis tests are also desirable for examining a measure's responsiveness. In the preceding two sections, we have discussed a wide array of strategies for marshaling evidence of a measure's responsiveness, including both anchor-based and distribution-based methods, and within-groups and between-groups approaches. Much like construct validity work, researchers who assess responsiveness by testing a variety of hypotheses about the nature and direction of changes on the focal measure are limited primarily by their imagination. The previously mentioned study in which the researchers compared responsiveness for four different versions of the RMDQ study (Macedo et al., 2011) provides an example of evidence triangulation. In addition to calculating the GRI for the four versions of the RMDQ, the researchers used three other approaches: They calculated ES_{Within} for each measure; they correlated change scores on the measures with ratings on the 11-point global rating scale; and they did ROC analyses that compared the ability of the different RMDQ versions to distinguish people who had or had not improved, according to their transition rating.

As with validation efforts, it is important to articulate in advance the hypotheses being tested. Most often, however, researchers fail to formally state the hypotheses, which must then be inferred. By stating explicit hypotheses, readers will be in a better position to understand which definition of responsiveness was used and to evaluate the suitability of the tests that were undertaken.

It is also prudent to formulate specific standards for acceptability of the hypotheses rather than relying on statistical significance or simply permitting an open-ended or post hoc interpretation. Revicki et al. (2008) have recommended that correlation coefficients as indicators of responsiveness should be at least .30 to .35. Others suggest correlations of .50 or higher (e.g., Crosby et al., 2003). Guyatt and colleagues (1999) offered qualitative descriptors for different correlation values. They calculated correlations between changes on the Chronic Respiratory Questionnaire (CRQ) and other relevant change measures, including the 6MWT and several transition scales. The researchers made a priori predictions about the expected magnitude of correlations and designated how coefficients would be interpreted: weak (*rs* from .20 to .35), moderate (.35 to .50) and strong (>.50). Many researchers use Cohen's standards of *small, moderate,* and *large* for ES or SRM estimates. However, they do not usually stipulate that the effects must be at least moderate (for example) in order for responsiveness to be considered acceptable. Standards can be stated either in absolute terms (e.g., the ES must be >.40) or in relative terms (e.g., certain correlations are expected to be ≥.20 higher than others).

When responsiveness assessment involves multiple hypothesis tests, it is also useful to set a priori goals for how many hypotheses need to be supported to be considered adequate evidence of responsiveness. For example, De Boer and colleagues (2006) tested six hypotheses regarding the responsiveness of the Vision-Related Quality of Life Core Measure (VCM1). The hypotheses were stated in relative terms (i.e., higher correlations were predicted for some change score relationships than for others). The researchers stated upfront that they would consider responsiveness as poor if four or more hypotheses were rejected. Three of the six hypotheses were supported, leading the researchers to conclude that the measure was moderately responsive.

18.4.b Study Design for a Responsiveness Assessment

Responsiveness assessments inherently require a longitudinal design. A sample of subjects must be measured with the focal instrument on at least two occasions, often over an interval of many weeks or months. A study of responsiveness is usually undertaken with finalized measures, with ones that have already yielded evidence of reliability and validity.

As we have seen, the study can adopt either a within-groups design in which change over time is measured for a single group or a between-groups design in which differences in change scores are compared for different groups. Both within- and between-groups analyses can be undertaken in a single study to marshal corroborating evidence. If a within-groups design is used, the analyses should be undertaken for everyone in the sample, not just for the people who changed. The study should be designed to yield various types of convergent, divergent, and discriminative information about the capacity of the measure to capture a change in the construct of interest.

The study should be designed using a population in which change is expected to occur over a specified interval. This may be a population in which deterioration is anticipated (e.g., patients with a progressive disease) or a population in which a treatment of widely acknowledged efficacy is administered, such as patients undergoing cataract surgery for measures of vision-related quality of life or patients getting hip replacement surgery for mobility outcomes. As noted previously, responsiveness should not be tested in a clinical trial of a new innovation whose effectiveness is unknown because of the risk of ambiguous results. Several authors have suggested that responsiveness could be assessed in a clinical trial of an intervention of known effectiveness (e.g., Husted et al., 2000; Revicki et al., 2008), but once an intervention is "known" to be efficacious, there may be little incentive to conduct a new trial, except perhaps with a new population, in which case efficacy would not be "known."

The time interval between measurements should be given careful consideration. Enough time should have elapsed that one could reasonably expect change to have occurred on the focal construct for a sizeable subset of the sample. However, very lengthy time periods may create several problems, including response shift (Chapter 17), which can undermine efforts to understand whether the construct itself has really changed. Lengthy time intervals are also likely to be associated with higher rates of attrition. Attrition usually results in a biased subset of respondents for the second measurement, so efforts to minimize attrition are important. The time interval should be the same for the target measure as for the comparator measures used in hypothesis testing.

Several strategies for identifying an appropriate time interval were discussed in Chapter 8 in the context of test–retest reliability. For example, a separate small study with the focal population could be undertaken in which a health transition scale could be administered at regular intervals to better understand when changes on the construct is most likely to occur. Experts involved in content validity work could also be asked to recommend an appropriate time interval (Polit, 2014).

When a known-groups approach to responsiveness assessment is adopted, a comparison group whose change trajectory is expected to differ from that of the target group is required. The group should be identified on the basis of a conceptual model, prior research, or well-established clinical knowledge. If continuous scores are dichotomized to create the "known groups," it is most defensible to use a well-established cutpoint. As in any other comparison-group design, care should be taken to minimize the effect of confounding variables, using either design strategies (e.g., matching) or analytic tools (statistically controlling confounders) to allow for appropriate interpretation of group differences.

The measurements for all key variables should be made independently at the two time points. If all measures are self-reports, the study participants should not be told what their score was at a prior measurement and should not be told how much change has occurred on any measure. If some variables are measured by means of ratings by others, the raters should be blinded to the scores on all other measures.

The data collection plan is a major component of the study design for a responsiveness study. For each hypothesis to be tested, a good measure of the relevant criterion or construct must be found. The measures should be appropriate for the target population, reliable, valid, and, ideally, responsive as well. It is a good idea to incorporate one or more global rating scale into the design of a responsiveness study to provide one piece of evidence as part of a broader strategy of triangulation. GRSs can also play a role in interpretations of change scores, as we discuss in the next chapter.

Decisions about the statistical analysis to be undertaken should be driven by the nature of the measurements for the hypotheses being tested (Table 18.1). If an effect size indicator is calculated to summarize the magnitude of a change, there is no consensus about which one is preferable. Some prefer the SRM to ES (e.g., Zou, 2005), but others prefer Cohen's ES. Norman and colleagues (2007), for example, have done a mathematical analysis of different responsiveness coefficients and concluded that the SRM should be interpreted with caution because "any measure based on variability in change scores can give misleading information" (p. 815), especially if the amount of change is similar among sample members because this would inflate the value of the SRM. There does not appear to be a justification for computing more than one index, which many researchers have done, because they are redundant in terms of their ability to offer supportive evidence for hypotheses designed to assess longitudinal construct validity. If both indices are computed, however, they should not be compared; the SRM and ES will invariably be different unless the T1 and T2 scores have a correlation of .50.

Although many of the examples we used in this chapter to illustrate the assessment of responsiveness were for measures developed using CTT, the methods we have described have also been used with measures created with item response theory (IRT) models, including measures that rely on computerized adaptive testing (CAT). For example, Cheville and colleagues (2012) assessed the responsiveness of the CAT for the Activity Measure for Post-Acute Care (a measure of functional decline) using data from monthly assessments of patients with late-stage lung cancer. They used several different anchors, including a GRS and an index of critical clinical events, and also computed distribution-based statistics such as the ES and SRM.

18.4.c Sampling in Responsiveness Assessment

As previously noted, the sample in a responsiveness study should be drawn from a relevant population in which change on the focal construct is expected to occur over the time interval of the measurements. As with any hypothesis-testing endeavor, large samples are preferred to small ones. The COSMIN group's scoring system for the quality of responsiveness studies awards a rating of "excellent" for samples of 100 or more for the item on sample size (Terwee et al., 2012). Yet, a sample of 100 might not be "excellent," depending on the expected size of the effects in the various hypothesis tests, and sample size needs should be estimated based on the anticipated smallest effect. Power analysis is geared to estimating sample size needs for statistically significant results, and although statistical significance is not the only criterion to consider in coming to conclusions about responsiveness, nonsignificant results tend to be ambiguous and therefore should be avoided, if possible, by using an adequate sample size.

18.4.d Comparative Studies of Responsiveness

Unlike the typical study to test reliability and validity, responsiveness studies are frequently undertaken by researchers who are not the original instrument developers. Many comparative studies have been designed to examine which of several different measures of the same construct exhibit the greatest degree of responsiveness.[8] Indeed, many of the studies cited

---

[8]In such comparative studies, the comparisons of different measures are often done qualitatively. However, Liang et al. (1990) have proposed the *relative efficiency index,* calculated by squaring the ratio of paired *t* test values for two measures, for making more formal comparisons.

in this chapter were comparative. For example, Eurich and coresearchers (2006) compared the responsiveness of several generic and specific measures of quality of life in heart failure using three external criteria and concluded that the Kansas City Cardiomyopathy Questionnaire was most responsive. Freeman et al. (2013) assessed the relative responsiveness of four mobility measures in a sample of patients with multiple sclerosis and concluded that the four measures were broadly comparable in detecting mobility changes.

There are also examples of comparative studies that compare responsiveness for measures developed using CTT and IRT models. For example, Fries, Krishnan, Rose, Lingala, and Bruce (2011) compared the responsiveness of six physical function instruments in a sample of patients with rheumatoid arthritis. Two were "legacy" instruments (the Physical Function [PF] subscale of the SF-36 and the Health Assessment Questionnaire Disability Index [HAQ]), two were "item improved" instruments that were adaptations of the PF and HAQ, and two were static 10- and 20-item IRT-derived PF measures developed as part of the Patient Reported Outcomes Measurement Information System (PROMIS®) project. Although changes over a 12-month period in this sample tended to be modest, the investigators concluded that the most responsive instrument was the PROMIS PF-20, which was also the instrument that had the greatest precision across the widest range of physical functioning (adequate standard errors from -4.0 SD units below the population mean on the latent trait to about $+0.5$ SD units).[9]

In such comparative studies, researchers often rely on the magnitude of the responsiveness coefficients to draw conclusions about the relative responsiveness of the "competing" measures. However, given our definition of responsiveness, it would be better to compare the overall pattern of hypothesis-testing results to identify the measure that offers the most persuasive aggregate evidence that the measure is truly capturing change in the underlying construct.

18.4.e Interpretation of Responsiveness Results

As is true regarding the interpretation of construct validity results, drawing conclusions about a measure's responsiveness is complex because in a well-designed study, there would be a lot of evidence to integrate. Contrary to what has sometimes been sought, there is no single "responsiveness coefficient" that can confirm that a measure has longitudinal validity. Greater confidence in a measure's responsiveness is achieved by amassing supporting evidence from multiple hypothesis tests. Because it is likely that not all hypotheses will be supported, it is wise to establish a priori standards for how much confirmatory evidence is considered sufficient to conclude that the instrument is responsive.

In developing standards and interpreting results, it is important to take into consideration that change scores are inherently less reliable than point-in-time scores (Chapter 17), which in turn means that expectations for hypothesis testing should be tempered accordingly. In a construct validity study, a researcher may demand a correlation of .70 or greater as evidence of excellent validity. In a responsiveness study in which both the focal measure and other measures are change scores, correlations of .70 might be difficult to achieve. As an illustration using a study already mentioned in this chapter, Schatz et al. (2011) used the mini-Asthma Quality of Life Questionnaire (mAQLQ) as the gold standard for the six-item Asthma Impact Survey (AIS-6). The correlation for the criterion validation was $-.85$, but the correlation for *changes* on both instruments 5 months later was $-.58$.

When the responsiveness hypothesis tests are not supported, the pattern of results requires careful interpretive effort to decipher whether the problem lies with the focal measure itself, the conceptualization, the research or sampling design, or the other measures

---

[9]Comparisons of the responsiveness of CTT and IRT measures sometimes suggest that the two are similar. For example Ko and colleagues (2013) compared raw scores on the Oxford Knee Score (OKS) with scores on the OKS from a Rasch-fitted model and found that they had comparable responsiveness.

used in the hypothesis tests. If the hypotheses seem reasonable and the study design was appropriate, then perhaps the instrument needs to be revised to better measure change on an attribute. Flaws in the design or the hypotheses might lead to a new study of the measure's responsiveness.

Like validity, responsiveness is not a fixed property of a measure. A measure's responsiveness can vary from one population (or context) to another. Researchers who use an instrument that has been reported as reliable, valid, and responsive should fully understand the population and context in the development sample before drawing conclusions about the measure's quality for new investigations.

18.4.f Reporting a Responsiveness Study

A measure's responsiveness is sometimes reported along with other psychometric properties, but it may also be reported independently. An independent report is clearly needed when researchers undertake a study to compare the responsiveness of several measures of the same construct.

Because responsiveness represents longitudinal validity, it is important to explain to readers the conceptual basis for any hypothesis tests and to formally state hypotheses that are being tested along with the criteria for confirming them. The comparator measures used in the tests should be described, including the constructs they measure, the rationale for selecting them, their psychometric properties, and their suitability for the focal population. Special care might be needed in defending a measure of a "gold standard" for a criterion-related responsiveness assessment. Other design decisions need to be explained and defended, including a justification for the sample design, the sample size, the time interval between measurements, and analytic approach. The paper should provide information about why the construct was expected to change over the specified interval, and the Results section should summarize how much change occurred (e.g., the percentage of patients who improved, remained stable, or deteriorated).

Some suggestions about presenting results for a construct validation presented in Chapter 13 are also relevant for presenting responsiveness findings. Ideally, information about both responsiveness and change score reliability (Chapter 17) would be presented in the same paper. Also, it is appropriate, as in all research, to use tentative language in reporting results. Responsiveness is never *confirmed*, *determined*, or *established*; it is supported to a varying degree. Because responsiveness, like cross-sectional validity, is not an "all or nothing" property of a measure, researchers writing a paper on a measure's responsiveness should present all the evidence and then—to expand on a statement from Cronbach and Meehl's (1955) influential paper on validity—indicate the *degree* of responsiveness that the measure appears to have based on the aggregated evidence.

18.4.g Evaluating a Responsiveness Study

Guidelines for evaluating responsiveness assessment studies have been offered by the COSMIN workgroup (Terwee et al., 2012). The COSMIN scoring system (Box I) includes ratings for various design and analysis decisions, such as the amount and handling of missing data, sample size, use of a longitudinal design, the time interval, and so on. A few of the elements in the rating scheme are evaluative with respect to study design decisions (e.g., was the sample size adequate?), but many items focus on whether relevant information was provided. For example, one item asks whether the time interval between measurements was stated, but no item asks whether the time interval was appropriate. Moreover, none of the items focus on the adequacy of the evidence itself (i.e., the system focuses primarily on the research rather than on measurement properties). A thorough evaluation of the evidence would encompass not only whether something was or was not reported but whether the decisions led to high-quality evidence that support an inference of responsiveness for the measure under study. The COSMIN scoring system is very useful for those preparing a report on a responsiveness study, that is, as a guide to what information should be provided, but may not be comprehensive as a guide to evaluating the responsiveness of the measures themselves.

As with construct validation, an evaluation of responsiveness must take into account numerous conceptual, methodologic, and statistical challenges. An important issue in evaluating a paper that describes a responsiveness assessment is whether the researchers were thorough and creative in developing relevant hypotheses to be tested. Did the researchers miss strategic opportunities to strengthen the evidence regarding a measure's responsiveness? The researchers' approach should be robust, and the interpretation of the findings should be well-grounded. The bottom line in an evaluation of a responsiveness study is whether the evidence is rigorous and whether the pattern of evidence suggests adequate longitudinal validity.

References

Beaton, D. E., Bombardier, C., Katz, J., & Wright, J. G. (2001). A taxonomy for responsiveness. *Journal of Clinical Epidemiology, 54*, 1204–1217.

Beaton, D. E., Hogg-Johnson, S., & Bombardier, C. (1997). Evaluating changes in health status: Reliability and responsiveness of five generic health status measures in workers with musculoskeletal disorders. *Journal of Clinical Epidemiology, 50*, 79–91.

Bellamy, M. (2012). *WOMAC 3.1 Osteoarthritis Index. User's guide.* Retrieved from http://womac.com

Cheville, A. L., Yost, K., Larson, D., Dos Santos, K., O'Byrne, M., Change, M., & Yang, P. (2012). Performance of an item response theory-based computerized adaptive test in identifying functional decline. *Archives of Physical Medicine & Rehabilitation, 93*, 1153–1160.

Cohen, J. (1988). *Statistical power analysis for the behavioral sciences* (2nd ed.). Hillsdale, MJ: Lawrence Erlbaum.

Cornelius, B. L., Groothoff, J., van der Klink, J., & Brouwer, S. (2013). The performance of the K10, K6 and GHQ-12 to screen for present state DSM-IV disorders among disability claimants. *BMC Public Health, 13,* 128.

Cronbach, L. J., & Meehl, P. E. (1955). Construct validity in psychological tests. *Psychological Bulletin, 5*, 281–302.

Crosby, R. D., Kolotkin, R., & Williams, G. R. (2003). Defining clinically meaningful change in health-related quality of life. *Journal of Clinical Epidemiology, 56*, 395–407.

Dauden, E., Herrera, E., Puig, L., Sanchez-Carazo, J., Toribio, J., Caloto, M. T., . . . Lara, N. (2012). Validation of a new tool to assess health-related quality of life in psoriasis: The PSO-LIFE questionnaire. *Health and Quality of Life Outcomes, 10*(56).

De Boer, M. R., Terwee, C. B., DeVet, H. C. W., Moll, A. C., Völker-Dieben, H., & van Rens, G. (2006). Evaluation of cross-sectional and longitudinal construct validity of two vision-related quality of life questionnaires: The LVQOL and VCM1. *Quality of Life Research, 15*, 233–248.

De Vriendt, T., Clays, E., Moreno, L. A., Bergman, P., Vicente-Rodriguez, G., Nagy, E., . . . De Henauw, S. (2011). Reliability and validity of the Adolescent Stress Questionnaire in a sample of European adolescents --the HELENA study. *BMC Public Health, 11*, 717.

DeVellis, R. F. (2012). *Scale development: Theory and application* (3rd ed.). Thousand Oaks, CA: Sage.

DeVet, H. C. W., Terwee, C., Mokkink, L. B., & Knol, D. L. (2011). *Measurement in medicine: A practical guide.* Cambridge, MA: Cambridge University Press.

Deyo, R. A., & Inui, T. S. (1984). Toward clinical applications of health status measures: Sensitivity of scales to clinically important changes. *Health Services Research, 19*, 275–289.

DunnGalvin, A., Cullinante, C., Daly, D., Flokstra-de Blok, B., Dubois, A., & Hourihane, J. (2010). Longitudinal validity and responsiveness of the Food Allergy Quality of Life Questionnaire-Parent Form in children 0-12 years following positive and negative food challenges. *Clinical & Experimental Allergy, 40*, 476–485.

DunnGalvin, A., Flokstra-de Blok, B., Burks, A. E., Dubois, A., & Hourihane, J. (2008). Food Allergy QoL Questionnaire for children 0-12 years: Content, construct, and cross-cultural validity. *Clinical & Experimental Allergy, 38*, 977–986.

Eurich, D. T., Johnson, J., Reid, K., & Spertus, J. (2006). Assessing responsiveness of generic and specific health related quality of life measures in heart failure. *Health and Quality of Life Outcomes, 4*, 89.

Feinstein, A. R. (1987). *Clinimetrics.* New Haven, CT: Yale University Press.

Freeman, J., Walters, R., Ingram, W., Slade, A., Hobart, J., & Zajicek, J. (2013). Evaluating change in mobility in people with multiple sclerosis: Relative responsiveness of four clinical measures. *Multiple Sclerosis Journal, 19*, 1632–1639.

Fries, J. F., Krishnan, E., Rose, M., Lingala, B., & Bruce, B. (2011). Improved responsiveness and reduced sample size requirements of PROMIS physical function scales with item response theory. *Arthritis Research & Therapy, 13*, R147.

Furr, R. M., & Bacharach, V. R. (2014). *Psychometrics: An introduction* (2nd ed.). Thousand Oaks, CA: Sage.

Goreshi, R., Okawa, J., Rose, M., Feng, R., Lee, L., Hansen, C., . . . Werth, V (2012). Evaluation of reliability, validity, and responsiveness of the CDASI and the CAT-BM. *Journal of Investigative Dermatology, 132*, 1119–1124.

Guyatt, G. H., Bombardier, C., & Tugwell, P. (1986). Measuring disease-specific quality of life in clinical trials. *Canadian Medical Association Journal, 134*, 889–895.

Guyatt, G. H., Deyo, R., Charlson, M., Levine, M., & Mitchell, A. (1989). Responsiveness and validity in health status measurement: A clarification. *Journal of Clinical Epidemiology, 42*, 403–408.

Guyatt, G. H., King, D. R., Feeny, D., Stubbing, D., & Goldstein, R. (1999). Generic and specific measurement of health-related quality of life in a clinical trial of respiratory rehabilitation. *Journal of Clinical Epidemiology, 52*, 187–192.

Guyatt, G. H., Osoba, D., Wu, A., Wyrwich, K., & Norman, G. (2002). Methods to explain clinical significance of health measures. *Mayo Clinic Proceedings, 77*, 371–383.

Guyatt, G. H., Walter, S., & Norman, G. (1987). Measuring change over time: Assessing the usefulness of evaluative instruments. *Journal of Chronic Diseases, 40*, 171–176.

Hays, R. D., & Hadorn, D. (1992). Responsiveness to change: An aspect of validity, not a separate dimension. *Quality of Life Research, 1*, 73–75.

Husted, J. A., Cook, R. J., Farewell, V., & Gladman, D. (2000). Methods for assessing responsiveness: A critical review and recommendations. *Journal of Clinical Epidemiology, 53*, 459–468.

Kirshner, B., & Guyatt, G. (1985). A methodological framework for assessing health indices. *Journal of Chronic Diseases, 38*, 27–36.

Ko, Y., Lo, N., Yeo, S., Yang, K., Yeo, W., Chong, H., & Thumboo, J. (2013). Comparison of the responsiveness of the SF-36, the Oxford Knee Score, and the Knee Society Clinical Rating System in patients undergoing total knee replacement. *Quality of Life Research, 22*, 2455–2459.

Liang, M. H. (2000). Longitudinal construct validity: Establishment of clinical meaning in patient evaluation instruments. *Medical Care, 38*(Suppl. II), S84–S90.

Liang, M. H., Larson, M., Cullen, K. E., & Schwartz, J. A. (1990). Comparisons of five health status instruments for orthopedic evaluation. *Medical Care, 28*, 632–642.

Liang, M. H., Lew, R., Stucki, G., Fortin, P., & Daltroy, L. (2002). Measuring clinically important changes with patient-oriented questionnaires. *Medical Care, 40*(Suppl. II), II45–II51.

Macedo, L. G., Maher, C., Latimer, J., Hancock, M., Machado, L., & McAuley, J. (2011). Responsiveness of the 24-, 18- and 11-item versions of the Roland Morris Disability Questionnaire. *European Spine Journal, 20*, 458–463.

McCaskey, M., Ettlin, T., & Shuster, C. (2013). German version of the Whiplash Disability Questionnaire: Reproducibility and responsiveness. *Health and Quality of Life Outcomes, 11*, 36.

Mokkink, L. B., Terwee, C., Patrick, D., Alonso, J., Stratford, P., Knol, D. L., . . . DeVet, H. C. W. (2010). The COSMIN study reached international consensus on taxonomy, terminology, and definitions of measurement properties for health-related patient-reported outcomes. *Journal of Clinical Epidemiology, 63*, 737–745.

Norman, G. R., Stratford, P., & Regehr, G. (1997). Methodological problems in the retrospective computation of responsiveness to change: Lessons of Cronbach. *Journal of Clinical Epidemiology, 50*, 869–879.

Norman, G. R., Wyrwich, K., & Patrick, D. (2007). The mathematical relationship among different forms of responsiveness coefficients. *Quality of Life Research, 16*, 815–822.

Nunnally, J., & Bernstein, I. H. (1994). *Psychometric theory* (3rd ed.). New York, NY: McGraw-Hill.

Paradowski, P. T., Witonski, D., & Roos, E. (2013). Cross-cultural translation and measurement properties of the Polish version of the Knee Injury and Osteoarthritis Outcome Score (KOOS) following anterior cruciate ligament reconstruction. *Health and Quality of Life Outcomes, 11*, 107.

Polit, D. F. (2014). Getting serious about test–retest reliability: A critique of retest research and some recommendations. *Quality of Life Research, 23*(6), 1713–1720.

Revicki, D. A., Cella, D., Hays, R., Sloan, J., Lenderking, W., & Aaronson, N. (2006). Responsiveness and minimal important differences for patient reported outcomes. *Health and Quality of Life Outcomes, 4*, 70.

Revicki, D. A., Hays, R. D., Cella, D., & Sloan, J. (2008). Recommended methods for determining responsiveness and minimally important differences for patient-reported outcomes. *Journal of Clinical Epidemiology, 61*, 102–109.

Rust, H., & Golombok, S. (2009). *Modern psychometrics: The science of psychological assessment* (3rd ed.). New York, NY: Routledge.

Samsa, G., Edelman, D., Rothman, M., Williams, G. R., Lipscomb, J., & Matchar, D. (1999). Determining clinical important differences in health status measures. *Pharmacoeconomics, 15*, 141–155.

Schatz, M., Zeriger, R. S., Yang, S., Chen, W., & Kosinski, M. (2011). Further validation and definitions of the psychometric properties of the Asthma Impact Survey. *Journal of Allergy and Clinical Immunology, 128*, 44–49.

Schwartz, C. E., & Rapkin, B. D. (2004). Reconsidering the psychometrics of quality of life assessments in light of response shift and appraisal. *Health and Quality of Life Outcomes, 2*, 16.

Schwartz, C. E., & Sprangers, M. A. G. (2010). Guidelines for improving the stringency of response shift research using the then test. *Quality of Life Research, 19*, 455–464.

Streiner, D. L., & Norman, G. R. (2008). *Health measurement scales: A practical guide to their development and use* (4th ed.). Oxford: Oxford University Press.

Terwee, C. B., Dekker, F., Wiersinga, W., Prummel, M., & Bossuyt, P. (2003). On assessing responsiveness of health-related quality of life instruments: Guidelines for instrument evaluation. *Quality of Life Research, 12*, 349–362.

Terwee, C. B., Mokkink, L. B., Knol, D. L., Ostelo, R., Bouter, L. M., & DeVet, H. C. W. (2012). Rating the methodological quality in systematic reviews of studies on measurement properties: A scoring system for the COSMIN checklist. *Quality of Life Research*, *21*, 651–657.

Testa, M. A., & Simonson, D. C. (1996). Assessment of quality of life outcomes. *New England Journal of Medicine*, *334*, 835–840.

Tseng, B., Gajewski, B., & Kluding, P. (2010). Reliability, responsiveness, and validity of the Visual Analog Fatigue Scale to measure exertion fatigue in people with chronic stroke. *Stroke Research and Treatment*, *2010*, 412964.

Wright, J. G., & Feinstein, A. R. (1992). A comparative contrast of clinimetric and psychometric methods for constructing indexes and rating scales. *Journal of Clinical Epidemiology*, *45*, 1201–1218.

Zou, G. Y. (2005). Quantifying responsiveness of quality of life measures without an external criterion. *Quality of Life Research*, *14*, 1545–1552.

The Interpretation of Change Scores

Chapter Outline

Over the past few decades, hundreds of articles have been written about the thorny issue of interpreting change scores. The literature on this topic relates not only to measurement but also to the profound challenges of interpreting clinical trial results and to the conceptualization of *clinical significance*.

As noted in our measurement taxonomy (Fig. 3.1), interpretation is not a measurement property but rather an aspect of measurement concerned with efforts to make numerical scores meaningful. For point-in-time scores, the interpretive question is What does a score mean? Is a particular score high or low, favorable or unfavorable? For a change score, researchers want to know not only if the value is real/reliable (Chapter 17) and responsive/valid (Chapter 18) but also whether the amount of change is trivial or important. Researchers and clinicians are no longer content to know whether a change resulting from health interventions or from a normal progression of a disease is statistically significant (which is strongly influenced by sample size) but also whether the change is meaningful for patients.

Many researchers have attempted to develop, explain, and promote quantitative guidelines for interpreting change scores, and the myriad perspectives and approaches have the potential to create more interpretive challenges than the change score values themselves. Like responsiveness, the interpretation of change scores is a topic fraught with controversy and disagreement. The literature is a rapidly evolving one, and perhaps greater consensus will emerge in the coming years. This chapter summarizes some of the major strategies and points of view relating to change score interpretation at this juncture.

19.1   Basic Issues in Interpreting Change Scores

Because of the complexity of the topic of interpretation, we begin by describing a few important issues that play a role in the debate.

19.1.a Benchmarks and the Representation of Change

Efforts to develop interpretive guidelines for a measure have focused on deriving **benchmarks** that designate how much change is "meaningful," "worthwhile," or "clinically important." The benchmarks represent a threshold of change (i.e., the amount of the change) at or beyond which an improvement or deterioration can be considered sufficiently large to be noteworthy.

As described in Chapter 17, change scores are typically represented as the difference between a baseline and a follow-up measurement derived through simple subtraction. Most often, researchers seek to establish an interpretive benchmark for change that is in the units of the measure itself; for example, a change of, say, 5 points on the SF-36 or an improvement of 4 points on the Center for Epidemiologic Studies Depression Scale (CES-D).

Sometimes, however, interpretive efforts involve representing measured change as percentages. Benchmarks of importance expressed as percentages have the advantage as being more readily interpreted than raw change score. For example, the Initiative on Methods, Measurement, and Pain Assessment in Clinical Trials (IMMPACT) convened a special panel on clinical significance, and one recommendation of the consensus review was that a 30% improvement in self-reported pain intensity (e.g., on a visual analog scale [VAS]) represented a benchmark for positive clinical change (Dworkin et al., 2005). Researchers in the field of psychopharmacology have advocated expressing the amount of improvement on key outcomes as percentage improvement (Hiller, Schindler, & Lambert, 2012).

Representing change and benchmarks as percentages allows for direct comparisons across measures. A clear disadvantage, however, is that the percentages have different meaning depending on the values of the baseline scores. For example, a 30% drop in pain levels on a 0 to 100 VAS could signify a large absolute improvement from 80 to 56 (24 points) or a small absolute improvement from 30 to 21 (9 points). This limitation has led some researchers and professional groups to develop benchmarks that combine percentage change with absolute change. For example, the Osteoarthritis Research Society International (OARSI) and the Outcome Measures in Rheumatology (OMERACT) network set criteria that would classify patients as *responders* to treatment if (for example) they had a 50% or greater improvement in pain or physical function and an absolute improvement of 20 or more points on a 0-to-100 point scale (Pham et al., 2003).

This chapter focuses primarily on the large body of conceptual and methodologic work that has been undertaken to establish benchmarks for change scores, not percentage change.

19.1.b Patient-Reported Outcomes Versus Other Types of Measures

Most of the efforts to develop interpretive guidelines for change scores have been undertaken in connection with patient-reported outcomes (PROs), and, in particular, for measures of health-related quality of life. However, the concepts and methods associated with interpretation of numerical scores are not *inherently* specific to PROs. One reason for the research focus on PROs is that clinicians often have "intuitive" understanding of how to interpret changes in widely used clinical measures (e.g., blood pressure) but lack such understanding for scores on the hundreds of PROs that are in use. Although many measurement examples in this chapter are for PROs, the concepts discussed here may be appropriate for interpreting change scores for biophysiologic, performance-based, and observational measures. Indeed, the methods used to facilitate interpretation in PROs are now also being applied to clinical outcomes, such as the work in establishing a benchmark for important change in forced expiratory volume in 1 second (FEV_1) at 100 ml (Donohue, 2005).

Despite some conceptual similarities across types of measures, the nature of the measure *can* affect how interpretive benchmarks are established. As noted in several earlier chapters, PROs fall along a continuum in terms of their objectivity/subjectivity. For PROs that measure how patients *feel*, interpretation must take into account the patients' perspective. For some PROs, however, the focal constructs can be independently evaluated. For example, dyspnea can be measured by patient reports but also can be evaluated clinically through spirometry. For many health outcomes, either patients or clinicians/researchers (or both) can offer interpretive direction. Thus, researchers who seek to establish interpretive guidance must come to a conclusion about whose perspective on meaningfulness matters.

19.1.c Individuals Versus Groups: Change Versus Difference

Interpreting meaningful change at the individual level has often been confused in the medical literature with interpreting clinically important mean group differences at the end of a trial. Although several writers have explicitly noted that it is inappropriate to establish benchmarks based on individual change and then interpret mean group differences in clinical trials in terms of those benchmarks (e.g., Dworkin et al., 2009; Guyatt, 2000; Testa, 2000), this is a commonplace practice.

The confusion may stem in part from terminology that has become widespread. A term that is frequently used in connection with the interpretation of change is *MCID*, which stands for the *minimal clinically important difference*.[1] The word *difference* suggests a group comparison rather than an individual change over time. Like the Consensus-based Standards for the selection of health Measurement Instruments (COSMIN) group (DeVet, Terwee, Mokkink, & Knol, 2011), we use terminology and acronyms that refer to the interpretation of *changes* rather than *differences* because this chapter focuses on change scores, most importantly the *minimal important change*. The thresholds discussed in this chapter relate primarily to the interpretation of changes in individual scores, although we discuss group-level interpretation at the end of this chapter.

19.1.d Benchmarks for Change Scores: Concepts and Methods

The main conceptual task in deriving benchmarks is to have a clear vision of what the benchmark for "meaningfulness" represents, and the main methodologic task is to operationalize that conceptualization. There has been no consensus on either concepts or methods.

Part of the turmoil in the literature on interpreting change is that several different types of benchmarks have been established, and they are not always carefully explained. Even when the operationalization of a benchmark has been specified, there is often some fuzziness

---

[1]Some researchers have argued for removing the "clinical" designation from the MCID term because of a desire to establish thresholds based solely on patients' (rather than clinicians') perspective (e.g., Juniper, Guyatt, Willan, & Griffith, 1994; Schünemann & Guyatt, 2005). Thus, the acronym *MID* (*minimal important difference*) is also found frequently in the literature, especially when the focal construct is quality of life.

about what the benchmark is intended to represent conceptually. In various combinations, the words "minimal," "smallest," "sufficient," "detectable," "perceivable," "important," "worthwhile," and "clinically significant" have been used by different writers in conjunction with these interpretive benchmarks, often without a definition or distinction being formally stated. Clearly, it matters a great deal if one emphasizes a *minimal* or *smallest* threshold versus an *important* or *clinically significant* one.

Several researchers have made efforts to compare various change score benchmarks. One such study was conducted by Beaton and colleagues (2011), who compared 13 different approaches to establishing benchmarks for change scores on the Disabilities of the Arm, Shoulder, and Hand (DASH) scale. Based on Beaton et al.'s study, we have created a classification with five broad benchmark categories, reflecting their conceptual meaning. As shown in Table 19.1, these include (A) values of reliable change, based on measurement error (discussed in Chapter 17); (B) minimal perceivable change (MPC); (C) minimal important change (MIC); (D) final state attainment; and (E) combination approaches that typically combine a measurement error criterion with a second criterion such as final state or MIC. Each of these thresholds will be described and illustrated in Section 19.2.

In terms of methods, many different approaches to quantifying the threshold for meaningful change have been proposed. The three most widely used approaches are shown in the column headings in Table 19.1. One method involves using an expert panel to establish the threshold, and the other two are anchor-based and distribution-based approaches. In brief, anchor-based methods for setting a benchmark use an external criterion to determine how large a change score must be to be viewed as meaningful. Distribution-based methods derive a threshold value on the basis of the distributional properties of a sample. These two approaches overlap with methods described in Chapter 18 on assessments of responsiveness. Indeed, one of the confusing aspects of the literature on change scores is that interpretation and responsiveness have often been confounded. The COSMIN group played an important role in distinguishing the two.

Table 19.1	A Classification of Benchmarks for Change Score Interpretation and Methods of Deriving Benchmark Values			
		Methods of Deriving Benchmark Value		
Interpretive Benchmark Category[a]	Acronym	Expert Panel/ Consensus	Anchor-Based Approach	Distribution-Based Approach
A. Change that is reliable, greater than measurement error	SDC, RCI, 1 *SEM*			X
B. Change that is minimally perceivable	MPC		X	X
C. Change that is minimally important	MIC	X	X	X
D. Final state/patient acceptable symptom state	PASS	X	X	X
E. Combination (Category A + C or A + D)	–	X	X	X

[a]This category scheme was developed by the authors on the basis of work done by Beaton et al. (2011).
SDC, smallest detectable change; RCI, reliable change index; *SEM*, standard error of measurement; MPC, minimal perceivable change; MIC, minimal important change; PASS, patient acceptable symptom state.

19.1.e Universal Versus Specific Interpretive Benchmarks

It would be extremely appealing to have interpretive benchmarks based on simple and universal rules rather than having to compute a different threshold of meaningfulness for every newly created measure and for every population. Several such benchmarks have been proposed, at least as a reasonable starting point or approximation for an important amount of change. As one example, Norman, Sloan, and Wyrwich (2003, 2004) proposed that a change of a half a standard deviation (0.5 SD for baseline scores) is a statistically and psychologically defensible benchmark for interpreting a change score as noteworthy. In terms of an effect size (ES), which is a mean change score divided by the baseline SD, a benchmark of 0.5 SD corresponds to a *moderate* effect using Cohen's (1988) standards. Another benchmark thought to have broad applicability, especially for quality of life measures, is a mean change of 0.5 per item on a 7-point scale; for example, a change of 3.0 points on a scale with six items (Jaeschke, Singer, & Guyatt, 1989; Juniper et al., 1994). Yet another recommendation is to use a change value equal to about 5% to 10% of the instrument range as an approximate rule of thumb for meaningful change (Ringash, O'Sullivan, Bezjal, & Redelmeier, 2007).

However, others have criticized both these specific suggestions and the broader notion that there could be a universal or semiuniversal benchmark (e.g., Farivar, Liu, & Hays, 2004; Wright, 2003). Those lobbying for measure-specific and group-specific standards often base their arguments on evidence that the amount of change that is important varies for people at different points on the scale at the baseline measurement or at different levels of disease severity (e.g., Beaton, Boers, & Wells, 2002; Stratford, Binkley, Riddle, & Guyatt, 1998; Tubach et al., 2005a). In other words, where a patient begins can influence the amount of change necessary for the change to be considered important. Moreover, there is evidence that the benchmark is often different for positive change (improvement) and negative change (deterioration). Several studies have found that the amount of change needed to detect important improvement is lower than the amount needed to detect important deterioration (Doyle, Crump, Pinitlie, & Oza, 2001; Hays & Wooley, 2000). There has also been some discussion of possible differences in threshold values on a measure for people with chronic versus acute illnesses (e.g., Norman et al., 2004; Wright, 2003; Wyrwich, 2004).

Several researchers have explored the degree to which different approaches to establishing thresholds yield similar values. Some researchers, especially those promoting a "universal" threshold, have found approximate comparability (e.g., Norman et al., 2003). Others have found, however, that different methods lead to dissimilar benchmarks (e.g., Beaton et al., 2011; Turner et al., 2010). In the Beaton et al. (2011) study, rather sizeable differences in change score threshold values were found when 13 calculation methods were compared, and there were also noteworthy disparities in the diagnostic accuracy of the thresholds. Indeed, this is not surprising when one considers that the benchmarks used in the analysis span the five categories in Table 19.1. Different conceptualizations of what the threshold should capture are unlikely to lead consistently to the same amounts of change needed to reach that threshold.

The two next sections describe different benchmark definitions and alternative methods of establishing them. The issue of triangulation across methods is discussed later in the chapter.

19.2 Conceptualizations of Interpretive Benchmarks

The work that has been done to define and operationalize interpretive benchmarks for change scores has its roots in a seminal paper by Jaeschke and colleagues (1989). These researchers advocated the development of strategies for interpreting change scores: "Translating changes in instrument score into clinically meaningful terms is crucial in the interpretation of study results" (p. 408). Although they referred to *changes* in scores in this statement, they went on to provide an often quoted definition that refers to *differences*: "The minimal clinically important difference (MCID) can be defined as the smallest difference in score in the domain of interest which patients perceive as beneficial and which would mandate, in the absence of troublesome side effects and excessive cost, a change in the patient's management" (p. 408).

This definition, in its entirety, has to our knowledge never been fully operationalized. Patients are often involved in establishing a threshold for what is "minimal" for PRO measures, but it is usually the researchers, not the patients, who decide on the cutpoint for what is deemed "beneficial" or "important." Side effects and costs are not typically taken into consideration in the thresholds. And "clinical" input on what amount of change in a score would result in a change in patient management is seldom sought in establishing the benchmark. Thus, although the Jaeschke et al. (1989) definition regarding change score benchmarks has been cited in hundreds of papers, researchers have gone in many different directions in translating and quantifying it.

Benchmarks are most often described in terms of the methods used to derive a benchmark value, and we review the primary strategies in the next section of this chapter. First, however, we look briefly at different conceptualizations using a classification system (and some terminology) that we developed. The categories are based loosely on our reading of the 13 methods used in the study by Beaton and colleagues (2011).

19.2.a Benchmarks Based on Measurement Error

In Chapter 17, we described methods of estimating whether a change score is "real" or reliable using the smallest detectable change (SDC) or reliable change index (RCI). A few researchers have used the SDC/RCI as a threshold for meaningful change (e.g., Wolinski et al., 1998), and Beaton and colleagues (2011) included an index of reliable change as one of the benchmarks in their comparative study of 13 MIC definitions.

In the gerontologic literature, Willis and others (e.g., Schaie & Willis, 1986; Willis, Jay, Diehl, & Marsiske, 1992) have proposed that one standard error of measurement (1 *SEM*) represents a crucial threshold for defining individual change. Wyrwich, Tierney, and Wolinsky (1999, 2002) have undertaken several studies that have found correspondence between 1 *SEM* and the MCID, as established using anchor-based methods, for measures of health-related quality of life among patients with chronic illnesses. Thus, change beyond a measurement error value is sometimes interpreted as a minimal threshold of importance.

Several commentators have noted that it may not make much sense to compute a threshold for important change at the individual level if that threshold is less than the value for a reliable change score. For example, Swartz and colleagues (2011) noted that "the measurement precision of the instrument should also be taken into account when defining an MID (minimal important difference)" (p. 1165). Combination approaches, described in Section 19.2.e, consider both measurement precision plus other criteria for setting a benchmark of importance.

19.2.b Minimal Perceivable Change

In our classification, we distinguish a benchmark that emphasizes the "minimal" amount of change that is detectable or discernible (Category B in Table 19.1) from one that emphasizes a change that is "important" (Category C). Most researchers who set out to establish a threshold for a particular measure do not make this distinction, and so there is often ambiguity in what the threshold actually represents until one reads the details of how the threshold was operationalized.

In our typology, we call the benchmark that focuses on the smallest change that is perceptible to patients or clinicians as the **minimal perceivable change (MPC)**. Only a handful of researchers, notably those who have done research on quality of life in patients with asthma, have used a similar term. Barber, Santanello, and Epstein (1996) appear to have been the first to designate a threshold as the *minimal patient perceivable improvement* (MPPI) and the *minimal patient perceivable deterioration* (MPPD).

Although only a few other researchers have used "perceivable" or a similar term to describe their thresholds (e.g., Broeders, Molema, Hop, Vermue, & Folgering, 2003; Santanello, Zhang, Seidenberg, Reiss, & Barber, 1999), many benchmarks are calibrated to detect the smallest amount of change that patients (or clinicians) are able to detect or perceive. In anchor-based methods, the MPC might correspond to a small amount of change (a report of "a little bit better") on a global rating scale (GRS). Using distribution-type methods such as a baseline *SD*, a minimal perceptible change might correspond to a *small effect* (0.2 *SD*) using Cohen's (1988) criterion for effect size. Some researchers have found that "small improvement" on a GRS yields a similar change score threshold to a small effect size (e.g., Kelleher, Pleil, Reese, Burgess, & Brodish, 2004). A few have proposed an ES of .20 as the definition of a meaningful change threshold, including a recent study that assessed several static IRT-based measures developed within the Patient Reported Outcomes Measurement Information System (PROMIS®) project (Bjorner et al., 2014).

19.2.c Minimal Important Change

The COSMIN group (DeVet et al., 2011) used the term **minimal important change (MIC)** for all change score benchmarks, whether the researchers focused primarily on the "minimal" or the "important" aspect of change. They defined MIC as "the smallest change in score in the construct to be measured which patients perceive as important" (p. 245), but they acknowledged that for non-PRO measures, a clinician's perspective could be relevant. As we shall see, however, patients' view about what is important is seldom taken into account.

Methodologists have disagreed about whether to emphasize a threshold that is "minimal" versus "important" in establishing a benchmark of meaningfulness. Revicki, Hays, Cella, and Sloan (2008), for example, have stated that "it is important to identify the subset of people who have experienced minimal change" (p. 104). Sloan (2005), on the other hand, noted that his definition of an interpretive threshold "represents a difference that holds some practical meaning to the appropriate stakeholders while not necessarily being, strictly speaking a *minimally* important difference" (p. 59, emphasis in the original). In our category scheme shown in Table 19.1, we define MIC (Category C) as *the smallest change score value for a change that is judged to be important or significant to a relevant stakeholder group*, usually patients, but sometimes clinicians or others. This threshold is higher than the MPC and could be operationalized using distribution methods (e.g., an *SD* of 0.5) or using anchors that require a greater amount of change than for the MPC. For example, instead of anchoring change scores on a GRS rating of "a little better," an MIC as we define it would anchor the threshold at "somewhat better" or "much better," as many researchers have done.

In the section on methods for establishing interpretive thresholds, we use the acronym MIC throughout (i.e., without distinguishing it from MPC) to be consistent with the COSMIN terminology but urge readers to attend to what the term represents when thresholds for particular instruments are being described. Particular attention needs to be paid to the nature of the threshold (how much is enough to be meaningful?) and the nature of any anchor (whose perspective was considered?).

19.2.d Final State Benchmarks

Unlike all the other types of benchmarks described thus far, "final state" benchmarks (Category D in Table 19.1) are not linked to change scores but rather to the patients' final status after a change on the focal construct is presumed to have occurred. This approach, which has been advocated by Tubach and colleagues (2005b, 2006), focuses on a threshold that signifies a successful patient outcome, the **patient acceptable symptom state (PASS)**. Patients whose score on a measure exceeded the PASS benchmark would be considered to have a desirable or satisfactory outcome, regardless of how much change was required to achieve that state.

Tubach and colleagues (2006) argued that patients are more interested in "feeling good" than in simply "feeling better" (although this hypothesis needs to be tested across diseases and conditions and across health constructs). For example, patients might be more interested in attaining a pain level below 30 (on a 0 to 100 scale) than in reducing their pain from 65 to 50. The study by Tubach et al. (2006) revealed that the PASS threshold was higher for patients whose baseline scores were less favorable, consistent with research that has found that the MIC varies for different levels of initial disease severity.

In their study, Tubach et al. (2006) estimated PASS threshold values for final-state measures of pain and physical function using an anchor-based approach. The anchor was whether patients with knee and hip osteoarthritis had attained a satisfactory state. Distribution-based approaches have also been used to operationalize "final state" criteria, as we illustrate in the next section.

Beaton and colleagues (2011), in their evaluation of 13 different thresholds, used diagnostic testing to classify individuals undergoing physical therapy as "responders" or "nonresponders" to treatment, based on change scores on the DASH scale. Their receiver operating characteristic (ROC) analysis used two patient-reported criteria for the responder classification: whether or not treatment goals were met and whether or not there was important improvement, based on patients' rating on a GRS as "much better." The researchers found that the final state thresholds had especially good classification accuracy compared to other methods of setting a benchmark of importance.

19.2.e Combination Benchmarks

A number of combination approaches are beginning to appear in the health care literature, and many involve using a measurement-error criterion plus a second criterion, usually "final state" or the MIC, for setting a benchmark of important change. One of the earliest combination methods originated in the psychotherapy literature.

In Chapter 17, we described the RCI that was proposed by Jacobson and Truax (1991) for evaluating whether a person's change score on a psychotherapy outcome was beyond measurement error. The RCI is actually the first component of a two-part process that Jacobson proposed for defining a clinically significant change for individuals. First, a person's change on the measure has to be reliable, as assessed by the RCI. And second, the person has to move from a "dysfunctional" status on the measure at baseline to a "normal" state following treatment. Thus, this combination or "hybrid" method combines reliable change with a threshold based on a patient's final state.

Jacobson and Truax (1991) and Jacobson, Roberts, Berns, and McGlinchey (1999) recognized the challenge of classifying patients based on the second criterion. They proposed three alternative methods of operationalizing whether a patient had achieved a classification of "normal," all based on a conceptualization of movement from a dysfunctional population to a normally functioning population:

■ *Method A.* The final score should fall outside the range of the dysfunctional population, defined as being at least 2 *SD*s from the mean for that population, in the direction of a better outcome.

■ *Method B.* The final score should fall within the range of the functional (normal) population, defined as being within 2 *SD*s of the mean for that population.

■ *Method C*. The final score should place the person closer to the mean of the functional population than to the mean of the dysfunctional population.

Jacobson and colleagues (1999) concluded that when the distributions for the two populations overlap, then Method C is the best criterion. Method C is also a simple cutoff value to compute, when relevant norms are available:

$$\text{Cutoff} = (\text{Mean}_{\text{Dysfunctional}} + \text{Mean}_{\text{Functional}}) \div 2$$

When norms for a healthy population are not available, however, Method A is the only viable alternative. Using the combined two criteria of the RCI plus final state, patients can be classified into various groups: (1) recovered (reliably changed and in a positive final state), (2) improved but not recovered (reliably changed, but failed to meet the final-state criterion), and (3) unchanged, or not reliably changed.

Jacobson's approach had not until recently gotten much attention in the medical literature, but there have been recent efforts to use it. For example, Mann, Gosens, and Lyman (2012) applied this approach, using Method C, with normative data for the Knee Injury and Osteoarthritis Outcome (KOOS) pain scale, the DASH scale, and the International Knee Documentation Committee (IKDC) measure. Beaton et al. (2011), in their comparative analysis of change score benchmarks for the DASH, used Methods B and C based on normative data for the U.S. general population on the DASH to define the boundaries of a healthy population. They noted that their study results "point to a combination of change greater than error and/or a final score within general population norms as being the most clinically sensible with strong diagnostic accuracy" (p. 487). Replication of their findings with other populations and measures will be helpful in understanding the generalizability of their conclusions.

Other "hybrid" approaches have been suggested, combining a measurement error criterion with MIC rather than a "final state." For example, Jordan, Dunn, Lewis, & Croft (2006) applied nine different benchmark definitions to change scores on the Roland–Morris Disability Questionnaire (RMDQ) with patients with low back pain. The nine definitions included one anchor-based method, four measurement-error (distribution) methods, and four combination methods with thresholds that met both a measurement error and an anchor-based minimum change threshold. They used the combination methods to derive a "rule" for determining clinical improvement on the RMDQ. As we shall see, triangulation among methods is becoming increasingly common, and although they are seldom described as "combination" methods, they do often take several criteria for establishing a threshold into account.

19.3 Methods of Establishing Interpretive Thresholds

Dozens of methods have been used to establish interpretive change score thresholds for health care measures, particularly among quality-of-life researchers. There is little agreement on which approach is preferable. In fact, there is not total agreement on whether so much effort should be devoted to deriving threshold values, with some arguing that any MIC value is better than none (Redelmeier, Guyatt, & Goldstein, 1996), while others recommending caution in search for the MIC "holy grail" (e.g., Hays & Woolley, 2000).

We think interpretive aids can be helpful but recognize that, at present, there is no "perfect" or ideal way to establish thresholds of meaningfulness. In this section, we review major options, which include consensus panels, anchor-based methods, and distribution-based methods.[2]

---

[2]Other methods, such as population-based approaches that identify subpopulations with different levels of health (e.g., Stewart et al., 1989) as a basis for establishing thresholds, are not described here but are reviewed in an article by Crosby, Kolotkin, and Williams (2003).

19.3.a Experts and Consensus Panels

A traditional approach to developing interpretive thresholds for health outcomes is to obtain input from a panel of health care experts, usually clinicians, but sometimes a combination of clinicians and patients. The panels often convene in face-to-face sessions, either at conference workshops or specially organized meetings. For example, a group of 36 international experts met at a workshop during the 8th International Forum on Primary Care Research on Lower Back Pain in Amsterdam in 2006 (Ostelo et al., 2008). The panel reviewed MIC values that were proposed in studies using anchor-based methods for five widely used measures of pain and function: the Numerical Rating Scale for pain, a VAS for pain, the Roland–Morris Disability Questionnaire (RMDQ), the Oswestry Disability Index, and the Quebec Back Pain Disability Questionnaire. After reviewing previously established MICs, the panel arrived at a consensus recommendation. Table 19.2, which summarizes the results, shows that the original MICs were highly variable across studies and provided divergent interpretive assistance for a change score. In the expert panel, the recommended MIC change score range was narrowed in an initial review, and further discussion led to specific MIC recommendations. The panel concluded that both absolute score change and percentage improvement were important for interpretive purposes. The percentage improvement from baseline across all measures was 30%, which is consistent with the recommendations of the IMMPACT consensus panel mentioned earlier (Dworkin et al., 2005) and also consistent with the finding in the study by Jordan and colleagues (2006), who used a combination approach to defining clinical significance for the RMDQ.

Methods other than face-to-face meetings have also been used to obtain expert feedback. For example, Burback, Molnar, St. John, and Man-Son-Hing (1999) surveyed geriatricians and neurologists in Canada and asked a question designed to estimate the MIC: "From your experience following demented patients, what are the smallest changes in the Folstein Mini-Mental State Examination (MMSE) scores that are compatible with a noticeable change in the patient's overall condition?" The mean and median value, based on responses from 161 physicians, was 3.72 and 3.00 points, respectively.

Wyrwich, Tierney, Babu, Kroenke, and Wolinsky (2005) used Delphi survey methods followed by a half-day face-to-face consensus panel meeting to derive MIC values on the

Table 19.2	Minimal Important Change (MIC) Values From Expert Panel for Measures Used in Research on Low Back Pain			
Measure	**Score Range**	**MIC Change Score Range, From Anchor-Based Studies[a]**	**MIC Change Score Value: Expert Consensus**	**MIC Percent Improvement: Expert Consensus**
Visual Analog Scale for pain	0–100	2–29 points	15 points	30%
Numerical Rating Scale for pain	0–10	1.0–4.5 points	2 points	30%
Roland–Morris Disability Questionnaire	0–24	2.0–8.6 points	5 points	30%
Oswestry Disability Index	0–100	4–15 points	10 points	30%
Quebec Back Pain Disability Questionnaire	0–100	8.5–32.9 points	20 points	30%

[a]Based on values obtained in several different studies, using different MIC methods; sources are available in Ostelo et al. (2008).
Adapted from tables in Ostelo, R., Deyo, R., Stratford, P., Waddell, G., Croft, P., & DeVet, H. C. W. (2008). Interpreting change scores for pain and functional status in low back pain. *Spine, 33*, 90–94.

SF-36 subscales for three groups of physicians with expertise in quality-of-life measurement in patients with chronic obstructive pulmonary disease (COPD), asthma, and heart disease, respectively. The researchers found that panel-derived MIC thresholds were different for the three disease groups, and in all cases, they were larger than the MIC values that had previously been established for the SF-36 in a study of patients with arthritis using five different anchors (Kosinski, Zhao, Dedhiya, Osterhaus, & Ware, 2000).

Thus, expert panels have been used both as an independent method of establishing an MIC or as a supplementary effort in conjunction with other approaches. Make, Casaburi, and Leidy (2005), in their introduction to a special issue on interpretive benchmarks in the journal *COPD*, urged that opinions about meaningful change should be sought from other health care experts (e.g., nurses, behavioral scientists) and from patients, in addition to medical experts.

19.3.b Anchor-Based Methods for Establishing a Minimal Important Change

The hallmark of an anchor-based approach to deriving the MIC of a measure is that an independent external criterion is used to establish the change score threshold that defines meaningfulness. The goal is to identify the number of score points on the focal measure that is typical for those who reach a desirable status on the criterion (e.g., a "much improved" status) or an important level of deterioration on the criterion.

In using this approach, researchers must make four critical decisions: (1) What is an appropriate criterion for the construct being measured? (2) How many criteria should be used? (3) How will the criterion or criteria be measured? and (4) How will "minimally meaningful" be defined? To illustrate, Table 19.3 presents some study examples that illustrate a range of different anchoring decisions that have been made in establishing MICs for various health measures.

In terms of selecting a criterion, an important issue is whose perspective to take into account. For many PROs, the patients' perspective, using a GRS that asks patient about change over a specified period, may be the best criterion. It does not make sense, for example, to ask clinicians to rate the degree to which their patients' level of fatigue has improved, worsened, or stayed the same. The clinicians would be basing their rating on patients' reports, so it is preferable to ask patients directly about change when establishing the MIC for a fatigue scale. In other cases, however, a clinician's assessment of change might be a better criterion, especially for PRO measures that are not totally subjective, such as physical function. A clinician's assessment can be based both on what their patients are telling them about changes and also on alterations on objective performance measures or physiologic tests. Sometimes change scores on clinical tests can themselves be used as the criterion for the MIC, and sometimes the criterion is a measure of an important life event (e.g., return to work). Thus, thought should be given to what would make an appropriate criterion for establishing that a change on the focal measure is meaningful, given the nature of the construct being measured and the population of interest.

Several factors other than perspective affect the choice of a suitable criterion. First, the criterion should be a measure that correlates highly with the focal measure. The stronger the relationship, the more confident one can be that an interpretation vis-à-vis the anchor is appropriate. In many cases, a suitable criterion has been identified as part of the measure's validation process, and evidence about the degree of correlation is likely to be available. Revicki and colleagues (2008) recommend that the correlation between the focal measure and the criterion be .30 to .35, at a minimum. Guyatt et al. (2000) suggested a minimum correlation of .50.

Second, the criterion should be a measure that itself has high interpretability. For example, if the MIC benchmark for a PRO was described as equivalent to (for example) a 20% improvement in FEV_1, or to a reduction in pain that patients themselves described as "much improved," the criterion would be immediately meaningful. It makes little sense to tie the MIC to change scores on another scale that is itself difficult to interpret. And third,

Table 19.3   Examples of Anchors and Cutpoints for Minimum Important Change or Minimum Perceivable Change

Focal Scale[a]	Anchor(s)[a]	Perspective on Amount of Change	Anchor Scale	Cutpoint on Anchor for Improvement Threshold	Threshold Term	Citation
King's Health Questionnaire	■ Change score (T2–T1) for perceived treatment benefit ■ Change score (T2–T1) in perceived disease impact	Patient	1–3 1–6	■ 1 scale point improvement (e.g., from "no" to "a little" benefit) ■ 1 scale point improvement (e.g., from causes "severe" to "moderate" problems)	MID	Kelleher et al. (2004)
Asthma diary symptom score	Perceived change in asthma	Patient	1–7	4 ("a little better")	MPPI	Santanello et al. (1999)
6-minute walk test	Perceived change in overall health	Patient	–7–+7	2 ("a little bit better")	MCID	Kwok, Pua, Mamum, and Wong (2013)
Roland–Morris Disability Questionnaire	Perceived change in pain	Patient and clinician (averaged)	–7–+7	5 ("quite a bit better")	MCID	Stratford et al. (1998)
Oswestry Disability Index	Perceived treatment benefit at 2-year follow-up	Patient	1–7	3 (intermediate scale labels not provided; 1 = "I am completely disabled", 7 = "I am completely recovered")	MIC	Johnsen et al. (2013)
Quebec Back Pain Disability Scale (QBPDS)	Global perceived effect of treatment	Patient	1–6	2 ("much improved")	MCIC	van der Roer, Ostelo, Bekkering, van Tulder, and DeVet (2006)
Functional Assessment of Cancer Therapy-Breast (FACT-B)	■ Change (T2–T1) in performance status rating ■ Change (T2–T1) in performance status rating	Physician Patient	0–4 0–4	■ 1 scale point change (e.g., "completely disabled" to "limited self-care") ■ 1 scale point change (e.g., "completely disabled" to "limited self-care")	MID	Eton et al. (2004)
Health Assessment Questionnaire (HAQ)-Disability	■ Change in swollen/tender joint count ■ Change in T2–T1 rating of how "patient is doing"	– Patient and physician	0%–50% 1–5	■ Improvement in 1%–19% of patient's joints ■ 1 scale level of improvement (e.g., from "fair" to "good")	MIC	Kosinski et al. (2000)

[a]Several studies established MIC values for multiple focal scales; in such cases, only one is shown in this table; other studies used multiple anchors, and not all are shown.
MCIC, minimal clinically important change; MCID, minimal clinically important difference; MIC, minimal important change; MID, minimal important difference; MPPI, minimal patient perceivable improvement.

the criterion would ideally be one that is highly valued by relevant audiences, or correlated with highly valued outcomes (e.g., reduced risk of rehospitalization).

Multiple anchors that rely on different perspectives may in some cases be attractive because of possible limitations with a single criterion. Indeed, Guyatt and others have been proponents of using multiple anchors in establishing MIC thresholds (e.g., Guyatt et al., 2000, 2002). Table 19.3 has several examples of studies that used more than one criterion to establish the MIC value on a focal measure (e.g., Eton et al., 2004; Kosinski et al., 2000).

A third decision in setting an MIC benchmark concerns how to measure the criterion. This is a particular concern for those using a GRS as their anchor. As we described in Chapter 18, the number of GRS score values can range from 3 (e.g., *got worse, stayed the same, got better*) to 15, with scores measuring the degree of perceived change. Some researchers obtain information using a single rating question, whereas others first ask the 3-point question on deterioration, stability, or improvement, and then ask a second question for *amount* of deterioration or improvement, if relevant (e.g., Jaeschke et al., 1989). In recent work, a widely used approach is a single 5- or 7-point rating question that asks about degree of change on the construct of interest (e.g., from *very much worse* to *very much better*). Another popular GRS is a 15-point scale whose values range from −7 (*a very great deal worse*) through 0 (*no change*) to +7 (*a very great deal better*).

Yet another way to measure the criterion is to ask a point-in-time status question twice and then compute a change score for the criterion. For example, one of the anchors used in a study by Kelleher et al. (2004) to define the MIC on King's Health Questionnaire (KHQ), a measure of quality of life for patients with lower urinary tract dysfunction, was the change in a patient's assessment of the perceived impact of the bladder condition. The 5-point rating question on perceived current disease impact was asked at baseline and then at follow-up. The researchers used a change of 1 point (e.g., from causing *moderate problems* to causing *minor problems*) as the anchor for the MIC on the KHQ (Table 19.3). Those who opt for this approach often mention problems such as recall bias as a reason for not asking a direct transition question, but change scores on a single 5- or 7-point rating item are susceptible to low reliability and are therefore problematic as well. A few researchers have used an anchor that requires a social comparison. Redelmeier et al. (1996) derived MIC values for the Chronic Respiratory Questionnaire based on patients' ratings of their own condition relative to that of others with the same condition. They found that these between-person comparisons yielded MIC threshold values similar to those obtained for the more traditional within-person comparisons.

The final decisions for anchor-based methods concern how much change is enough to be considered meaningful and whose viewpoint will be used in making that determination. As described earlier, the interpretive threshold can be set to capture "minimal change," corresponding to an anchor of a small but discernible change (e.g., "slightly improved"), which we have called "minimal perceivable change." Many researchers use this lowest degree of change as the anchor for the MIC, and examples are shown in Table 19.3 (e.g., Kwok et al., 2013). Others, however, use a higher cutpoint on the criterion, such as "moderately" or "much" improved (e.g., Stratford et al., 1998; van der Roer et al., 2006).

The literature on the MIC has tended to stress that the MIC represents a change that *patients* perceive as beneficial, drawing on the previously quoted definition in the groundbreaking paper by Jaeschke et al. (1989). To illustrate researchers' emphasis on patients' perspectives, at least conceptually, Table 19.4 presents some examples of how "minimal importance" has been defined. As this table shows, definitions overwhelmingly suggest that patients should be the ones to evaluate what is important. However, in the vast majority of cases in which the MIC is calculated using the anchor-based approach, it is the researchers, not the patients, who have decided how much change was enough to be considered meaningful. That is, patients describe the *amount* of change they have experienced, but researchers designate the amount that is important. Ferreira and colleagues (2012), for

Table 19.4	Selected Definitions of "Minimally Important" in Relation to Patients' Perceptions	
Citation	**Term Used in Reference**	**Definition**
Jaeschke et al. (1989)	MCID	"The smallest difference in score ... which patients perceive as **beneficial. ...**" (p. 408)[a]
Fritz and Irrgang (2001)	MCID	"The smallest change in a scale that is **important** to patients" (p. 778)
Guyatt et al. (2002)	MID	"The smallest difference in score ... that patients perceive as **important**, either beneficial or harmful. ... (p. 377)
Barrett, Brown, Mundt, and Brown (2005)	MID	"The smallest amount of **benefit** that patients can recognize and value" (p. 250)
Schünemann and Guyatt (2005)	MID	"The smallest difference in score ... that informed patients or informed proxies perceive as **important**, either beneficial or harmful" (p. 594)
Jordan et al. (2006)	MID	"A change in an individual's score that either the patient or the clinician would identify as being an **important** change" (p. 45).
Revicki et al. (2008)	MID	"The smallest score or change in score that would likely be **important** from the patient's or clinician's perspective" (p. 103)

[a]The Jaeschke et al. (1989) definition has been used in dozens of other studies.
MID, minimal important difference; MCID, minimal clinically important difference.

example, reviewed studies that had established the MIC for measures relating to low back pain, and in all 24 studies that had used an anchor-based approach, the cutpoint on the anchor to establish the MIC was decided by the researchers.

The goal of the body of research on change score interpretation is to help with conclusions about whether a change score is trivial or meaningful. It is possible, however, that patients perceive minimal change ("slight improvement") as insignificant, despite the frequent use of minimal change as a cutpoint to anchor the MIC.[3] Some research on this issue suggests that patients need to feel "much better" (not a little better) to be satisfied with a treatment (Ferreira, Ferreira, Herbert, & Latimer, 2009). In another study in which researchers asked patients with low back pain to rate how much was the minimum improvement in pain and activities of daily living (ADL) ability they would consider worthwhile to undergo treatment, the median percentage improvement was 25% to 30%, suggesting that more than "slight" improvement would be meaningful to them (Yelland & Schluter, 2006). These studies are consistent with the previously mentioned work of Tubach and colleagues (2005b, 2006), who proposed the PASS as more appropriate than the MIC because it establishes a threshold value on a final state measure indicating that patients "feel good" rather than "feel better." However, it is possible that feeling "a little better" is more important to patients with a chronic illness than to those with an acute illness, who desire a return to full health and capacity.

---

[3]It has been suggested that some patients may rate their status as "slightly improved" even when they have not perceived a change simply to be agreeable or to please their clinician (Ostelo et al., 2008). Some patients, however, may say that they have not changed, even if they *have* changed because they are dissatisfied with their degree of improvement or final state.

To achieve a threshold that is important and not just discernible, researchers may need to obtain more information from patients (or clinicians, or both) about whether a "slight" improvement is simply a "perceivable" change or an important and meaningful one. Alternatively, researchers can directly use an anchor that embodies the concept of satisfactory or meaningful change. Here are a few examples of this approach:

- In the Kelleher et al. (2004) study to establish an MIC threshold for the King's Health Questionnaire, one anchor involved changes in patients' perceptions of treatment *benefit*.

- Ten Klooster, Drossaers-Bakker, Taal, and van de Laar (2006) asked patients to rate their pain levels at baseline and 2 weeks after a local corticosteroid injection on a VAS for pain. Their anchor was a GRS whose categories were *worse, unchanged, unsatisfactory improved, satisfactory improved,* and *good to very good improved.* The cutpoint for the VAS pain benchmark was based on those who reported satisfactory improvement.[4]

- Tubach et al. (2005b) used as their anchor for establishing the PASS threshold for pain and function scales a simple question of whether patients were "satisfied" with their current state.

- Riddle, Stratford, and Binkley (1998) used as an anchor for the Roland–Morris Back Pain Questionnaire a physical therapist's rating of whether a patient had or had not met treatment goals.

It appears that more work is needed for many PROs to ensure that operationalizations of "minimal importance" correspond to conceptual definitions of the MIC and that patients are included in the decision about what amount of change is meaningful.

Once decisions have been made about which anchor or anchors to use, how to measure them, and what anchor cutpoints will signify minimal importance, researchers then must use the anchor to establish how many change score points on the focal measure correspond to the designated point on the anchor. The majority of researchers have used one of two strategies: (1) calculating the mean change score at the selected anchor cutpoint or (2) using receiver operating curve (ROC) analysis.

The simplest procedure is to compute the mean change score on the focal scale for subgroups based on responses on the criterion. Figure 19.1 presents an example for a fictitious ADL scale. In this example, let us suppose that patients completed the ADL scale at baseline (T1) and 3 months later (T2), and during the interval, both positive and negative changes were expected to occur. At T2, patients were also asked to respond to a 7-point GRS about their perceived degree of change in their physical functioning. Figure 19.1 shows the mean change scores on the ADL scale for seven subgroups with different amounts of perceived change on the GRS. In this example, the MIC for improvement would be 3.89 change score points if the benchmark was set at the "much better" response or at 2.17 if the benchmark was set at the "little better" response. Note that the MIC values for deterioration, in this example, would be different than the MIC for improvement, but not by much (e.g., 3.89 vs. −4.03 for "much" change). The subgroup means in Figure 19.1 are idealized; in reality, the differences in subgroup means on the criterion are not always perfectly linear and consistent with expectations, especially if some subgroups are small.

Another approach is to treat the focal scale as a diagnostic test for discriminating between improved and unchanged patients (or between unchanged and deteriorated patients) and to undertake an ROC analysis. In this situation, the anchor is used as the "gold standard." Sensitivity is the number of patients that are "correctly" identified as improved on the basis of change scores on the focal scale, divided by the number of patients categorized as improved on the basis of the anchor. Specificity is the number correctly identified as unchanged by the change scores on the focal scale, divided by the number of patients

---

[4]Ten Klooster et al. (2006) used a different term for their threshold: patient-perceived satisfactory improvement (PPSI). Their stated goal was to derive "information on relevant changes from the patient's perspective" (p. 155), noting that the MIC as usually established does not meet this objective.

Please rate the changes you have experienced in the past three months with regard to *your ability to perform regular activities of daily living*, such as standing up from a sitting position or taking a bath or shower:

GRS rating	Mean change score on ADL scale (Posttest – Baseline)
1. Very much better	5.50
2. Much better	3.89
3. A little better	2.17
4. No change	0.75
5. A little worse	-1.89
6. Much worse	-4.03
7. Very much worse	-5.98

Highlighted categories indicate possible MIC thresholds for improvement.

Figure 19.1

Example: A global rating scale anchor used to establish a minimal important change (improvement) on a fictitious activities of daily living (ADL) scale.

classified as unchanged on the anchor. The ROC curve analysis plots each change score value against the sensitivity and specificity of predicting the anchor. The MIC is then defined as the change score that yields the lowest amount of misclassification.

The use of an ROC approach requires researchers to divide the sample into two subgroups based on the anchor, and so again a decision must be made regarding how to define "meaningfully improved." In the example in Figure 19.1, patients who gave a rating of either 1 or 2 (i.e., "very much better" or "much better") could be contrasted with all other patients to define an "improved" or "not improved" group for the ROC analysis. Or, the threshold could be set at 3 ("a little better") to distinguish *any* improvement (ratings of 1 to 3) from all others (ratings of 4 to 7). Another decision is whether to contrast "improved" versus "not improved" patients (e.g., a rating of 1 to 2 vs. a rating of 3 to 7 on the GRS) or to contrast "improved" versus "unchanged" patients. If the latter is desired, two cutpoints are needed: one to define patients who have improved on the criterion (e.g., a rating of 1 to 2) and another to define patients who are unchanged (e.g., a rating of 3 to 5).

Anchor cutpoints are often set a priori by researchers, presumably reflecting their own conceptualization of how to define importance, or their desire to be consistent with other research teams. It is usually advisable, however, to verify the appropriateness of the cutpoint decision by testing the significance of differences in mean change scores on the focal scale for people in different subgroups on the criterion. For example, van der Roer and colleagues (2006) used an ROC analysis to establish the MIC for three pain-related scales that contrasted an *improved* group (defined as those who reported they were "much improved" or "completely recovered" on a GRS) with an *unchanged* group (defined as those who reported they were unchanged, slightly improved, or slightly worse). They found that the mean change scores on the focal scales for the "slightly improved" and "unchanged" subgroups were not significantly different and concluded that their decision about collapsing subgroups was justified. As a caution, however, it may be difficult to have confidence in nonsignificant differences if the subgroup sizes are modest.

19.3.c Distribution-Based Methods for Establishing a Minimal Important Change

The major alternative to an anchor-based approach to setting an MIC value is what has been called *distribution-based methods*. Distribution methods are based on the statistical characteristics of a sample, and they express the MIC as a standardized metric. The most frequently used metric is based on Cohen's (1988) effect size index (ES), operationalized at the individual level in terms of a fraction of the *SD* in baseline scores.

Various thresholds for minimally important change based on the ES/SD have been offered in the literature, the most frequent being a threshold of 0.5 (i.e., one-half an SD in the distribution of baseline scores; Norman et al., 2003, 2004). Norman and colleagues found that there was "remarkable" (2003) and "truly remarkable" (2004) consistency supporting a threshold equivalent to an SD of 0.5. They argued that this consistency was unlikely to be a coincidence but rather could be tied to theory and evidence on the psychology of human discrimination. Norman and colleagues computed ES values for dozens of measures for which the MIC had been calculated using anchor-based methods, with the MIC value in the numerator and the baseline SD in the denominator. After removing a few studies for various reasons, they found that the mean ES was 0.495, and that the distribution of ES values was approximately normal. They further found that the mean effect size was not significantly different for studies that used a patient GRS versus a more clinically oriented anchor, for scales that had a 7-point scale for response options versus a different scale, or for measures that were general or disease specific. Unfortunately, these researchers did not examine the extent to which the ES value might be sensitive to anchor cutpoints emphasizing "minimal" versus "important."

Unlike anchor-based methods, the SD/ES and other similar methods do not directly yield an MIC threshold value in change score units. However, it is easy to compute what that threshold value should be for any scale for which baseline distribution information is available. For example, if the baseline SD for a scale were 8.0, then the MIC using the 0.5 criterion would be 4.0. This value, like any MIC, could be used as the benchmark to classify individual patients as having or not having clinically meaningful change. Several researchers have defined an MIC for their measure on the basis of the 0.5 SD benchmark. For example, De Morton and Lane (2010) created a Rasch-based index for measuring mobility in older people across a broad spectrum of abilities, the De Morton Mobility Index or DEMMI, and used 0.05 SD to calculate the benchmark for important change.

Other SD values have been proposed as the MIC benchmark. For example, an ES/SD of .20 (traditionally considered a "small" effect using Cohen's criteria) has been suggested as a threshold for minimal change (Bjorner et al., 2014; Kelleher et al., 2004; Samsa et al., 1999). Beaton et al. (2011) used an SD of 0.2 as one of the 13 MIC methods in their comparative study. Values in the range of 0.30 to 0.33 SD have also been used to set the MIC threshold (e.g., Eton et al., 2004; Twiss, Doward, McKenna, & Eckert, 2010).

An alternative distribution-based method, as noted earlier, is to establish the MIC threshold value on the basis of measurement error. In particular, a number of researchers have cited 1 SEM as their operationalization of the MIC threshold (e.g., Hilliard et al., 2013; Tsiligianni et al., 2012). Norman et al. (2003) noted that for measures with a test–retest reliability of .75, the 0.5 SD threshold is exactly equivalent to 1 SEM. As discussed in Chapter 17, the SDC or RCI based on a 95% confidence interval sets a rather stringent standard for coming to conclusions about "real" change for individual patients. Wyrwich (2004) maintained that "the 1 SEM threshold is well beyond the necessary 'more than likely' or 51 percent level of confidence that change occurred at the individual level" (p. 586).

19.3.d Comparison of Methods for Establishing Benchmarks

Commentators have disagreed about which method yields the most trustworthy and helpful benchmark for interpreting change scores, but most people agree that none of the approaches is ideal. The anchor-based approach, which is preferred by the COSMIN group and by the U.S. Food and Drug Administration, adds more work to the already burdensome program of research required of instrument developers. Identifying an appropriate and reliable anchor is not easy, and, in fact, one of the biggest criticisms of the anchor-based approach is that a single GRS is a poor choice of a criterion because of weak reliability and the problem of recall bias. Gatchel et al. (2010) have argued that basing the MIC for a PRO "on another related self-report rating is both circular in logic and fraught with potential bias" (p. 1740). On the other hand, the use of alternative anchors (such as clinical indicators of change or clinicians' perceptions of change) has little appeal among those who believe that changes on PROs must be interpreted from a patient's perspective. Also, anchor-based approaches can sometimes cause confusion in the literature. The use of alternative criteria, different operationalizations of the criteria, and different cutpoints to establish meaning-fulness can result in the derivation of many different MIC values for the same measure. On the positive side, anchor-based approaches may yield MICs that are easier to communicate to clinicians and patients (e.g., "Patients whose score increased by four or more points on this scale were more likely than others to have reported great improvement in pain levels").

Distribution approaches have been advocated by some (e.g., Norman et al., 2003; Samsa et al., 1999). MICs based on distribution approaches are easy to compute and thus have particular appeal for new scales. Moreover, the use of distributional methods may not re-quire a separate study; information about a measure's standard error of measurement or about a distribution of baseline scores is usually available without special effort or expense. However, it may be difficult to communicate what a distribution-based MIC represents to nonresearch audiences. A persistent criticism of distribution methods is that they yield val-ues that are not linked to any clinical yardstick. In and of themselves, they do not embed any notion of "meaningfulness" or "importance." Clinicians may be no better off interpreting an MIC based on an *SD* (or 1 *SEM*) than they would be with raw change scores. Another problem with MICs based on *SD*s is that the value is clearly dependent on the heterogene-ity of the population under study. This is less likely to be an issue with a 1 *SEM* threshold. Those who have suggested distribution-based MICs, however, usually emphasize that they are a "good place to start" (Samsa et al., 1999, p. 150) or "an approximate rule of thumb in the absence of more specific information" (Norman et al., 2003, p. 590) rather than an absolute or rigid guideline for setting the MIC.

Because of the problems with the two primary methods of establishing interpretive benchmarks, many researchers have pursued more complex approaches, as discussed next.

19.3.e Triangulation of Methods

The absence of a "gold standard" method for establishing interpretive thresholds has led sev-eral experts to argue for a triangulation of methods (e.g., Leidy & Wyrwich, 2005; Revicki et al., 2008). Many researchers have, in fact, chosen a path of triangulation, which can occur in a single study or across studies in efforts to integrate threshold recommendations.

Many approaches to triangulation within a study can be adopted, including using mul-tiple anchors and blending anchor-based and distribution methods. Often, these efforts are not viewed as a "combination" approach (Method E in Table 19.1) in which the MIC value is based on meeting two criteria (e.g., a measurement error criterion and an anchor-based criterion) but rather an effort to "converge" on a reasonable estimate for the MIC through different approaches.

Some triangulation studies involve methods that are sophisticated but laborious. For example, DeVet and colleagues (2007) developed an innovative visual approach, called the *anchor-based MIC distribution method*, which graphically integrates a distribution-based and anchor-based approach. They claimed that their method leads to better decisions about defining *minimal importance* on an anchor, but the complexities of the method make it a procedure that is unlikely to be widely adopted.

Most efforts at triangulation rely on applying multiple methods to compute an MIC. Certain types of triangulation seem to have particular appeal. One type that appears to be gaining favor is to combine *SEM* and *SD* methods with an anchor-based method. An ex-ample of a study that combined multiple anchors and multiple approaches was undertaken by Patel and colleagues (2013), who sought to establish the MIC for King's Brief Interstitial Lung Disease Questionnaire (K-BILD). These researchers used two distribution methods (1 *SEM* and 0.3 *SD*), a clinical anchor (a forced vital capacity [FVC] change of at least 7%

from baseline), and patients' responses on four GRSs (a change of ±2 or ±3 on a GRS whose scores could range from −7 to +7). Integrating all information, the researchers established the MIC on the K-BILD at 8 points.

For those who pursue such triangulated strategies, advice about how to reach a conclusion is scarce. That is, once a research team follows a path of triangulation in a study, how should they proceed to integrate the MIC information? Many writers have recommended presenting a range of MIC values rather than a single value. However, an MIC range may be confusing for those wishing to interpret change scores and who may struggle to grasp which part of the range is most appropriate to their situation, unless the range is presented in connection with explicit guidelines, such as suggesting different MIC values for people with different baseline scores.

Some researchers report both a range and a suggested single value for the MIC benchmark using a variety of methods to derive the single value. Patel and colleagues (2013), for example, *averaged* across their various methods to arrive at the MIC value of 8 points on the K-BILD measure. Other researchers have stated as their rule the selection of whatever MIC value is largest, thus yielding the most conservative value. For example, Hsieh and colleagues (2007) used the 1 *SEM* and an anchor-based method to calculate the MIC for the Barthel Index in patients with stroke. They established a priori that the larger of the two MIC values would establish the benchmark. Such an approach has the virtue of ensuring that reliable change and "important" change is taken into account. Other researchers do not formally state their method of integrating MIC information but seem to use an "eyeball" approach to land on a value that is based on several possible MICs. For example, Eton and colleagues (2004) used multiple anchors that included both the patients' and the clinicians' perspective and combined the anchor-based MICs with distribution methods (1 *SEM*, 0.33 *SD*, and 0.5 *SD*) to conclude that there was sufficient convergence to recommend an MIC of 7 to 8 points on the Functional Assessment of Cancer Therapy-Breast (FACT-B) scale. None of the proposed methods of integration seem especially appropriate, however, when the MIC values from different approaches are conspicuously divergent, as they were in the Beaton et al. (2011) comparative study.

For any given measure, no single study is likely to provide the final word on what an MIC value should be, especially because the value is likely to vary across populations and applications. Some advice has emerged about integrating MIC evidence as a progression of activities. Sloan (2005) recommended using a simple calculation of the MIC using distribution-based methods, such as 0.5 *SD*, as a starting point. Next, explorations of the appropriateness of this estimate, using multiple anchors, can be used to validate or modify the initial estimate. Finally, feedback from clinicians or patients (e.g., by means of a special panel) would be used to further refine the MIC. Revicki and colleagues (2008) recommended starting by establishing an MIC on the basis of multiple relevant anchors and then examining various distribution methods for "supportive information" (p. 103). Regardless of the starting point, there seems to be some agreement that finding a defensible MIC for widely used and psychometrically sound measures involves a process of evaluating and integrating evidence, which can occur through systematic reviews or in the context of a dedicated consensus exercise by a panel of experts. As Revicki et al. noted, confidence in a specific MIC value "evolves over time and is confirmed by additional research evidence" (p. 103). As measures "mature" and become more widely used in clinical trials or in clinical settings, interpreting change may become increasingly less daunting.

19.4 Interpretation at the Group Level

All of the anchor-based methods for establishing MIC values discussed in this chapter are based on individual change scores. These methods seek to determine how much change must occur for a patient to pass a threshold value of meaningful improvement or deterioration on a focal measure. Yet, despite the clear connection between benchmarks and *individual* change scores, the thresholds have often been used to interpret group differences at a single point in time, most often postintervention outcomes in a clinical trial.

Several writers have noted that it is inappropriate to interpret the mean differences in an intervention and control group in relation to the MIC. For example, if the mean difference on a measure between groups is 2.0 and the MIC for that measure is 4.0, it should not be concluded that the effect is not clinically important simply because the mean difference is only half the value of the MIC. Because of the heterogeneity of treatment effects, mean effects can mask individual benefit. A mean group difference of 2.0 could be consistent with a sizeable percentage of the target group achieving a meaningful benefit (e.g., an improvement of 4.0 or greater) from an intervention. Conversely, if the mean group difference between a treatment and control group is greater than 4.0, it does not mean that every patient benefited from the treatment.

MIC thresholds can, however, be used to create new outcomes that aid in the interpretation of clinical trial results. Once a threshold for meaningful change is established, researchers can classify individual subjects in all arms of a clinical trial in terms of their having attained the threshold. In particular, study participants can be classified as *responders* or *nonresponders* to treatment based on an established threshold of important change. Then, a **responder analysis** that compares the percentage of responders in treatment and control groups can be undertaken. A distinct advantage of responder analyses is that they are readily understandable, and they can facilitate comparisons across trials, or across different outcomes in a trial.

In its guidelines on the use of PROs in clinical trials to support labeling claims, the U.S. Food and Drug Administration (2009) avoided any reference to MIC or minimal important difference. They advocated the use of a responder analysis for clinical trial interpretation and stressed that the evidence for establishing the threshold for classification as a *responder* be derived from anchor-based methods. As an alternative to a responder analysis, the FDA suggested presenting a *cumulative distribution function* to depict change scores (and hence the effect of an intervention) for all arms of a trial, "avoiding the need to pick a responder criterion" (p. 25). Wyrwich, Norquist, Lenderking, and Acaster (2013) presented such a graph, showing change scores for patients in three different arms of a trial to test the effects of different doses of Aricept® on cognitive functioning. The X-axis of the graph represented change scores on the test, and the Y-axis represented the cumulative percentage of patients achieving the change. The X-axis designated points along the change score continuum that represented an important change threshold, and so the graph portrayed both responder information and overall differences in group change.

Hopefully, as researchers gain familiarity with MIC benchmarks, they will come to appreciate the importance of applying them to individuals and extrapolating them to groups rather than using the threshold to understand mean group differences. Dworkin and colleagues from the IMMPACT group (2009) pointed out that drawing inferences about the clinical meaningfulness of group differences in clinical trials involves consideration of a wide range of factors. These include the results of traditional tests of statistical significance, responder analyses using interpretive thresholds, and other key factors such as cost, convenience, patient adherence, and patient safety.

19.5   Developing and Evaluating Minimal Important Change Benchmarks

This section describes some issues to consider in designing studies to establish a measure's MIC, in reporting the information, and in evaluating the work of other researchers.

19.5.a   Study Design and Sampling for Establishing the Minimal Important Change

Studies that are undertaken to establish a benchmark for interpreting change scores require a longitudinal design. A sample of subjects must be measured with the focal instrument on at least two occasions, over an interval of several weeks or months. Sometimes, the work is done during a responsiveness assessment, but often, it is done as a completely separate endeavor and not always by the people who developed the measure.

Much of the advice we offered in Chapter 18 regarding study design for assessments of responsiveness also apply to efforts to develop interpretive guidelines for change scores. The study must gather data from a population in which variation in change scores over the time interval is anticipated. Both improvement and deterioration on the construct of interest might be expected. This, in turn, means that attention should be paid to baseline floor and ceiling effects on the focal measure.

The length of time between measurements should be selected based on some knowledge about the trajectory of change on the construct for the population of interest. The time interval should be large enough for change to have occurred for at least some people, but not so long as to risk problems with attrition and response shift, as discussed in Chapter 18. The time interval should be the same for the focal measure and for the period designated on any anchors.

If changes on the focal construct evolve slowly and the time interval required for measuring a change on the construct is long, then concerns about response shift are likely to increase, especially for constructs of a highly subjective nature. To be safe, it might be prudent to include a then test (Chapter 17) in the design of the study. If there is evidence of response shift, researchers should be careful to explain the implications for using MIC values.

For an anchor-based approach to establishing MIC benchmark, key decisions are what the criteria will be, how to measure them, and what the cutpoint will be to define meaningfulness, as discussed in Section 19.3.b. Multiple anchors are often attractive, and combining anchors that include patient input with ones of a more clinical nature may be particularly helpful for different audiences of interpreters. Interpretation might also be enhanced by including as an anchor a question about patient satisfaction with treatment or satisfaction with the amount of change experienced. If possible, the anchors should be ones for which evidence of validity and reliability is available.

In terms of sampling, it is always desirable to recruit a sample that is representative of the target population. If one of the methods for establishing the MIC is linked to sample heterogeneity, such as 0.5 *SD*, baseline variability on the focal measure will obviously affect its value. One should not artificially constrain variability in baseline scores to reduce the MIC, but it might be prudent to exclude extreme outliers or at least to do a sensitivity test with outliers excluded.

Sample size is an especially critical issue when an anchor-based approach is used. Subgroups created on the basis of the chosen cutpoint should be sufficiently large that mean values on the focal measure are stable. If categories have to be collapsed because of small *N*s in certain cells, the unfortunate result may be that the cutpoint is established as a result of inadequate sample size rather than for conceptual reasons (e.g., if "slight" and "moderate" improvement have to be combined to achieve a stable mean on the focal measure).

In performing the analyses to establish the MIC, it is prudent to perform calculations separately for improvement and deterioration. It is also a good practice to examine the generalizability of the MIC across important groups within the sample, such as people with different degrees of illness severity or different levels of the focal construct at baseline. When different MICs are reported for people with different baseline scores, they are often reported for tertiles of the baseline distribution (i.e., those with the lowest, middle, and highest scores) or for quartiles of the distribution. For example, Hart, Wang, Stratford, and Miolduski (2008) used a GRS to calculate the MIC for an IRT-based computerized adaptive test of functional status for patients with foot or ankle impairments undergoing rehabilitative therapy. The MIC ranged from 5 points (on a 0- to 100-point scale) for patients in the top quartile at intake to 12 points for those in the bottom quartile.

Triangulation of methods is an increasingly popular approach to establishing MIC values. When an anchor-based approach is used, it is easy to combine this with one or two distribution approaches. If multiple methods will be used to derive MIC values, the rules for integrating different MIC values should be formulated upfront. We think it is especially prudent to take measurement error into account in coming to conclusions about the MIC. It makes little sense to derive a threshold of importance if that threshold has a fairly high possibility of being achieved simply as a result of random fluctuations of measurement. In other words, the MIC should ideally be larger than the SDC, or at least larger than 1 *SEM*. Thus, whenever the MIC is established for a measure, it is important to also have information about its standard error of measurement.

19.5.b Reporting Minimal Important Changes

Because MIC values for a measure are sensitive to both population and context, it is important to describe the sample and circumstances in a report on the MIC. Sample characteristics should be sufficiently detailed so that readers can understand the relevance of the MIC benchmark for a new application. In terms of context, a specific rationale should be provided for why change on the measure was expected and why the selected time interval was chosen.

The report should provide a judicious rationale for all major decisions, particularly for the chosen criteria and cutpoint in anchor-based methods. If the MIC relied on a cutpoint on a GRS indicating "slight" change, an explicit discussion should be offered for why small changes were considered to be meaningful. In other words, the conceptualization of the MIC should be explained in the report's introduction, and it should correspond to the operationalization described in the Method section. If the MIC definition in the report suggests that the goal was to obtain patients' perspective on importance, then it is prudent to provide some evidence that patients did, in fact, consider the cutpoint as signifying nontrivial (meaningful) change.

In triangulated studies, researchers are likely to obtain a range of MIC values. If a range is presented in a report, it is advisable to offer guidance for how the range should be interpreted. For a responder analysis, a single MIC value is usually adopted, but it would also be possible to use different MICs for patients with different baseline scores on the focal measure. The MIC is often used for estimating sample size requirements in a new trial, so a single "best estimate" of the MIC is likely to prove valuable.

19.5.c Evaluating Minimal Important Changes in a Report

When evaluating a report describing the derivation of a benchmark for interpreting change scores on a measure, it is important to assess whether the researchers provided a conceptual definition of what they considered important change and whether that definition is congruent with the cutpoint on an anchor. If the conceptual definition points to the primacy of patients' view on importance, for example, were patients actually involved in deciding which threshold to use? If the researchers themselves decided to emphasize "minimal change" rather than "important change," the rationale for that decision should be evaluated.

If only distributional methods were used, the report should explain why this approach was considered adequate. And, if only an anchor-based approach was used, it is useful to examine what the report said about measurement error and reliable change. For example, if the calculated MIC is less that the SDC, or less that one *SEM*, then the report should caution readers about interpreting a change score that might surpass the MIC benchmark but may not be reliable.

If multiple anchors were used in an anchor-based method, or if multiple different methods were triangulated, the authors of the report should provide a good rationale for the method they used to combine the information. Ideally, the report would also say something about whether the MIC benchmark could be applied along the full range of values on the focal measure.

References

Barber, B. L., Santanello, N., & Epstein, R. (1996). Impact of the global on patient perceivable change in an asthma specific QOL questionnaire. *Quality of Life Research, 5*, 117–122.

Barrett, B., Brown, D., Mundt, M., & Brown, R. (2005). Sufficiently important difference: Expanding the framework of clinical significance. *Medical Decision Making, 25*, 250–261.

Beaton, D. E., Boers, M., & Wells, G. A. (2002). Many faces of the minimal clinically important difference (MCID): A literature review and directions for future research. *Journal of Rheumatology, 14*, 109–114.

Beaton, D. E., van Erd, D., Smith, P., van der Velde, G., Cullen, K., Kennedy, C., & Hogg-Johnson, S. (2011). Minimal change is sensitive, less specific to recovery; a diagnostic testing approach to interpretability. *Journal of Clinical Epidemiology, 64*, 487–496.

Bjorner, J. B., Rose, M., Gandek, B., Stone, A., Junghaenei, D., & Ware, J. (2014). Method of administration of PROMIS scales did not significantly impact score level, reliability, or validity. *Journal of Clinical Epidemiology, 67*, 108–113.

Broeders, M., Molema, J., Hop, W., Vermue, N., & Folgering, H. (2003). Does the inhalation device affect the bronchodilatory dose response curve of salbutamol in asthma and chronic pulmonary disease patients? *European Journal of Clinical Pharmacology, 59*, 449–495.

Burback, D., Molnar, F., St. John, P., & Man-Son-Hing, M. (1999). Key methodological features of randomized controlled trials of Alzheimer's disease therapy. *Dementia and Geriatric Cognitive Disorders, 10*, 534–540.

Cohen, J. (1988). *Statistical power analysis for the behavioral sciences* (2nd ed.). Hillsdale, MJ: Lawrence Erlbaum.

Crosby, R. D., Kolotkin, R., & Williams, G. R. (2003). Defining clinically meaningful change in health-related quality of life. *Journal of Clinical Epidemiology, 56*, 395–407.

De Morton, N. A., & Lane, K. (2010). Validity and reliability of the De Morton Mobility Index in the subacute hospital setting in a geriatric evaluation and management population. *Journal of Rehabilitation Medicine, 42*, 956–961.

DeVet, H. C. W., Ostelo, R., Terwee, C., van der Roer, N., Knol, D. L., Beckerman, H., & Bouter, L. (2007). Minimally important change determined by a visual method integrating an anchor-based and a distribution-based approach. *Quality of Life Research, 16*, 131–142.

DeVet, H. C. W., Terwee, C., Mokkink, L. B., & Knol, D. L. (2011). *Measurement in medicine: A practical guide.* Cambridge, MA: Cambridge University Press.

Donohue, J. F. (2005). Minimal clinically important difference in COPD lung function. *COPD, 2*, 111–124.

Doyle, C., Crump, M., Pinitlie, M., & Oza, A. (2001). Does palliative chemotherapy palliate? Evaluation of expectations, outcomes and costs in women receiving chemotherapy for advanced ovarian cancer. *Journal of Clinical Oncology, 19*, 1266–1274.

Dworkin, R. H., Turk, D., Farrar, J., Haythornethwaite, J., Jensen, P., Katz, N., . . . Witter, J. (2005). Core outcome measures for chronic pain clinical trials: IMMPACT recommendations. *Pain, 113*, 9–19.

Dworkin, R. H., Turk, D., McDermott, M., Peirce-Sandmer, S., Burke, L., Cowan, P., . . . Sampaio, C. (2009). Interpreting the clinical importance of group differences in chronic pain clinical trials: IMMPACT recommendations. *Pain, 146*, 238–244.

Eton, D. T., Cella, D., Yost, K., Yount, S., Peterman, A., Neuberg, D., . . . Wood, W. (2004). A combination of distribution- and anchor-based approaches determined minimally important differences (MIDs) for four endpoints in a breast cancer scale. *Journal of Clinical Epidemiology, 57*, 898–910.

Farivar, S. S., Liu, H., & Hays, R. (2004). Half standard deviation estimate of the minimally important difference in HRQOL scores? *Expert Review of Pharmacoeconomics & Outcomes Research, 4*, 515–523.

Ferreira, M. L., Ferreira, P., Herbert, R., & Latimer, J. (2009). People with low back pain typically need to feel "much better" to consider intervention worthwhile: An observational study. *Australian Journal of Physiotherapy, 55*, 123–127.

Ferreira, M. L., Herbert, R., Ferreira, P., Latimer, J., Ostelo, R., Nascimento, D., & Smeets, R. (2012). A critical review of methods used to determine the smallest worthwhile effect of interventions for low back pain, *Journal of Clinical Epidemiology, 65*, 253–261.

Fritz, J., & Irrgang, J. (2001). A comparison of a modified Oswestry Low Back Pain Disability Questionnaire and the Quebec Back Pain Disability Scale. *Physical Therapy, 81*, 776–788.

Gatchel, R. J., Lurie, J., & Mayer, T. (2010). Minimal clinically important difference. *Spine, 35*, 1739–1743.

Guyatt, G. H. (2000). Making sense of quality-of-life data. *Medical Care, 38*(9, Suppl.), II175–II179.

Guyatt, G. H., Osoba, D., Wu, A., Wyrwich, K., Norman, G. (2002). Methods to explain the clinical significance of health status measures. *Mayo Clinical Proceedings, 77*, 371–383.

Hart, D. L., Wang, Y., Stratford, P., & Miolduski, J. (2008). Computerized adaptive test for patients with foot or ankle impairments produced valid and responsive measures of function. *Quality of Life Research, 17*, 1081–1091.

Hays, R. D., & Woolley, J. M. (2000). The concept of clinically meaningful difference in health-related quality of life research. *Pharmacoeconomics, 19*, 419–423.

Hiller, W., Schindler, A., & Lambert, M. (2012). Defining response and remission in psychotherapy research: A comparison of the RCI and the method of percent improvement. *Psychotherapy Research, 22*, 1–11.

Hilliard, M. E., Lawrence, J., Modi, A., Anderson, A., Crume, T., Dolan, L., . . . Hood, K. K. (2013). Identification of minimal clinically important difference scores of the PedsQL in children, adolescents, and young adults with type 1 and type 2 diabetes. *Diabetes Care, 36,* 1891–1897.

Hsieh, Y. W., Wang, C., Wu, S., Chen, P., Sheu, C., & Hsieh, C. (2007). Establishing the minimal clinically important difference of the Barthel Index in stroke patients. *Neurorehabilitation and Neural Repair, 21,* 233–238.

Jacobson, N. S., Roberts, L., Berns, S., & McGlinchey, J. (1999). Methods for defining and determining the clinical significance of treatment effects: Description, application, and alternatives. *Journal of Consulting and Clinical Psychology, 67,* 300–307.

Jacobson, N. S., & Truax, P. (1991). Clinical significance: A statistical approach to defining meaningful change in psychotherapy research. *Journal of Consulting and Clinical Psychology, 59,* 12–19.

Jaeschke, R., Singer, J., & Guyatt, G. H. (1989). Measurement of health status: Ascertaining the minimal clinically important difference. *Controlled Clinical Trials, 10,* 407–415.

Johnsen, L. G., Hellum, C., Nygard, O., Storheim, K., Brox, J., Rossvol, I., Grotle, M. (2013). Comparison of the SF6D, the EQ5D, and the Oswestry Disability Index in patients with chronic low back pain and degenerative disc disease. *BMC Musculoskeletal Disorders, 14,* 148.

Jordan, K., Dunn, K., Lewis, M., & Croft, P. (2006). A minimal clinically important difference was derived for the Roland-Morris Disability Questionnaire for low back pain. *Journal of Clinical Epidemiology, 59,* 45–52.

Juniper, E. F., Guyatt, G. H., Willan, A., & Griffith, L. E. (1994). Determining a minimal important change in a disease-specific quality of life questionnaire. *Journal of Clinical Epidemiology, 47,* 81–87.

Kelleher, C. J., Pleil, A., Reese, P., Burgess, S., & Brodish, P. (2004). How much is enough and who says so? The case of the King's Health Questionnaire and overactive bladder. *BJOG, 111,* 605–612.

Kosinski, M., Zhao, S., Dedhiya, S., Osterhaus, J., & Ware, J. (2000). Determining minimally important changes in generic and disease-specific health-related quality of life questionnaires in clinical trials of rheumatoid arthritis. *Arthritis & Rheumatism, 43,* 1478–1487.

Kwok, B. C., Pua, Y., Mamum, K., & Wong, W. (2013). The minimal clinically important difference of six-minute walk in Asian older adults. *BMC Geriatrics, 13,* 23.

Leidy, N. K., & Wyrwich, K. (2005). Bridging the gap: Using triangulation methodology to estimate minimal clinically important differences (MCIDs). *COPD, 2,* 157–165.

Make, B., Casaburi, R., & Leidy, N. (2005). Interpreting results from clinical trials: Understanding minimal clinically important differences in COPD outcomes. *COPD, 2,* 1–5.

Mann, B. J., Gosens, T., & Lyman, S. (2012). Quantifying clinically significant change: A brief review of methods and presentation of a hybrid approach. *The American Journal of Sports Medicine, 40,* 2385–2393.

Norman, G. R., Sloan, J., & Wyrwich, K. W. (2003). Interpretation of changes in health-related quality of life: The remarkable universality of half a standard deviation. *Medical Care, 41,* 582–592.

Norman, G. R., Sloan, J., & Wyrwich, K. W. (2004). The truly remarkable universality of half a standard deviation: Confirmation through another look. *Expert Review of Pharmacoeconomics & Outcomes Research, 4,* 581–586.

Ostelo, R., Deyo, R., Stratford, P., Waddell, G., Croft, P., & DeVet, H. C. W. (2008). Interpreting change scores for pain and functional status in low back pain. *Spine, 33,* 90–94.

Patel, A., Siegert, R., Keir, G., Bajwah, S., Barker, R., Maher, T., . . . Birring, S. (2013). The minimal important difference of the King's Brief Interstitial Lung Disease Questionnaire (K-BILD) and forced vital capacity in interstitial lung disease. *Respiratory Medicine, 107,* 1438–1443.

Pham, T., Van der Heijde, D., Lassere, M., Altman, R., Anderson, J., Bellamy, N., . . . Dougados, M. (2003). Outcome variables for osteoarthritis clinical trials: The AMERACT-OARSI set of responder criteria. *Journal of Rheumatology, 30,* 1648–1654.

Redelmeier, D. A., Guyatt, G. H., & Goldstein, R. (1996). Assessing the minimal important difference in symptoms: A comparison of two techniques. *Journal of Clinical Epidemiology, 49,* 1215–1219.

Revicki, D., Hays, R., Cella, D., & Sloan, J. (2008). Recommended methods for determining responsiveness and minimally important differences for patient-reported outcomes. *Journal of Clinical Epidemiology, 61,* 102–109.

Riddle, D. L., Stratford, P., & Binkley, J. (1998). Sensitivity to change of the Roland-Morris Back Pain Questionnaire, Part 2. *Physical Therapy, 78,* 1197–1207.

Ringash J., O'Sullivan, B., Bezjal, A., & Redelmeier, D.A (2007). Interpreting clinically significant changes in patient-reported outcomes. *Cancer, 100,* 196–202.

Samsa, G., Edelman, D., Rothman, M., Williams, G., Lipscomb, J., & Matchar, D. (1999). Determining clinically important differences in health status measures. *Pharmacoeconomics, 15,* 1410155.

Santanello, N. C., Zhang, J., Seidenberg, B., Reiss, T. F., & Barber, B. L. (1999). What are minimal important changes for asthma measures in a clinical trial? *European Respiratory Journal, 14,* 23–27.

Schaie, K., & Willis, S. (1986). Can decline in adult intellectual functioning be reversed? *Developmental Psychology, 22,* 223–232.

Schünemann, H., & Guyatt, G. H. (2005). Commentary—Goodbye M(C)ID! Hello MID, where do you come from? *Health Services Research, 40,* 593–597.

Sloan, J. S. (2005). Assessing the minimally clinically significant difference: Scientific considerations, challenges, and solutions. *COPD, 2,* 57–62.

Stewart, A. L., Greenfield, S., Hays, R., Wells, K., Rogers, W., Berry, S., . . . Ware, J. (1989). Functional status and well-being of patients with chronic conditions: Results from the Medical Outcomes Study. *Journal of the American Medical Association, 262,* 907–913.

Stratford, P. W., Binkley, J. M., Riddle, D., & Guyatt, G. H. (1998). Sensitivity to change of the Roland-Morris Back Pain Questionnaire. *Journal of Physical Therapy, 78,* 1186–1196.

Swartz, R. J., Schwartz, C., Basch, E., Cai, L., Fairclough, D., McLeod, L., . . . Rapkin, B. (2011). The king's foot of patient-reported outcomes: Current practices and new developments for the measurement of change. *Quality of Life Research, 20,* 1159–1167.

Ten Klooster, P. M., Drossaers-Bakker, K., Taal, E., & van de Laar, M. (2006). Patient-perceived satisfactory improvement (PPSI): Interpreting meaningful change in pain from the patient's perspective. *Pain, 121,* 151–157.

Testa, M. A. (2000). Interpretation of quality-of-life outcomes: Issues that affect magnitude and meaning. *Medical Care, 38*(9, Suppl.), II166–II174.

Tsiligianni, I., van der Molen, T., Moraitaki, D., Lopez, I., Kocks, J., Karagiannis, K., . . . Tsanakis, N. (2012). Assessing health status in COPD: A head-to-head comparison between the COPD Assessment Test (CAT) and the Clinical COPD Questionnaire (CCQ). *BMC Pulmonary Medicine, 12,* 20.

Tubach, F., Dougados, M., Falissard, B., Baron, G., Logeart, I., & Ravaud, P. (2006). Feeling good rather than feeling better matters more to patients. *Arthritis & Rheumatism, 55,* 526–530.

Tubach, F., Ravaud, P., Baron, G., Falissard, B., Logeart, I., Bellamy, N., . . . Dougados, M. (2005a). Evaluation of clinically relevant changes in patient reported outcomes in knee and hip osteoarthritis: The minimal clinically important improvement. *Annals of the Rheumatic Diseases, 64,* 29–33.

Tubach, F., Ravaud, P., Baron, G., Falissard, B., Logeart, I., Bellamy, N., . . . Dougados, M. (2005b). Evaluation of clinically relevant states in patient reported outcomes in knee and hip osteoarthritis: The patient acceptable symptom state. *Annals of the Rheumatic Diseases, 64,* 34–37.

Turner, D., Schünemann, H., Griffith, L., Beaton, D., Griffiths, A., Critch, J., & Guyatt, G. H. (2010). The minimal detectable change cannot reliably replace the minimal important difference. *Journal of Clinical Epidemiology, 63,* 28–36.

Twiss, J., Doward, L., McKenna, S., & Eckert, B. (2010). Interpreting scores on multiple sclerosis-specific patient reported outcome measures (the PRIMUS and U-FIS). *Health and Quality of Life Outcomes, 8,* 117.

U.S. Food and Drug Administration. (2009). *Guidance for industry patient-reported outcome measures: Use in medical product development to support labeling claims.* Washington, DC: U.S. Department of Health and Human Services.

van der Roer, N., Ostelo, R., Bekkering, G., van Tulder, M., & DeVet, H. C. W. (2006). Minimal clinically important change for pain intensity, functional status, and general health status in patients with nonspecific low back pain. *Spine, 31,* 578–582.

Willis, S., Jay, G., Diehl, M., & Marsiske, M. (1992). Longitudinal change and prediction of everyday task competence in the elderly. *Research on Aging, 14,* 216–243.

Wolinsky, F. D., Wan, G., & Tierney, W. (1998). Changes in the SF-36 in 12 months in a clinical sample of disadvantaged older adults. *Medical Care, 36,* 1589–1598.

Wright, J. G. (2003). Interpreting health-related quality of life scores: The simple rule of seven may not be so simple. *Medical Care, 41,* 597–598.

Wyrwich, K. W. (2004). Minimal important difference thresholds and the standard error of measurement: Is there a connection? *Journal of Biopharmaceutical Statistics, 14,* 97–110.

Wyrwich, K. W., Norquist, J., Lenderking, W., & Acaster, S. (2013). Methods for interpreting change over time in patient-reported outcome measures. *Quality of Life Research, 22,* 475–483.

Wyrwich, K. W., Tierney, W. M., Babu, A., Kroenke, K., & Wolinsky, F. (2005). A comparison of clinically important differences in health-related quality of life for patients with chronic lung disease, asthma, or heart disease. *Health Services Research, 40,* 577–591.

Wyrwich, K. W., Tierney, W. M., & Wolinsky, F. (1999). Further evidence supporting an SEM-based criterion for identifying meaningful intra-individual changes in health-related quality of life. *Journal of Clinical Epidemiology, 52,* 861–873.

Wyrwich, K. W., Tierney, W. M., & Wolinsky, F. (2002). Using the standard error of measurement to identify important intra-individual change on the asthma quality of life questionnaire. *Quality of Life Research, 11,* 1–7.

Yelland, M. J., & Schluter, P. (2006). Defining worthwhile and desired responses to treatment of chronic low back pain. *Pain Medicine, 7,* 38–45.

GLOSSARY

acquiescence response set A bias in self-report scales that occurs when respondents characteristically agree with statements ("yea-say"), independent of item content.

adaptive measure A measuring approach that uses responses to early questions to guide the selection of subsequent questions; most often administered by a computer. See also *computerized adaptive testing*.

adjusted goodness of fit index (AGFI) A statistic used to evaluate the goodness of fit of a proposed model to the data (e.g., in confirmatory factor analysis); a value greater than .90 is often considered as an adequate fit.

agreement, ICC The type of intraclass correlation assessment that concerns the extent to which the scores on a measure are identical across multiple measurements; ICC formulas for agreement have both random and systematic error in the denominator.

alpha (α) In measurement, an index of internal consistency (i.e., Cronbach's alpha).

anchor-based approach An approach to estimating a measure's responsiveness, and to developing a benchmark of importance for interpreting change scores, that relies on a "gold standard" or criterion.

anonymity Protection of participants' confidentiality such that even the researcher cannot link individuals with the data they provided.

area under the curve (AUC) In an ROC analysis, an index of the performance of a diagnostic or screening measure vis-à-vis diagnostic accuracy, summarized in a single value that typically ranges from .50 (no better than random classification) to 1.0 (perfect classification).

assimilatory bias An observational bias in which the observer distorts observations in the direction of identity with previous inputs, in the direction of greater orderliness and regularity than is present.

assumption A principle that is accepted as being true based on logic or reason, without proof.

attenuation The effect that low reliability of a measure has on depressing correlation coefficients between measures.

attrition The loss of participants over the course of a study, which can create bias by changing the composition of the sample initially drawn.

AUC See *area under the curve*.

back translation The translation of a translated text (i.e., from a forward translation) back into the original language so that original and back-translated versions can be compared to assess semantic equivalence.

Bartlett's test of sphericity A statistical test used in factor analysis and other multivariate analyses that tests the null hypothesis that the correlation matrix is an identity matrix (i.e., one in which all correlations are zero).

baseline data Data collected at an initial measurement (e.g., prior to an intervention) so that changes can be evaluated.

benchmark A threshold value on a measure that has significance, such as a threshold for interpreting whether a change in scores on a measure is meaningful or clinically important.

between-subjects design A research design in which separate groups of people are compared (e.g., smokers and nonsmokers; intervention and control group subjects).

bias Any influence that distorts the results of a study and undermines validity.

Bland–Altman plot A graphic depiction of the degree of agreement between two sets of scores for people who have been measured twice on the same continuous measurement scale; the plot highlights random differences between the two measurements through the construction of a parameter called the *limits of agreement*.

blinding The process of preventing those involved in a study (participants, intervention agents, data collectors, or health care providers) from having information that could lead to a bias; also called *masking*.

carryover effect In a test–retest or intrarater reliability context, the biasing effect that an initial administration of a measure has on responses in a second administration, for example, through a practice or rehearsal effect or memory of earlier responses.

case–mean imputation An approach to imputation of missing values that involves imputing a missing value with the mean of other relevant variables from the case with the missing value (e.g., using the mean of nine nonmissing items on a scale to impute the value of the 10th item, which is missing).

categorical variable A variable with "scores" that are discrete values (e.g., gender) rather than values along a continuum (e.g., weight).

category response curve (CRC) In item response theory analyses of polytomous items, a graphical display of the probability of a person's response in each response category, given the person's latent trait.

ceiling effect The effect of having scores restricted at the upper end of a score continuum, which limits discrimination at the upper end of the measurement, constrains true variability, and restricts the amount of upward change possible.

centered translation A translation of an instrument into another language wherein the wording in the original is maintained and forms the standard against which the translation is compared. See also *decentered translation*.

central tendency bias An observational bias in which observers distort observations in the direction of uniformity and a middle ground.

change score A person's score difference between two measurements on the same measure, calculated by subtracting the value at one point in time from the value at the second point.

chi-square goodness of fit statistic (χ^2_{GOF}) A statistic used to evaluate the goodness of fit of a proposed model to the data (e.g., in confirmatory factor analysis); a nonsignificant chi-square suggests a good fit.

classical test theory (CTT) A measurement theory that has traditionally been used in the development of multi-item scales; in CTT, any score on a measure is conceptualized as having a "true score" component and an error component, and the goal is to approximate the true score.

clinical impact method A method used to select items for a clinimetric measure; the method involves a substudy to find which items in the item pool are most relevant and important to patients (or clinicians).

clinimetrics An approach to the quantitative measurement of clinical phenomena such as symptoms and signs; an alternative approach to psychometrics for health measurement.

closed-ended question A question that offers respondents a set of specific response options; also referred to as a *fixed alternative question*.

coefficient alpha The most widely used index of internal consistency that indicates the degree to which the items on a multi-item scale are measuring the same underlying construct; also referred to as *Cronbach's alpha*.

cognitive interview An interview sometimes used in a pretest of an instrument in which respondents are asked to explain the process by which they answer questions; basic approaches include a *think-aloud* method and the use of targeted *probes*; also used in connection with content validity work.

cognitive test A performance test designed to assess cognitive skills or cognitive functioning (e.g., an IQ test).

Cohen's *d* See *effect size*.

Cohen's kappa See *kappa*.

common factor variance A measure of the variance that two or more measures share in common, as in a factor analysis of multiple items; also referred to as *communality*.

communality In a factor analysis, a measure of a variable or item's shared variance with other variables; also referred to as *common factor variance* and sometimes symbolized as h^2.

comparative fit index (CFI) A statistic used to evaluate the goodness of fit of a proposed model to the data (e.g., in a confirmatory factor analysis or IRT analysis), involving the comparison of the proposed model with a null model; a value greater than .95 is often considered as indicative of a good fit.

composite scale A measure of an attribute involving the aggregation of information from multiple items into a single numerical value that places people on a continuum with respect to the attribute.

computerized adaptive testing (CAT) An approach to measuring a latent trait in which computer algorithms are used to tailor a set of questions to individuals, usually using questions from an item bank created using item response theory; with CAT, highly precise measures of a trait can typically be secured with a small set of targeted items.

concept analysis A systematic process of analyzing a concept or construct, with the aim of identifying the boundaries, definitions, and dimensionality for that concept.

conceptual definition The abstract or theoretical meaning of the construct being studied.

conceptual equivalence The extent to which a construct of interest exists and is comparable in another culture; of relevance in the translation or cultural adaptation of an instrument.

conceptual map A schematic representation of a theory or conceptual model that graphically represents key constructs and linkages among them.

concurrent validity A type of criterion validity that concerns the degree to which scores on a measure are correlated with an external criterion (a "gold standard"), measured at the same time.

confidence interval (CI) The range of values within which a population parameter is estimated to lie at a specified probability (e.g., 95% CI).

confirmatory factor analysis (CFA) An analytic method, based on structural equation modeling, that examines covariances among variables; useful for testing hypotheses about the structural validity of a multi-item measure.

consistency, ICC The type of intraclass correlation assessment that concerns the extent to which the ranking of people is consistent across multiple measurements; ICC formulas for consistency have only random (and not systematic) error in the denominator.

construct An abstraction or concept that is inferred from human behavior or human traits.

construct validity The degree to which evidence about a measure's scores in relation to other scores supports the inference that a construct has been appropriately represented; the degree to which a measure captures the focal construct.

content equivalence The extent to which the individual items on a translated or adapted measure are relevant within a new culture.

content validity The degree to which a multi-item instrument has an appropriate set of relevant items reflecting the full content of the construct domain being measured.

content validity index (CVI) An index summarizing the degree to which a panel of experts agrees on an instrument's content validity (i.e., the relevance, comprehensiveness, and balance of items comprising a scale). See also *item-level content validity index* and *scale-level content validity index*.

continuous variable A variable that can take on an infinite range of values along a specified continuum (e.g., height); less strictly, a variable measured on an interval or ratio scale.

convergent validity A type of construct validity concerning the degree to which scores on a focal measure are correlated with scores on measures of constructs with which there is a hypothesized correlation (i.e., whether there is conceptual convergence).

COSMIN The **Co**nsensus-based **S**tandards for the selection of health **M**easurement **In**struments, an initiative that developed an important measurement taxonomy and sought to standardize the definitions of measurement properties.

criterion-referenced An assessment or classification that indicates whether a person did well or poorly on some attribute in relation to an established criterion but not relative to others in the population (*norm-referenced*).

criterion validity The extent to which scores on a measure are an adequate reflection of (or predictor of) a criterion (i.e., a "gold standard" measure).

Cronbach's alpha See *coefficient alpha*.

cross-cultural validity The degree to which the items on a translated or culturally adapted scale perform adequately and equivalently, individually and in the aggregate, in relation to their performance on the original instrument; an aspect of construct validity.

cutpoint The point in a distribution of scores used to classify or divide people into different groups, such as cases and noncases for a disease or health problem (e.g., the cutpoint for classifying newborns as being low birthweight is 5.5 pounds [2,500 grams]).

data saturation See *saturation*.

decentered translation A translation of an instrument into another language wherein the translation could result in wording modifications to items on the original instrument. See also *centered translation*.

Delphi survey A technique for obtaining judgments from an expert panel about an issue of concern; experts are questioned individually in several rounds, with a summary of the panel's views circulated between rounds, to achieve some consensus.

diagnostic accuracy The degree to which a measure is accurate in diagnosing or predicting "caseness" and "noncaseness" for a condition, as established by a gold-standard criterion. See also *sensitivity* and *specificity*.

dichotomous item An item or test question with two alternatives (e.g., yes/no, true/false, correct/incorrect); also called a *binary* item.

differential item functioning (DIF) The extent to which an item functions differently for one group or culture than for another, despite the groups being equivalent with respect to the underlying latent trait.

difficulty See *item difficulty*.

disacquiescence response set A bias in self-report scales created when respondents characteristically disagree with statements ("nay-say"), independent of content.

disattenuation correction A formula used to "correct" a correlation coefficient by removing the effect of imperfect reliability or internal consistency on one or both measures.

discriminant validity See *divergent validity*.

discriminative validity See *known-groups validity*.

distribution-based methods An approach to estimating a measure's responsiveness, and to developing a benchmark of importance for interpreting change scores, that relies on distributional properties of the data, often the distribution of change scores.

divergent validity An approach to construct validation that involves gathering evidence that the focal measure is not a measure of a different construct, distinct from the focal construct; also referred to as *discriminant validity*.

domain sampling model The model underpinning scale development in the classical test theory framework, which conceptually involves the random sampling of a homogeneous set of items from a hypothetical universe of items relating to the construct.

effect size (ES) An index summarizing, in standardized units, the magnitude of change in a group or the amount of difference in two groups on a measure; calculated by dividing the mean difference in scores by an index of variability, usually the baseline *SD*; sometimes referred to as *Cohen's d* or the *standardized mean difference*; sometimes used as evidence of a measure's responsiveness.

eigenvalue The value equal to the sum of the squared weights for a linear composite, such as a factor in a factor analysis, indicating how much variance in the solution is accounted for.

endogenous variable In a structural equations model or path analysis, a variable whose variation is determined by other variables within the model.

enhancement of contrast effect An observational bias in which observers distort observations in the direction of dividing content into clear-cut entities.

equivalence In the context of instrument translation, the degree to which the translated and original measures are comparable; equivalence can be evaluated on many levels, including conceptual equivalence, content equivalence, semantic equivalence, technical equivalence, measurement equivalence, and factorial equivalence.

error of leniency An observational bias reflecting the tendency for an observer to rate things too positively.

error of measurement (X_E) In classical test theory, the difference between a hypothetical true score (X_T) and an obtained score (X_O) on a measure of a construct. See also *measurement error*.

error of severity An observational bias reflecting the tendency for an observer to rate things too harshly.

error term The mathematical expression (e.g., in a regression analysis) that represents all unknown or unmeasurable attributes that can affect a variable of interest.

exogenous variable In a structural equations model or path analysis, a variable whose determinants lie outside the model.

exploratory factor analysis (EFA) An analysis undertaken to explore the underlying dimensionality of a set of items, typically without firm *a priori* hypotheses about the structure of the focal construct.

extreme response bias A bias resulting in consistent selection of extreme alternatives (e.g., *strongly agree* or *strongly disagree*) to scale items, regardless of item content.

face validity The extent to which an instrument looks as though it is a measure of the target construct.

factor analysis A statistical procedure for disentangling complex interrelationships among items and identifying the items that "go together" as a unified dimension.

factor correlation matrix In factor analysis with oblique rotation, the factor × factor matrix that shows the correlations among the factors.

factor extraction The first phase of a factor analysis, which involves extracting as much variance as possible through the successive creation of linear combinations of the items or variables in the data set.

factor loading In factor analysis, the weight associated with an item or variable in relation to a given factor.

factor matrix In a factor analysis of scale items, a matrix with items on one dimension and factors on the other, with matrix entries being factor loadings of the items on the factors; factor matrices can be either *rotated* or *unrotated*.

factor rotation The second phase of factor analysis, during which the reference axes for the factors are pivoted to more clearly align items or variables with a single factor.

factor score A person's score on a latent variable (factor), derived by summing score values on contributing items, sometimes using item weighting.

factorial equivalence The extent to which the dimensionality of a construct is similar for an adapted measure and original measure; also referred to as *factorial invariance*, which includes several types of invariance such as *dimensional*, *configural*, *metric*, and *scalar invariance*.

fixed alternative question An item or question that offers respondents a set of prespecified response options; also referred to as a *closed-ended question*.

floor effect The effect of having scores restricted at the lower end of a score continuum, which limits the ability of the measure to discriminate at the lower end, constrains true variability, and limits the amount of downward change possible.

focus group interview An interview with a small group of individuals assembled to provide feedback on a given topic, usually guided by a moderator using a semi-structured topic guide.

formative index A multi-item measure whose items are viewed as "causing" or defining the construct of interest rather than being the effects of the construct; sometimes called a *heterogeneous measure*. See also *reflective scale*.

forward translation The translation of an item (or any text, such as scale instructions) from an original source language into a target language. See also *back translation*.

fully crossed design In measurement, a design in which every person or object is rated by every observer or rater and every observer rates every person.

generic scale A measure of a construct (e.g., quality of life) that is broadly applicable across different clinical or nonclinical populations.

global rating scale (GRS) A single item designed to provide a summary measurement of a person's status on a construct or his or her perception of change on a construct over a specified interval; also referred to as a *health transition rating*.

goodness of fit index (GFI) A statistic used to evaluate the goodness of fit of a proposed model to the data (e.g., in confirmatory factor analysis); a value greater than .90 is often considered as an adequate fit.

graded response model (GRM) A two-parameter item response theory model for polytomous items.

Guyatt's responsiveness index (GRI) An index summarizing, in standardized units, the amount of change in a group on a measure; calculated by dividing the mean score change for a group expected to change by the standard deviation for change in a group not expected to change; used to provide evidence of responsiveness.

halo effect An observational bias reflecting the tendency of an observer to be influenced by one characteristic in judging other, unrelated characteristics.

health transition scale A single item, often on a 7-point scale, that asks people to rate the extent to which they have improved/deteriorated (e.g., slightly, moderately, greatly) or stayed the same with regard to a focal attribute.

hypothesis-testing validity The extent to which it is possible to corroborate hypotheses regarding how scores on a measure function in relation to other variables; an important aspect of construct validity.

identification In model testing (e.g., in structural equation modeling or confirmatory factor analysis), a proposed model is *identified* if the known information available implies that there is one best value for each model parameter whose value is unknown.

imputation methods A broad class of methods used to address missing values problems by estimating (imputing) the missing values.

incremental fit index (IFI) A statistic used to evaluate the goodness of fit of a proposed model to the data (e.g., in confirmatory factor analysis), involving the comparison of the proposed model with a null model; a value greater than .95 is often considered as indicative of a good fit.

incremental validity The extent to which each item or component of a measure contributes something unique to the assessment of an attribute.

index A multi-item measure, by convention differentiated from the term *scale* in that the term *index* is used for a formative (rather than a reflective) measure.

infit statistic An indicator of an item's fit to a Rasch model that captures unexpected responses to an item with a difficulty level near the person's trait level.

information In item response theory, a term often used in lieu of *reliability* to indicate measurement precision;

information can be estimated both for individual items and for a scale or test.

instrument A device used to collect data (e.g., a questionnaire, test, or observation schedule).

inter-item correlation coefficients The correlation coefficients in a matrix that show the correlations between all items being considered for inclusion in a multi-item scale.

internal consistency The degree to which the subparts of a composite scale (i.e., the items) are interrelated and are all measuring the same attribute or dimension; a measurement property within the reliability domain.

interpretability The degree to which it is possible to assign qualitative meaning to an instrument's scores or change scores.

interrater (inter-observer) reliability The extent to which two raters or observers, working independently, assign the same score values for an attribute being measured.

interval measurement A measurement level in which an attribute of a variable is rank ordered on a scale that has equal distances between points on that scale but no rational zero point (e.g., Fahrenheit degrees).

interview A data collection method in which an interviewer asks questions of a respondent, either face-to-face or by telephone.

intraclass correlation coefficient (ICC) The statistical index used to assess the reliability (e.g., test–retest reliability) of a measure; the ICC estimates the proportion of total variance in a set of scores that is attributable to true differences among the people or objects being measured.

intrarater reliability The extent to which a rater or observer assigns the same score values for an attribute being observed on two separate occasions, as an index of self-consistency.

invariance The property of remaining unchanged, regardless of the conditions of measurement; an assumption in item response theory, with regard to sample and item independence.

item A single question or element on an instrument.

item analysis A broad collection of statistical procedures associated with scale construction in classical test theory as a preliminary assessment of the degree to which items are tapping the same construct—for example, examination of inter-item correlations and item-total correlations.

item bank A large collection of previously tested items, usually with the aim of using the items in computerized adaptive testing (e.g., the PROMIS® item bank established by NIH).

item characteristic curve (ICC) In item response theory, a graphic representation of an item's performance that models the relationship between people's responses to the item and their level of the latent trait; typically, an ICC is approximately S-shaped, and different parts of the curve yield information about different item parameters, such as difficulty and discrimination.

item difficulty A parameter in item response theory or Rasch models indicating the amount of a latent trait a respondent must possess in order to "pass" (or endorse) an item; also referred to as *item location*.

item discrimination A parameter in item response theory models that indicates the degree to which an item can differentiate between people with different levels of the latent trait.

item information function (IIF) A transformation of an item response function in item response theory that graphically displays how much *information* an item provides and where on the trait continuum information is at its maximum.

item-level content validity index (I-CVI) An index summarizing the degree to which experts agree on the relevance of an individual item on a scale.

item location A parameter in all item response theory or Rasch models indicating the amount of a latent trait a respondent must possess in order to "pass" (or endorse) an item; also referred to as *item difficulty*.

item pool The initial collection of items amassed for further assessment early in the process of developing a multi-item scale.

item response function (IRF) A mathematical function that indicates the probability that a person with a given latent trait (or ability) will endorse an item (or answer a test question correctly); displayed as an *item characteristic curve.*

item response theory (IRT) A "modern" measurement perspective that is gaining favor in lieu of classical test theory in developing highly precise measures of latent traits; in IRT, the focus is on understanding item characteristics, independent of the people who complete the items.

item-scale correlation The correlation between scores on an individual item under consideration for a scale and total scale scores, either *uncorrected* (when the total score includes the item) or *corrected* (when the item in question has been removed in computing the total score).

Kaiser-Meyer-Olkin (KMO) test A test, used to assess the sampling adequacy of items in a factor analysis, which compares the magnitude of correlation coefficients to the sizes of partial correlation coefficients (i.e., correlations after controlling for the effects of all other variables). The closer the value of the KMO statistic is to 1.0, the greater the degree of factorability.

kappa A statistical index of chance-corrected agreement or consistency between two nominal (or ordinal) measurements, often used to assess interrater or intrarater reliability.

known-groups validity A type of construct validity that concerns the degree to which a measure is capable of discriminating between groups known or expected to differ with regard to the construct of interest; also called *discriminative validity* or *contrast validity.*

KR-20 An index of internal consistency that can be used when the items on a scale are scored dichotomously; also called *Kuder–Richardson equation 20.*

latent trait A human trait or variable that is not manifest or directly observable but that can be inferred from people's behavior or their responses to a set of questions; term often used in the context of an item response theory analysis, confirmatory factor analysis, and structural equations analysis; sometimes referred to as *theta.* See also *construct.*

latent trait theory A measurement theory that is more often referred to as item response theory, but which also encompasses Rasch models.

level of measurement A system of classifying measurements according to the nature of the measurement and the type of permissible mathematical operations; the levels are nominal, ordinal, interval, and ratio.

likelihood ratio (LR) For a screening or diagnostic measure, the relative likelihood that a given result is expected in a person with (as opposed to one without) the target attribute; LR indexes summarize the relationship between specificity and sensitivity in a single number.

Likert scale Traditionally, a type of scale to measure attitudes, involving the summation of scores on a set of items that respondents rate for their degree of agreement or disagreement; more loosely, the name is attributed to many summated rating scales.

limits of agreement (LOA) An estimate of the range of differences in two sets of scores that could be considered random measurement error, typically with 95% confidence; graphically portrayed on Bland–Altman plots.

local independence An assumption in item response theory in which it is assumed that the latent trait being measured is the sole influence on a person's response to an item.

location See *item location.*

manifest variable An observed, measured variable that serves as an indicator of an underlying construct (i.e., a latent variable); terms used most often in a confirmatory factor analysis or structural equations analysis.

marginal homogeneity Equality between one or more of the row marginal proportions and the corresponding column proportions, based on the absence of statistical significance on a test such as McNemar's test.

marker variable In factor analysis, a variable (item) that is highly correlated with only one factor and that helps to define the underlying dimensionality of the factor.

maximum variation sampling A purposive sampling approach used by qualitative researchers involving the purposeful selection of cases with a wide range of variation on dimensions of importance.

mean substitution A relatively weak technique for addressing missing data problems that involves substituting missing values on a variable with the mean for that variable for all cases.

measure A device whose purpose is to obtain information to quantify an attribute or construct. See also *instrument*.

measurement The process of assigning numbers to represent the amount of a construct or attribute that is present in a person (or object), according to specified rules.

measurement equivalence In a translation or adaptation of an instrument, the comparability of various measurement properties (e.g., reliability, internal consistency) in the original and translated versions.

measurement error The systematic and random error of a person's score on a measure, reflecting factors other than the construct being measured and resulting in an observed score that is different from a hypothetical true score; a measurement property within the reliability domain.

measurement model In confirmatory factor analysis, the model that stipulates the hypothesized relationships among the manifest variables (e.g., items) and latent variables (constructs).

measurement parameter A statistical index that quantifies a measurement property of a measure within a population (e.g., Cronbach's alpha is a measurement parameter for the property of internal consistency).

measurement property A characteristic reflecting a distinct aspect of the measure's quality; properties include reliability, validity, reliability of change, and responsiveness.

measurement theory A framework for conceptualizing how scores generated by items on a measure represent the unobservable constructs or latent traits that they represent.

methods factor In an exploratory factor analysis, a factor that reflects correlations resulting from methodologic rather than substantive aspects of items.

minimal clinically important difference (MCID) See *minimal important change*.

minimal detectable change (MDC) See *smallest detectable change*.

minimal important change (MIC) A benchmark for interpreting change scores that represents the smallest change that is important or meaningful to patients or clinicians.

minimal perceivable change (MPC) A benchmark for interpreting change scores that represents the smallest change that is perceptible to patients or clinicians.

missing completely at random (MCAR) Values that are missing from a data set in such a manner that missingness is unrelated either to the value of the missing data or to the value of any other variable; the subsample with missing values is a totally random subset of the original sample.

missing not at random (MNAR) Values that are missing from a data set in such a manner that missingness *is* related to the value of the missing data and, usually, to values of other variables as well.

missing values Values missing for certain variables for some participants as a result of such factors as refusals, skips, question irrelevance, or researcher error.

moderacy bias A bias resulting in the consistent selection of midrange or neutral alternatives (e.g., "neither agree nor disagree") to scale items, regardless of item content; also called a *midpoint bias* or *end-aversion bias*.

monotonicity An assumption in item response theory modeling that concerns consistently increasing probability of endorsing an item with increasing levels of the latent trait.

multidimensional scale A scale that measures multiple facets of a broad and complex construct, typically yielding separate subscale scores for each dimension.

multiple imputation (MI) The gold standard approach for dealing with missing values, involving the imputation of multiple (m) estimates of the missing value, which are later pooled and averaged in estimating parameters.

multirater kappa The kappa-like statistic that is computed when there are more than two raters or observers.

multitrait–multimethod matrix method A method of assessing an instrument's construct validity using multiple measures for a set of people; the target instrument is valid to the extent that there is a strong relationship between it and other measures of the same attribute (convergent validity) and a weak relationship between it and measures purporting to measure a different attribute (divergent validity).

naysayers bias A bias in self-report scales created when respondents characteristically disagree with statements ("nay-say"), independent of content.

negative predictive value (NPV) A measure of the usefulness of a screening/diagnostic measure that can be interpreted as the probability that a negative test result is correct; calculated by dividing the number with a negative test who do not have the disease by the number with a negative test.

nested design In measurement, a design in which there is an implicit hierarchy, most often when raters or observers are nested within the people or objects being measured.

nominal measurement The lowest level of measurement involving the assignment of "scores" based on categorical classifications (e.g., males = 1; females = 2).

nonnormed fit index (NNFI) A statistic used to evaluate the goodness of fit of a proposed model to the data (e.g., in confirmatory factor analysis), involving the comparison of the proposed model with a null model; a value greater than .95 is often considered as indicative of a good fit; also referred to as the *Tucker Lewis* index or *TLI*.

normed fit index (NFI) A statistic used to evaluate the goodness of fit of a proposed model to the data (e.g., in confirmatory factor analysis), involving the comparison of the proposed model with a null model; a value greater than .95 is often considered as indicative of a good fit.

norm-referenced An assessment or classification that estimates the position of a person with regard to the trait being measured, relative to others within a defined population; the contrast is *criterion referenced*.

norms Performance standards based on score information on a measure from a large, representative sample.

oblique rotation In factor analysis, a rotation of factors such that the reference axes are allowed to move to acute or oblique angles, and hence the factors are allowed to be correlated.

observation A method of collecting information and measuring constructs by directly watching and recording behaviors and characteristics.

observational bias A bias in making and recording observations that tends to be systematic, reflecting characteristics of the observer (e.g., the error of leniency or severity).

observational checklist A formal instrument that observers use to record the presence or absence of specific traits, behaviors, or events under scrutiny.

observational rating scale A formal instrument that observers use to indicate the intensity or frequency of specific behaviors or events under scrutiny.

observed (obtained) score The actual score or numerical value assigned to a person on a measure.

one-parameter logistic (1-PL) model An item response theory model that estimates only the item difficulty (location) parameter; mathematically similar to the Rasch model.

open-ended question A question in an interview or questionnaire that does not restrict respondents' answers to preestablished alternatives.

operational definition The definition of a construct or variable in terms of the procedures by which it is to be measured.

operationalization The process of translating research or clinical concepts into measurable phenomena.

ordinal measurement A measurement level that rank orders phenomena along some dimension.

orthogonal rotation In factor analysis, a rotation of factors such that the reference axes are kept at right angles, and hence the factors remain uncorrelated.

outfit statistic An indicator of an item's fit to a Rasch model that captures unexpected responses to items that are at the extremes of the trait continuum.

outlier A value that lies outside the normal range of values on a measure, especially in relation to other cases in a data set.

parallel test An alternate form of a measure that in theory yields the same true score as the original for those being measured; within a domain sampling framework, two parallel tests can be created by randomly sampling two sets of items from a hypothetical universe of items.

parallel test reliability The extent to which scores for people who are administered two parallel tests are the same for both measures.

patient acceptable symptom state (PASS) A threshold for interpreting "final state" scores on a measure, signifying a desirable or satisfactory outcome for a patient.

patient-reported outcome (PRO) A health outcome that is measured by directly asking the patient for information.

patient-specific measure A measure of an attribute that allows patients to make decisions about which questions to answer.

pattern matrix In factor analysis, the matrix that presents partial regression coefficients between variables and factors; in oblique rotation, the matrix used to interpret the meaning of the factors.

percentile A value indicating the percentage of people who score below a particular score value on a measure; the 50th percentile is the median for the distribution of scores.

performance test A measure designed to assess a person's physical or cognitive abilities or achievements.

person–item map A graphic display of information from a Rasch analysis that shows the distribution of respondents along one side of a latent trait continuum or "ruler" and the distribution of items on the other side.

person reliability In Rasch model analysis, an index (ranging from 0.0 to 1.0) that indicates how effectively a set of items can discriminate among a group being measured.

person separation index (PSI) In Rasch analysis, an index (typically ranging from 1.0 to 3.0) that provides an estimate of the ratio of true variance to error variance and indicates how much "separation" among a group of people is possible.

polytomous item An item with three or more response options (e.g., a Likert-type item).

positive predictive value (PPV) A measure of the usefulness of a screening/diagnostic test that can be interpreted as the probability that a positive test result is correct; calculated by dividing the number with a positive test who have the disease by the number with a positive test.

precision In measurement, the degree to which an obtained score (trait estimate) closely approximates a true score; precision corresponds to low errors of measurement and is usually expressed in terms of the width of the confidence interval.

predictive validity A type of criterion validity that concerns the degree to which a measure is correlated with a criterion measured at a future point in time.

pretest The trial administration of a newly developed measure to identify flaws or to gain better understanding of how the construct in question is conceptualized by respondents.

principal components analysis (PCA) An analysis that is considered by some a type of factor analysis; PCA analyzes all variance in the observed variables, not just common factor variance, with 1s on the diagonal of the correlation matrix.

principal factors (PF) method A method of factor analysis that analyzes only common factor variance using estimates of the communality on the diagonal of the correlation matrix; sometimes called *principal-axis factoring*.

probe In cognitive interviews, a question designed to get detailed and reflective information from a respondent regarding how a question was processed and answered.

profile A verbal or graphic summary of a set of scores for a person on a set of related characteristics (e.g., a profile of health status based on subscale scores on the SF-36).

projective test A measure designed to elicit information about a person's innermost feelings and emotions through the presentation of vague stimuli (e.g., the Rorschach inkblot test).

proportion of agreement In assessing agreement/consistency between two nominal or ordinal measurements, the proportion of cases for which there is total agreement.

proximity effect A response bias resulting from the tendency to be influenced in responding to an item by the response to the previous item.

proxy report Responses about a person provided on his or her behalf by another person (a proxy) presumed to be sufficiently knowledgeable to supply needed information (e.g., a spouse, parent, or family caretaker).

psychometric assessment An evaluation of the quality of an instrument in which its measurement properties (i.e., its reliability, validity, and responsiveness) are estimated.

psychometrics A field of inquiry concerned with the theory of measurement of abstract psychological constructs and the application of the theory in the development of measuring tools.

purposive sampling A sampling approach used primarily in qualitative research in which the researcher uses judgments to make decisions about which participants will yield the best information based on the informational needs of the study and what has already been learned in prior interviews or observations.

qualitative research The investigation of phenomena, typically in an in-depth and holistic fashion, through the collection of rich narrative materials.

questionnaire A document or instrument used to gather self-report data via self-administration of questions.

random error (of measurement) An error resulting from simple and usually small fluctuations that occur by chance or haphazardly in no systematic fashion.

Rasch model A latent trait model, used to evaluate items for a scale or test, that estimates only item difficulty (location) parameters; mathematically similar to a one-parameter (1-PL) IRT model.

rating scale A scale that requires ratings of an object or concept along a continuum.

ratio measurement A measurement level with equal distances between scores and a true meaningful zero point (e.g., a person's weight).

readability The ease with which materials (e.g., items on a scale) can be read by people with varying reading skills, often empirically evaluated through readability formulas.

recall bias An error of retrieved recollections as a result of various cognitive and emotional forces; the bias can make it risky to measure change by asking retrospective questions.

receiver operating characteristic (ROC) curve A statistical technique that involves plotting specificity against sensitivity for different scores on a measure and so can be used to determine the best cutoff score for "caseness"; also used to generate an index (the *area under the curve*) that has relevance for assessing validity and responsiveness in some situations.

reference range A tool for interpreting measurements, usually from laboratory values, that involves establishing the score interval within which 95% of the values from a very large sample (the reference group) fall.

reflective scale A multi-item scale whose items are conceptualized as having been "caused" by the underlying trait that is being measured; items are viewed as "effect indicators" because they are the effects of an underlying construct; sometimes called a *homogeneous scale*. See also *formative index*.

regression to the mean A statistical phenomenon in which a score that is extreme at an initial measurement tends to be closer to the mean on a second measurement.

reliability The extent to which a measurement is free from measurement error; more broadly, the extent to which scores for people who have not changed are the same for repeated measurements; statistically, the proportion of total variance in a set of scores that is attributable to true differences among those being measured.

reliability coefficient A quantitative index, usually ranging in value from 0.00 to 1.00, that provides an estimate of how reliable an instrument is (e.g., the intraclass correlation coefficient).

reliable change index (RCI) An index used (especially in psychotherapy) to estimate the threshold for a "real" change in scores (i.e., a change that, with 95% confidence, is beyond measurement error); similar in concept to the *smallest detectable change* but based on a different formula.

reproducibility The extent to which scores can be reproduced on repeated administrations of the measure on two or more occasions. See also *test–retest reliability*.

responder analysis An analysis that compares people who are *responders* to an intervention, based on their having reached a benchmark on a change score (e.g., the minimal important change), compared to people who are nonresponders (have not reached the benchmark).

response bias An influence that leads a person to select a response option that does not correspond to his or her hypothetical "true score" for an item.

response options The prespecified list of possible answers to a closed-ended question or item; also called *response alternatives*.

response rate The rate of participation in a study, calculated by dividing the number of people who participate (i.e., who provide data) by the number of people who were sampled.

response set bias The systematic bias resulting from the tendency of some individuals to respond to items in characteristic ways (e.g., always agreeing), independently of item content.

response shift A shift over time in a person's cognitive appraisal of his or her attributes, resulting in changes in responses to questions, even when the attribute (construct) itself has not changed; the shift, triggered by a catalyst such as a health change, can result in recalibrations or reprioritizations that make it difficult to measure true change.

responsiveness The ability of a measure to detect change over time in a construct that has changed, commensurate with the amount of change that has occurred.

ROC curve See *receiver operating characteristic curve*.

root mean square error of approximation (RMSEA) An index used to evaluate how well a hypothesized model fits the data (e.g., in a confirmatory factor analysis or IRT modeling); an RMSEA of $<.06$ is considered an indicator of adequate fit.

rotated factor matrix The factor matrix of items and factors after rotation of the factor axes to better align items on the factors, with the goal of enhancing interpretability.

saturation The point at which a sense of closure is attained in the collection of qualitative data as a result of obtaining redundant information.

scale A composite measure of an attribute or trait involving the aggregation of information from multiple items into a single numerical value that places people on a continuum with respect to the trait. See also *reflective scale*.

scale-level content validity index (S-CVI) An index summarizing the degree to which experts agree on the relevance of all the items on a multi-item scale or subscale.

score A numerical value derived from a measurement that communicates *how much* of an attribute is present in a person or whether the attribute is present or absent.

scree test One approach to deciding the appropriate number of factors to extract in a factor analysis, which involves plotting eigenvalues against factors on a graph; discontinuities in the scree plot suggest where factoring should stop.

self-report A method of collecting data that involves a direct verbal report of information by the person being measured (e.g., by interview, questionnaire).

semantic equivalence In a translation or adaptation of an instrument, the extent to which the meaning of an item is the same in the target culture after the item is translated as it was in the original.

semi-structured interview An interview in which the researcher has a list of topics to cover rather than specific questions to ask.

sensibility The overall quality criterion for evaluating clinimetric measures as proposed by Feinstein, covering properties such as content and face validity, item clarity, acceptability to patients, feasibility of use in clinical settings, and sensitivity to treatment.

sensitivity The ability of a screening or diagnostic instrument to correctly identify a "case" (i.e., to correctly diagnose a condition).

smallest detectable change (SDC) An index that estimates the threshold for a "real" change in scores (i.e., a change that, with 95% confidence, is beyond measurement error); the SDC is a change score that falls outside the limits of agreement on a Bland–Altman plot.

social desirability response bias A bias in self-report instruments created when participants have a tendency to misrepresent their opinions in the direction of answers consistent with prevailing social norms.

Spearman–Brown prophecy formula A formula used to predict the value of an internal consistency estimate for different numbers of items (or for projecting how many items are needed to attain a certain level of internal consistency).

specificity The ability of a screening or diagnostic instrument to correctly identify noncases for a condition.

specific scale A multi-item measure that is designed for a specific population or purpose; notably for specific diseases (e.g., diabetes), behaviors (e.g., medication compliance), sites (e.g., shoulder), or age (e.g., children).

split-half reliability The degree of internal consistency of a multi-item scale, as assessed by correlating scores on two half-tests of the scale (e.g., odd items versus even items).

standard error of estimate (SEE) An index that quantifies the degree of accuracy of predictions made with a regression line; in measurement, sometimes used in a regression-based approach to building confidence intervals around an estimated true score.

standard error of measurement (SEM) An index that quantifies the amount of "typical" error on a measure and indicates the precision of individual scores.

standardized response mean (SRM) An index summarizing, in standardized units, the amount of change in a group or the amount of difference in change in two groups on a measure; calculated by dividing mean difference in scores by the standard deviation for change scores; sometimes used to provide evidence of responsiveness.

standardized root mean square residual (SRMR) An index used to evaluate how well a hypothesized model fits the data (e.g., in a confirmatory factor analysis); an SRMR of <.08 is considered an indicator of adequate fit.

standard scores Scores expressed in terms of standard deviations from the mean, with the raw scores typically transformed to have a mean of zero and a standard deviation of one; sometimes called *z-scores*.

static measure A fixed-length measure that is administered in the same fashion for everyone who is measured.

stem In an item for a scale, the portion of the item (either a question or declarative statement) designed to elicit a response.

structural equation modeling (SEM) A statistical method for testing and estimating causal relations among a set of variables.

structural validity The extent to which an instrument captures the hypothesized dimensionality of the broad construct; an aspect of construct validity.

structure matrix The matrix that contains the correlations between variables on the one hand and linear composites (e.g., factor scores or canonical variate scores) on the other.

subscale A measure of one aspect or dimension of a multidimensional construct.

summated rating scale A scale consisting of multiple items that are added together to yield an overall, continuous measure of an attribute (e.g., a Likert scale).

systematic error (of measurement) Typically, a measurement error that reflects a systematic bias or distortion of measurements (e.g., a leniency or severity bias of raters/observers).

T score A standard score in which raw scores are transformed such that the mean of the distribution equals 50 and the standard deviation equals 10.

technical equivalence In a translation or adaptation of an instrument for another culture, the equivalence of assumptions about the methods of instrument administration (e.g., equivalence in the norms about self-disclosure or privacy).

test information function (TIF) In item response theory, the aggregate amount of *information* present in a set of items, derived by adding together item information functions (IIFs); the TIF graphically displays the location on the trait continuum where precision on the scale is at its maximum and measurement error is lowest.

test–retest reliability The type of reliability that concerns the extent to which scores for people who have not changed are the same when a measure is administered twice; an assessment of a measure's stability.

then test A method of assessing response shift, which involves a comparison of a person's present appraisal of a construct with a retrospective appraisal of the same construct at an earlier point, to arrive at a measure of change that presumably reflects the same "yardstick."

think-aloud method A qualitative method used to collect data about cognitive processes, in which people's reflections on decisions are captured as they are being made; sometimes used as part of a cognitive interview during a pretest of a new instrument.

topic guide A list of broad question areas to be covered in a semi-structured interview or focus group interview.

transient error Measurement error that results from time-related fluctuations in people's moods, physiological states, or information processing mechanisms

triangulation The use of multiple methods to collect and interpret data so as to converge on an accurate representation of a phenomenon (e.g., the triangulation of evidence about a measure's construct validity).

true score A hypothetical score that would be obtained if a measure were infallible (i.e., without measurement error); theoretically, a true score is the mean of an infinite number of measurements of a person or object, taken under identical circumstances.

two-parameter logistic (2-PL) model An item response theory model that estimates both the item difficulty (location) parameter and the item discrimination parameter.

unidimensional scale A scale that measures only one construct, or a unitary aspect or facet of a construct.

unique variance In a factor analysis, the variance associated with an item or variable that is partly item-specific and partly error variance and is distinct from common factor variance.

unrotated factor matrix The factor matrix of items and factors resulting from the factor extraction stage of a factor analysis prior to any rotation of the axes.

validity In a measurement context, the degree to which an instrument is measuring the construct it purports to measure.

verbal report A method of collecting data that involves the provision of information by the person being measured, usually in the form of responses to questions.

visual analog scale (VAS) A scaling procedure used to measure certain clinical symptoms (e.g., pain, fatigue) by having people indicate on a straight line the intensity of the symptom; usually measured on a 100-mm scale with values from 0 to 100.

weighted kappa A kappa-type statistic used to assess agreement or consistency between two raters when the measurement scale is ordinal; the weights give partial credit to ratings that are in close proximity.

weighting Differential emphasis given to different items on a measure, commensurate with the differential importance of the item in measuring a given construct (or, in IRT, differential amounts of discrimination).

within-subjects design A research design in which a single group of subjects is compared under different conditions or at different points in time (e.g., before and after surgery).

yea-sayers bias A bias in self-report scales created when respondents characteristically agree with statements ("yea-say"), independent of content.

z-score A standard score, expressed in terms of standard deviations from the mean; raw scores are transformed such that the mean equals zero and the standard deviation equals 1.

Z test A test used in connection with item response theory measures for evaluating the significance of individual change scores on a latent trait.

Index

Note: Page numbers in **bold** denote Glossary entries.